Therapies for Nail Disorders
A Quick Guide to Best Practice

T0332029

Edited by

Nilton Di Chiacchio, MD, PhD

Head, Dermatologic Clinic
Hospital do Servidor Público Municipal de São Paulo
São Paulo, Brazil

Antonella Tosti, MD

Fredric Brandt Endowed Professor of Dermatology
Dr. Phillip Frost Department of Dermatology and Cutaneous Surgery
University of Miami Miller School of Medicine
Miami, Florida, USA

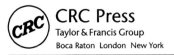

CRC Press
Taylor & Francis Group
Boca Raton London New York

CRC Press is an imprint of the
Taylor & Francis Group, an **informa** business

CRC Press
Taylor & Francis Group
6000 Broken Sound Parkway NW, Suite 300
Boca Raton, FL 33487-2742

International Standard Book Number-13: 978-1-138-37036-4 (Paperback)
978-1-138-37039-5 (Hardback)

**Visit the Taylor & Francis Web site at
http://www.taylorandfrancis.com**

**and the CRC Press Web site at
http://www.crcpress.com**

Contents

Contributors

Azhar Abbas Ahmed
Department of Dermatology
King Fahad General Hospital
Medina, Saudi Arabia

Aurora Alessandrini
Department of Dermatology, Experimental,
 Diagnostic and Specialty Medicine
University of Bologna
Bologna, Italy

Azzam Alkhalifah
Unaizah College of Medicine
Qassim University
Buraydah, Saudi Arabia

Hind M. Almohanna
Department of Dermatology and Dermatologic
 Surgery
Prince Sultan Military Medical City
Riyadh, Saudi Arabia

Roberto Arenas-Guzmán
Mycology Section
Dr. Manuel Gea González General Hospital
Mexico City, Mexico

Sarah Azarchi
Ronald O. Perelman Department of
 Dermatology
New York University School of Medicine
New York City, New York

Cristina Diniz Borges Figueira de Mello
Discipline of Dermatolgy
Department of Internal Medicine
Medical School of Sciences
Campinas State University (UNICAMP)
São Paulo, Brazil

Brandon Burroway
Dr. Phillip Frost Department of Dermatology and
 Cutaneous Surgery
University of Miami
Miami, Florida

Patricia Chang
Dermatology Service
Social Security General Hospital (IGSS)
Guatemala City, Guatemala

Leah Cohen
Herbert Wertheim College of Medicine
Florida International University
Miami, Florida

Carlton Ralph Daniel, III
Department of Dermatology
University of Mississippi
Jackson, Mississippi

and

University of Alabama
Birmingham, Alabama

Florence Dehavay
Dermatology Department
Brugmann, Saint-Pierre and Queen Fabiola
 Children's University Hospitals
Université Libre de Bruxelles
Brussels, Belgium

Nilton Di Chiacchio
Dermatologic Clinic
Hospital do Servidor Público Municipal de São
 Paulo
São Paulo, Brazil

Nilton Gioia Di Chiacchio
Faculdade de Medicina do ABC
Santo André, Brazil

and

Hospital do Servidor Público Municipal
 de São Paulo
São Paulo, Brazil

Judith Dominguez-Cherit
Department of Dermatology
Instituto Nacional de Ciencias Medicas y
 Nutricion "Salvador Subirán"
Mexico City, Mexico

Sabrina Escandón-Pérez
Social Medical Service
Anáhuac University
Mexico City, Mexico

Rachel Fayne
Department of Dermatology and Cutaneous
   Surgery
University of Miami Miller School
   of Medicine
Miami, Florida

Tatiana Villas Boas Gabbi
Department of Dermatology
Medical School
University of São Paulo
São Paulo, Brazil

Stamatis Gregoriou
1st Department of Dermatology and
   Venereology
National and Kapodistrian University of
   Athens Medical School
A. Sygros Hospital
Athens, Greece

Jacob Griggs
Dr. Phillip Frost Department of Dermatology
   and Cutaneous Surgery
University of Miami
Miami, Florida

Eckart Haneke
Private Dermatology Practice
Freiburg, Germany

and

Department of Dermatology
Inselspital, University of Bern
Bern, Switzerland

and

Centro de Dermatología Epidermis
Insttituto CUF
Matosinhos, Portugal

Matilde Iorizzo
Private Dermatology Practice
Bellinzona, Switzerland

Nathaniel J. Jellinek
Dermatology Professionals, Inc.
East Greenwich, Rhode Island

and

Department of Dermatology
Warren Alpert Medical School at Brown
   University
Providence, Rhode Island

and

Department of Dermatology
University of Massachusetts Medical School
Worcester, Massachusetts

Eder R. Juárez-Durán
Social Medical Service, Mycology Section
Dr. Manuel Gea González General Hospital
Mexico City, Mexico

Thomas Knackstedt
Department of Dermatology
MetroHealth Hospital
Cleveland, Ohio

Shari R. Lipner
Department of Dermatology
Weill Cornell Medicine
New York City, New York

Walter Refkalefsky Loureiro
Department of Dermatology
University of the State of Pará
Pará, Brasil

Suelen Montagner
Private Dermatology Practice
Campinas, Brazil

Sonali Nanda
Department of Dermatology and Cutaneous
   Surgery
University of Miami Miller School of Medicine
Miami, Florida

Leandro Fonseca Noriega
Department of Dermatology
Hospital do Servidor Público Municipal de São
   Paulo
São Paulo, Brazil

Jorge Ocampo-Garza
Dermatology Department
University Hospital Dr. José Eleuterio González
Universidad Autónoma de Nuevo León
Monterrey, Mexico

Emerson Henrique Padoveze
São Leopoldo Mandic Medical School
and
University of Campinas (UNICAMP)
Campinas, Brazil

Adriana Guadalupe Peña-Romero
Department of Dermatology
Hospital Angeles León
León, Mexico

Bianca Maria Piraccini
Department of Dermatology, Experimental,
    Diagnostic and Specialty Medicine
University of Bologna
Bologna, Italy

Eftychia Platsidaki
1st Department of Dermatology and Venereology
National and Kapodistrian University
    of Athens Medical School
A. Sygros Hospital
Athens, Greece

Bertrand Richert
Dermatology Department
Brugmann, Saint-Pierre and Queen Fabiola
    Children University Hospitals
Université Libre de Bruxelles
Brussels, Belgium

Evan A. Rieder
Ronald O. Perelman Department of
    Dermatology
New York University School of Medicine
New York City, New York

Dimitris Rigopoulos
1st Department of Dermatology and Venereology
National and Kapodistrian University of Athens
    Medical School
A. Sygros Hospital
Athens, Greece

Michela Starace
Department of Dermatology, Experimental,
    Diagnostic and Specialty Medicine
University of Bologna
Bologna, Italy

Glaysson Tassara Tavares
Federal University of Minas Gerais
Belo Horizonte, Brazil

Curtis T. Thompson
CTA Lab
and
Departments of Dermatology and Pathology
Oregon Health and Sciences University
Portland, Oregon

Antonella Tosti
Dr. Phillip Frost Department of Dermatology and
    Cutaneous Surgery
University of Miami Miller School of Medicine
Miami, Florida

Tracey C. Vlahovic
Department of Podiatric Medicine
Temple University of School of Podiatric
    Medicine
Philadelphia, Pennsylvania

Martin N. Zaiac
Department of Dermatology
Herbert Wertheim College of Medicine
Florida International University
Miami, Florida
and
Greater Miami Skin and Laser Center
Mount Sinai Medical Center
Miami Beach, Florida

1

Acute Paronychia

Jorge Ocampo-Garza and Patricia Chang

1.1 Introduction

Paronychia is the inflammation of one or more nail folds (proximal or lateral) of the fingers or toes.[1] It is usually the result from a breakdown of the protective barrier between the nail and the nail folds, which leads to bacterial or fungal infection.[2] Paronychia is divided, depending on its duration, into acute (<6 weeks) or chronic (>6 weeks).[3]

Acute paronychia usually occurs after injury or minor trauma (manicure, use of artificial nails, prick from a thorn, a torn hangnail, onychocryptosis, or onychophagia).[4] It is characteristically caused by *Staphylococcus aureus* and less commonly by *Streptococcus beta-haemolyticus* and gram-negative enteric bacteria.[5] Anaerobes and *Candida albicans* infection are often associated with repeated exposure of the fingers to wetness or oral flora.[6] Pseudomonas infections are characterized by a greenish discoloration in the nail bed.[3]

Acute paronychia is characterized by a rapid onset of erythema, edema, heat, and pain of the proximal or lateral nail folds (Figure 1.1), often with purulent secretion, and in some cases it can form a subungual abscess, which can cause transient or permanent dystrophy of the nail plate.[7,8] Untreated infections may lead to the formation of granulation tissue around the nail fold.[7] Acute paronychias usually involves only one digit at a time, and it regularly appears 2–5 days after the initial trauma (Figure 1.2).[2]

1.2 How to Confirm the Diagnosis

The diagnosis of acute paronychia is based on the physical examination of the nail folds and the patient's history. Imaging and laboratory tests are usually not needed for diagnosis of acute paronychia.[2] Culture of the expressed fluid is often nondiagnostic.[3] The digital pressure test can be helpful to identify the presence and extent of paronychial abscesses. The test is performed by having the patient oppose the thumb and affected finger or by applying light pressure to the distal volar aspect of the affected digit and observing for blanching in the area of the paronychia, which may indicate the presence of an abscess.[9]

Differential diagnosis should be made with other periungual inflammations such as chronic eczema, herpes simplex, psoriasis, Reiter syndrome, and pemphigus vulgaris.[4] Recurrent episodes of acute paronychia should raise suspicion for herpetic whitlow, which is a manifestation of herpes simplex infection and presents as a single or group of blisters with a honeycomb appearance close to the nail. The diagnosis is made by Tzanck testing or viral culture.[10] Reiter syndrome and psoriasis may involve the proximal nail fold and can mimic acute paronychia.[11]

1.3 Evidence-Based Treatment

The treatment of acute paronychia is determined by the degree of inflammation and whether an abscess is present. To date, there are no high-quality studies evaluating the use of oral versus topical antibiotics

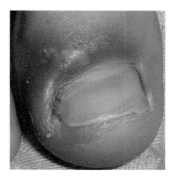

FIGURE 1.1   Acute paronychia of the lateral nail fold.

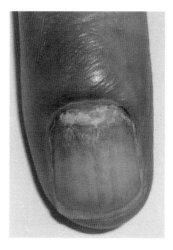

FIGURE 1.2   Acute paronychia of the right middle finger with onychomadesis.

for uncomplicated paronychia or the use of oral antibiotics in addition to surgical incision and drainage for acute paronychia with abscess.

In patients with minimal inflammation and no abscess formation, soaks in warm water, aluminum acetate (Burrow solution),[13] vinegar,[14] a dilute povidone–iodine solution,[15] or chlorhexidine, multiple times per day, may be effective (see Table 1.1, Evidence E). Soaking can lead to desquamation.

Mild cases may be treated with an antibiotic cream, such as mupirocin (Evidence E), gentamycin (Evidence D), bacitracin/neomycin/polymyxin B (Evidence E), fusidic acid (Evidence D), alone or in combination with a topical corticosteroid. A single nonrandomized study compared the efficacy of fusidic acid and betamethasone versus gentamycin ointment for acute paronychia, resulting in a reduction of the inflammatory score in the fusidic acid/betamethasone group (Evidence D).[16] Neomycin-containing compounds have the risk of allergic reactions (approximately 10%).

For severe cases or persistent lesions, empiric oral antibiotic therapy may be needed. An antistaphylococcal agent such as dicloxacillin (250 mg four times daily) or cephalexin (500 mg three to four times daily) is an effective first-line therapy (Evidence E). In areas where local methicillin-resistant *S. aureus* (MRSA) penetration is greater than 10%, agents such as trimethoprim–sulfamethoxazole (one to two double-strength tablets twice daily), clindamycin (300–450 mg four times per day), or doxycycline (100 mg twice daily) are the first-line of treatment (Evidence E).[17] In patients suspecting infection with oral flora (nail biting or finger sucking), the antibiotic coverage should include *S. aureus*, *Eikenella corrodens*, *Haemophilus influenzae*, and beta-lactamase-producing oral anaerobic bacteria such as amoxicillin–clavulanate (875/125 mg twice daily) (Evidence E). Or the combination of doxycycline (100 mg twice

TABLE 1.1

Treatments and Levels of Evidence

Treatment	Level of Evidence
Topical Treatment	
Soaks in warm water, aluminum acetate (Burrow solution), vinegar, a dilute povidone–iodine solution, or chlorhexidine	E[13–15]
Mupirocin cream	E[16]
Gentamycin	D[16]
Bacitracin/neomycin/polymyxin B	E[16]
Fusidic acid cream (alone or with topical corticosteroid)	D[16]
Systemic Treatment	
Dicloxacillin and cephalexin	E[17]
Trimethoprim–sulfamethoxazole	E[17]
Amoxicillin–clavulanate	E[17]
Combination of doxycycline, or trimethoprim–sulfamethoxazole, or penicillin VK, or cefuroxime, or ciprofloxacin, or moxifloxacin; plus metronidazole or clindamycin	E[10]
Surgical Treatment	
Abscess drainage	B[18]
Swiss roll technique (reflection of the proximal nail fold)	E[19]
Partial nail plate removal	E[14]

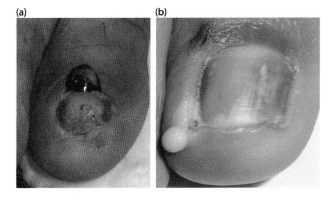

FIGURE 1.3 (a) Drainage of the proximal nail fold. (b) Drainage with needle of the lateral nail fold.

daily), or trimethoprim–sulfamethoxazole (1 double strength tablet twice daily), or penicillin VK (500 mg four times daily), or cefuroxime (500 mg twice daily), or ciprofloxacin (500–750 mg twice daily), or moxifloxacin (400 mg once daily); plus, metronidazole (500 mg three times daily), or clindamycin (450 mg three times daily) (Evidence E).[10]

Surgical management of acute paronychia is reserved for patients with abscess, failure of topical or oral treatment, or extensive involvement of the eponychium. Several surgical techniques have been described; however, there is no consensus or studies that describe the best procedure or the need for topical or systemic antibiotic therapy following the abscess drainage.[12] To drain an abscess, a No. 11 or 15 scalpel blade (with the sharp edge pointed away from the nail), a nail elevator, a 23- or 21-gauge needle, or a small hemostat is inserted into the nail sulcus and beneath the nail fold until the abscess is decompressed (Evidence B).[18] If spontaneous drainage does not occur, the digit can be massaged to express the fluid from the opening.

Extensive abscesses or those not immediately adjacent to the nail sulcus may require the creation of skin incisions, under local anesthesia, to drain the lesions (Figure 1.3a,b). If the entire eponychium is involved, the Swiss roll technique (reflection of the proximal nail fold) can be performed (Evidence E).[19]

Partial nail plate removal is usually performed for the treatment of paronychia associated with an ingrown toenail or in patients with an abscess extending to the nail bed (Evidence E).[14]

In a prospective study, 46 patients (26 with paronychia with abscess, 17 with paronychia and felon, and 3 with felon) were treated with incision and drainage without oral antibiotics. Forty-five patients were healed without complications at 45 days. The authors concluded that systemic antibiotics do not improve cure rates after incision and drainage of cutaneous abscesses (Evidence B).[20]

REFERENCES

1. Zaias N. *The Nail in Health and Disease*, 2nd ed. Norwalk, CT: Appleton and Lange; 1990.
2. Shafritz AB, Coppage JM. Acute and chronic paronychia of the hand. *J Am Acad Orthop Surg*. 2014 March;22(3):165–174.
3. Leggit JC. Acute and chronic paronychia. *Am Fam Physician*. 2017 July 1;96(1):44–51.
4. Chang P. Diagnosis using the proximal and lateral nail folds. *Dermatol Clin*. 2015 April;33(2):207–241.
5. Baran R, de Berker DA, Holzberg M et al., (eds). *Baran & Dawbers Diseases of the Nails and Their Management*. Oxford, UK: John Wiley & Sons, Ltd; 2012, pp. 623–625.
6. Brook I. Paronychia: a mixed infection. Microbiology and management. *J Hand Surg* 1993;18:358–359.
7. Lomax A, Thornton J, Singh D. Toenail paronychia. *Foot Ankle Surg*. 2016 December;22(4):219–223.
8. Jebson PJ. Infections of the fingertip. Paronychias and felons. *Hand Clin*. 1998;14(4):547–555.
9. Turkmen A, Warner RM, Page RE. Digital pressure test for paronychia. *Br J Plast Surg*. 2004;57(1):93–94.
10. Rigopoulos D, Larios G, Gregoriou S, Alevizos A. Acute and chronic paronychia. *Am Fam Physician*. 2008 February 1;77(3):339–346.
11. Baran R, Barth J, Dawber RP. *Nail Disorders: Common Presenting Signs, Differential Diagnosis, and Treatment*. New York, NY: Churchill Livingstone; 1991, pp. 93–100.
12. Shaw J, Body R. Best evidence topic report. Incision and drainage preferable to oral antibiotics in acute paronychial nail infection? *Emerg Med J*. 2005;22:813.
13. Daniel CR III. Paronychia. *Dermatol Clin*. 1985;3(3):461–464.
14. Jebson PJ. Infections of the fingertip: Paronychias and felons. *Hand Clin*. 1998;14(4):547–555, viii.
15. Stevanovic MV. Acute infections. In Wolfe SW, Pederson WC, Hotchkiss RN, Kozin SH (eds), *Green's Operative Hand Surgery*. Philadelphia, PA, Elsevier; 2011, pp. 41–84.
16. Wollina U. Acute paronychia: Comparative treatment with topical antibiotic alone or in combination with corticosteroid. *J Eur Acad Dermatol Venereol*. 2001;15(1):82–84.
17. Tosti R, Ilyas AM. Empiric antibiotics for acute infections of the hand. *J Hand Surg Am*. 2010;35(1):125–128.
18. Ogunlusi JD, Oginni LM, Ogunlusi OO. DAREJD simple technique of draining acute paronychia. *Tech Hand Up Extrem Surg*. 2005; 9:120.
19. Pabari A, Iyer S, Khoo CT. Swiss roll technique for treatment of paronychia. *Tech Hand Up Extrem Surg*. 2011; 15(2):75–77.
20. Pierrart J, Delgrande D, Mamane W et al. Acute felon and paronychia: Antibiotics not necessary after surgical treatment. Prospective study of 46 patients. *Hand Surg Rehabil*. 2016;35:40.

2

Bowen Disease

Leah Cohen and Martin N. Zaiac

2.1 Introduction

Squamous cell carcinoma (SCC) is the second most common cutaneous cancer, with an estimated 700,000 cases per year diagnosed in the United States.[1] Recognition and differentiation of common nail pathologies are essential for identifying tumors such as SCC, the most frequent malignancy of the nail.[2,3]

Bowen disease (BD) is an intraepidermal squamous cell carcinoma, or equivalently, squamous cell carcinoma in situ (SCCis).[4] Histologically, it is characterized by full-thickness epidermal dysplasia with intraepidermal distribution of atypical keratinocytes, without disruption of the basement membrane.[5] Often asymptomatic and grossly variable in presentation, the diagnosis of BD of the nail is often delayed an average of 5 years.[2,4] In this chapter we review general characteristics of BD of the nail, as well as discuss the variety of treatment strategies and their efficacy.

SCC is the most frequent malignant neoplasm of the nail unit, occurring twice as frequently in males, mainly in the fifth to sixth decades.[4] As an indolent entity, BD takes approximately 5–10 years to progress to invasive SCC.[3] The annual U.S. incidence of cutaneous BD was estimated to be 15 per 100,000 adjusted to the white population of the 1980s census.[6] However, the diagnosis of BD of the nail is rarely made.[2,3] For this reason, the incidence of BD of the nail is not well established or predicted. Literature regarding BD of the nail is limited and consists mainly of case series, with a total of approximately 300 reported cases to date in literature.[2,5,7,8]

BD and SCC of the nail share risk factors including ionizing radiation, tobacco use, arsenic, pesticides, immunosuppression, dyskeratosis congenita, traumas, and human papillomavirus (HPV) infections.[2,4,9–11] Although ultraviolet (UV) irradiation is often discussed as a cause of cutaneous BD, the nail plate is an effective UV filter, allowing only minimal transmission of UVB radiation to the nail plate.[12]

HPV has been suggested to be responsible for up to 60% of SCC of the nail cases.[4] Serotypes found include 2, 6, 11, 16, 18, 26, 31, 34, 35, 56, 58, and 73. Specifically, HPV16 has been detected in over 50 cases of BD of the nail[8,13–16] and is present in 75% of cases tested.[17] The strong HPV association suggests that genitodigital transmission plays an important role in the development of SCC and BD of the nail.[16,18] Nearly one-third of patients who develop SCC of the nail have a documented history of HPV-associated genital disease, including genital warts, dysplasia, and cervical or anogenital cancer.[4] It is approximated that time of onset between genital HPV disease and HPV-related disease of the nail is 12 years.[4] Of note, it seems immune status is not correlated with aggressive or multiple form of HPV-associated SCC of the nail.[4]

SCC of the nail mostly commonly affects one digit, namely, the thumb. Although less common, second finger, third finger, or multiple digit involvement has been observed.[9,19,20] BD and SCC of the digit most commonly arise in the lateral nail folds or distal groove, and over time grow to involve the nail bed and matrix by extension.[21–23] BD of the nail grows slowly and asymptomatically for years to decades before transforming into invasive SCC.[2] The progression into invasive SCC, which happens in 3%–5% of cases, can be asymptomatic or can be associated with pain, ulceration, bleeding, or development of a nodule.[24] BD of the nail has been documented to behave more aggressively than cutaneous BD, and more frequently is found to have histologic features of invasive SCC.[25] Despite its aggressive appearance, BD of the nail is less likely to become metastatic than cutaneous SCC from other sites.[25] For example, nodal involvement in patients with subungual SCC is reported in less than 2% of cases.[21]

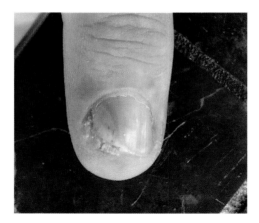

FIGURE 2.1   Bowen disease of the nail unit. (Courtesy of Martin N. Zaiac, MD.)

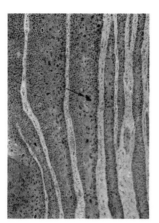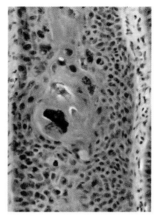

FIGURE 2.2   Mohs histology. (Courtesy of Martin N. Zaiac, MD.)

BD of the nail can develop in any part of the nail unit or periungual tissue. It has a wide presentation morphology, including hyperkeratosis, verrucous or warty lesion, erosions or ulcerations, oozing, scaling, periungual swelling, onycholysis, or paronychia. Most commonly, BD is found in the lateral nail folds, presenting as a hyperkeratotic or verrucous band that is associated with onycholysis and occasionally marginal band of melanonychia (Figure 2.1).[4,5] Subungual involvement is the most common cause for presentation.[20,26] If the matrix is involved, changes in the texture of the nail plate can be seen, along with loss of transparency and nail sheen.[3] In cases associated with HPV56 and darker-skinned individuals, ungual BD can be pigmented and may cause melanonychia.[3]

Histologically, BD of the nail demonstrates classic characteristics of carcinoma in situ, including loss of uniform stratification throughout all layers of the epidermis without disruption of the basement membrane or dermis. Dyskeratosis, large clumped cells with hyperchromic nuclei, atypical mitoses, and possibly even perinuclear vacuolization indicative of HPV infection can be seen (Figure 2.2).[3] Microinvasion is extremely common in long-standing BD.[21]

2.2 How to Confirm the Diagnosis

As a painless and indolent lesion, many patients do not have a high level of concern regarding these lesions. When detected on clinical exam, the differential diagnosis of BD of the nail includes viral warts, paronychia, eczema, nail deformity, onychomycosis, onychopapilloma, onychomatricoma, and other benign lesions.[9,19,20] Because misdiagnosis is so common, multiple treatments are often attempted before biopsy is performed.[2] The average delay to the first medical diagnosis of BD of the nail unit has been reported between 4.9 and 6 years.[2,7,8]

Due to the three-dimensional nature of the nail bed, the histopathologic diagnosis of SCC and BD of the nail are difficult. Incisional biopsy specimen may only reveal an in situ carcinoma, while an invasive component may be coexisting at the time of diagnosis.[2,27] Therefore, experts have suggested that a diagnosis of BD of the nail should be treated as if it may harbor a microinvasive component.[2,27]

2.3 Evidence-Based Treatment

Due to the unique anatomic structure of the nail unit, individualized treatment strategies are required to treat tumors of the nail. Foregoing treatment is generally not recommended unless the patient is elderly with multiple comorbidities and a history of poor wound healing. Treatment choice must consider many factors including the evidence of benefit, ease of use or time required for procedure, wound healing, cosmetic result, availability, and cost. Specifically, if the nail bed or matrix must be accessed, in the case of subungual neoplasm, partial or total nail plate avulsion will be required.[22] The British Association of Dermatologists (BAD) have created guidelines for the management of cutaneous BD.[24] Its guidelines acknowledge that there is no single modality that is regarded as superior than others for cutaneous BD management. However, some modalities have a higher level of evidence to support their use.

Knowing this, we will discuss the accepted treatments for cutaneous BD and how they apply to BD of the nail where limited literature exists. Treatments are categorized generally as surgical, nonsurgical destructive, and nonsurgical (Table 2.1). Surgical treatment includes surgical excision and Mohs micrographic surgery (MMS). Destructive treatments include curettage, cautery or electrodesiccation, and cryotherapy. Nonsurgical treatment encompasses a spectrum of options including topical therapies fluorouracil and imiquimod, photodynamic therapy, ablative lasers, and radiation.

2.3.1 Surgical

2.3.1.1 Surgical Excision (Evidence Level C)

A diagnosis of BD of the nail should raise high suspicions that an area with invasive properties may also exist within the same tumor. For this reason, surgical excision is considered. Local excision of small lesions with adequate surgical margins (approximately 4–6 mm) is usually sufficient and superior to amputation of the distal phalanx.[24] These defects can then undergo healing through secondary intention, tissue graft, or repair with a bridge flap.[3,24] Side effects of surgical excision include pain, poor wound healing, infection, and bleeding.

TABLE 2.1

Treatments and Levels of Evidence

Treatment	Level of Evidence
Nonsurgical Therapies	
5-Fluorouracil	E[24,30–33]
Imiquimod	E[33,35]
Photodynamic therapy	E[22,29,31,33,36–38]
Ablative laser	E[39–41]
Radiation therapy	E[34,40,42,44–47]
Curettage, cautery, or electrodesiccation	E[24]
Cryotherapy	E[29,30]
Surgical Therapies	
Surgical excision	C[3,24,28]
Mohs micrographic surgery	C[22]

Prior to the popularization of MMS, amputation of the distal phalanx was commonly utilized for definitive treatment of SCC of the nail. If bony invasion is suspected (and thereby invasive SCC), or visualized on imaging workup, amputation proximal to the interphalangeal joint is still recommended.[28]

2.3.1.2 Mohs Micrographic Surgery (Evidence Level C)

A primary concern when considering surgical excision of a nail unit tumor is the lack of nearby tissue, complicating reconstruction. MMS mitigates this issue by preserving maximal healthy tissue while addressing the full scope of the neoplasm. Although surgical excision and MMS have similar cure rates, MMS offers maximal preservation of normal tissues and lower likelihood of unnecessary physical deformity or psychological affect.[22]

The histopathology of tumors arising in the nail unit resembles that of other cutaneous neoplasms. However, the histology of the nail unit varies distinctly from normal skin, requiring the Mohs surgeon to have an in-depth understanding of this distinctive histology to accurately decipher residual tumor. Recurrence rates for MMS at the nail unit are higher than MMS in other locations, which can be attributed to difficulties in histologic interpretation from surgeons less familiar with the nail unit.[7]

For both surgical treatment modalities, if the surgical defect spares the nail matrix, it can be left to heal by secondary intention, closed primarily, or closed by flap or graft reconstruction. If the nail matrix is involved, resulting nail plate deformities are inevitable. If the surgeon is able, avoiding the nail matrix will provide the best cosmetic and functional results. If a portion of the nail matrix is affected, it may be best to remove the remaining matrix to avoid future cosmetic issue or ingrown nails.[21]

2.3.2 Nonsurgical Destructive Treatments

2.3.2.1 Curettage, Cautery, or Electrodesiccation (Evidence Level E)

Curettage is a simple and cost-effective method to treat cutaneous BD and periungual BD. The downside of treatment via curettage is that there is no confirmation of histologic margins, theoretically allowing for higher risks of tumor recurrence as compared to MMS. When compared to cryotherapy, lesions heal slightly faster, are less painful, and have lower recurrence rates.[24] Side effects of curettage are limited, but rarely include poor wound healing or scarring.

2.3.2.2 Cryotherapy (Evidence Level E)

Like curettage, cryotherapy is among the most simple, inexpensive, and efficient ways of treating cutaneous BD, especially when multiple lesions are present. Cryotherapy is an option for periungual BD. However, in the case of subungual lesions, this method is not generally applicable. Adequate cryotherapy has been described as using a single freeze–thaw cycle (FTC) of 30 seconds, two FTCs of 20 seconds separated by a period for thawing, or up to three treatments for 20 seconds over a course of several weeks.[29,30] Clearance rates for cryotherapy vary widely and are operator dependent. Side effects of cryotherapy include erythema, burning, irritation, and pain.

2.3.3 Nonsurgical Therapies

In general, nonsurgical treatments are considered less reliable as compared to surgical treatments.[3] Depending on the location of the lesion, they can often be difficult or impossible to apply without lifting the nail plate. For this reason, subungual lesions are less likely to be treated by these modalities.

2.3.3.1 Topical Therapies

2.3.3.1.1 5-Fluorouracil (Evidence Level E)

Topical fluorouracil (5-FU), a thymidylate synthase inhibitor that halts DNA synthesis, although not approved for the treatment of BD, is a commonly recognized treatment option for BD. Topically applied

5-FU is commercially available in a 5% cream; application generally consists of once or twice daily application for 2–8 weeks depending on BD location.[24,30] With this regimen, small randomized trials have found clinical cure rates of 48%–56% for cutaneous BD.[24,30] A systematic review in 2013 found that 5-FU is equivalent to cryotherapy for cutaneous BD.[31] One case series describes seven cases BD of the nail bed and periungual area, in which six cases were treated by MMS, and one treated with 5-FU.[32] Two of six lesions recurred after MMS, 1 and 2 years after surgery, while the lesion treated with topical 5-FU had residual BD found at 6 weeks post-treatment and subsequently underwent MMS for definitive treatment.[32] The most frequent side effects of 5-FU include erythema, pain, irritant dermatitis, and pruritus.[33] Patient adherence should be considered when prescribing a topical therapy, as daily application is usually required.

2.3.3.1.2 Imiquimod (Evidence Level E)

Imiquimod stimulates the immune system causing antitumor and antiviral activity. Off-label use of 5% imiquimod cream for BD and SCC has been tried. According to a 2009 systematic review, studies using daily (or five times weekly) topical imiquimod in the treatment of cutaneous BD were found to demonstrate clearance rates between 73% and 88%.[33–35] The authors of the review, however, do not recommend imiquimod for treatment of BD or SCC due to the limited number of studies, poor quality data, and lack of long-term follow-up data. No reports of imiquimod for BD of the nail specifically were found. Side effects of imiquimod therapy are numerous and common, including erythema, edema, weeping, pruritus, hypopigmentation, crusting/scabbing/scaling, erosion, burning, and pain, among other less common side effects.[33]

2.3.3.2 Photodynamic Therapy (Evidence Level E)

As a highly proliferative and superficial neoplasm, BD will easily concentrate topically applied photosensors and absorb a high amount of light energy and is therefore suited for photodynamic therapy (PDT).[36] Red light, aminolevulinic acid (ALA), and methyl-ALA (or MAL-PDT) are the most frequently used and investigated forms of PDT for the treatment of BD.[33]

Treatment of cutaneous BD with PDT has demonstrated cure rates of 68%–71% at 24-month follow-up.[29,37] A 2013 systematic review with a total of 363 participants found that there is limited evidence to suggest MAL-PDT is an effective treatment.[31] However, when comparing MAL-PDT with cryotherapy, MAL-PDT was significantly more efficacious.[31] No significant difference was found when comparing MAL-PDT to FU.[31] One study found significant difference in favor of ALA-PDT when compared to FU.[31] However, the authors stated that although cosmetic outcomes appear favorable with PDT, 5-year follow-up data is needed.[31]

Limited literature addresses treatment of subungual BD with PDT specifically. It is proposed that PDT can be a less invasive and equally successful way to treat subungual BD as compared with surgery.[22] One case report demonstrated the use of ALA-PDT for subungual BD showed no evidence of clinical recurrence with a follow-up of 30 months.[22] Interestingly, ALA-PDT may have dual functionality, not only clearing BD of the nail lesions, but also reducing high-risk HPV-infected tissue itself, as it has been shown to treat viral warts.[38] The most common side effects of PDT include immediate pain or burning sensation during therapy.

2.3.3.3 Ablative Laser (Evidence Level E)

The efficacy of lasers in treatment of BD is limited to case reports and small series. Likewise, literature for laser therapy for BD of the nail is minimal. One case report outlines successful treatment of periungual pigmented BD with CO_2 laser without permanent nail damage after unsuccessful treatment with imiquimod.[39] Several papers have discussed combination use of PDT and laser therapy for BD, outlining ablation of the epidermis with laser therapy prior to PDT application, with excellent treatment results.[40,41] Side effects of laser therapy include pain during treatment, erythema, swelling, pruritus, and pigmentary changes.

2.3.3.4 Radiation Therapy (Evidence Level E)

The use of radiation therapy for malignancies of the nail is an attractive nonsurgical option for many patients. External beam radiation therapy (EBRT) for cutaneous BD has demonstrated equivalent recurrence rates when compared to surgical excision, with impressive local control rates between 93% and 100% for BD.[34,40,42–44] Several reports exist describing the treatment of periungual or subungual SCC or BD with radiotherapy with success.[34,42,45] However, there is limited data on tolerance doses for digits and nails.[42] The anatomy of the nail unit is not well-suited for EBRT and therefore puts the patient at risk for unacceptable toxicity of the surrounding tissues, as well as nonuniform distribution of radiation.

To account for this, water bath photon irradiation for the treatment of BD of the nail has been used to provide uniform surface dosing. This was appropriate for the treatment of multiple BD lesions of the hand, digits, and nail bed seen in a case study, leading to complete clinical resolution for 20-month follow-up after water bath irradiation.[46] However, when the goal is to apply precise radiation to small lesions, high-dose-rate electronic surface brachytherapy (ESB) has been demonstrated to be efficacious.[47] With applicator sizes between 5 and 50 mm, lesions of the nail unit can be isolated and addressed, and the risk of toxicity to surrounding tissues is limited. Compared with EBRT, ESB requires only twice-a-week treatment to a cumulative total of eight fractions. The side effects of all types of radiation therapy include erythema, dry desquamation, moist desquamation, pigmentary changes, and risk of anonychia with variable regrowth, as well as risk of inducing secondary neoplasms in the field of radiation.[40] Long-term data using the varied types of radiotherapy in treating BD of the nail must still be determined.

2.4 Summary and Recommendations

Despite SCC being the most common neoplasm of the nail, the diagnosis of BD of the nail is rarely made. Subsequently, there is limited high-quality literature addressing BD of the nail. This can be explained by the clinical indolence of the lesion, as well as the mimicry of other common diagnoses of the nail. Clinicians should keep BD of the nail in their differential diagnosis and consider biopsy when evaluating a chronic, nonhealing, verrucous, hyperkeratotic lesion of the nail. The treatment of choice for BD of the nail is primarily MMS, as histologic confirmation may be achieved and healthy tissue may be spared. Nonsurgical therapies such as treatment with 5-FU, imiquimod, photodynamic therapy, laser ablation, and radiation have been utilized for BD of the nail, but no trials comparing the efficacy of these techniques as compared to MMS have been published as of 2018.[5] These therapies should be considered on a case-by-case basis, weighing the pros and cons of each modality for each patient.

REFERENCES

1. Rogers HW, Weinstock MA, Harris AR et al. Incidence estimate of nonmelanoma skin cancer in the United States, 2006. *Arch Dermatol.* 2010;146(3):5.
2. Lecerf P, Richert B, Theunis A, André J. A retrospective study of squamous cell carcinoma of the nail unit diagnosed in a Belgian general hospital over a 15-year period. *J Am Acad Dermatol.* 2013 August;69(2):253–261.e1.
3. Haneke E. Important malignant and new nail tumors: CME article. *JDDG: Journal der Deutschen Dermatologischen Gesellschaft.* 2017 April;15(4):367–386.
4. Richert B, Lecerf P, Caucanas M, André J. Nail tumors. *Clin Dermatol.* 2013 September;31(5):602–617.
5. Wollina U. Bowen's disease of the nail apparatus: A series of 8 patients and a literature review. *Wien Med Wochenschr.* 2015 October;165(19–20):401–405.
6. Chute CG. The subsequent risk of internal cancer with Bowen's disease. A population-based study. *JAMA.* 1991 August 14;266(6):816–819.
7. Young LC, Tuxen AJ, Goodman G. Mohs' micrographic surgery as treatment for squamous dysplasia of the nail unit: Mohs surgery for nail unit dysplasia. *Australas J Dermatol.* 2012 May;53(2):123–127.
8. Perruchoud DL, Varonier C, Haneke E et al. Bowen disease of the nail unit: A retrospective study of 12 cases and their association with human papillomaviruses. *J Eur Acad Dermatol Venereol.* 2016 September;30(9):1503–1506.

9. Lambertini M, Piraccini BM, Fanti PA, Dika E. Mohs micrographic surgery for nail unit tumours: An update and a critical review of the literature. *J Eur Acad Dermatol Venereol*. 2018 October;32(10):1638–1644.

10. Dika E, Piraccini BM, Balestri R et al. Mohs surgery for squamous cell carcinoma of the nail: Report of 15 cases. Our experience and a long-term follow-up: Mohs surgery for SCC of the nail. *Br J Dermatol*. 2012 December;167(6):1310–1314.

11. Dika E, Fanti PA, Misciali C, Vaccari S, Piraccini BM. Mohs surgery for squamous cell carcinoma of the nail unit: 10 years of experience. *Dermatol Surg*. 2015;41(9):1015–1019.

12. Parker SG, Diffey BL. The transmission of optical radiation through human nails. *Br J Dermatol*. 1983;108:11–16.

13. Ikenberg H, Gissmann L, Gross G, Grussendorf-Conen E-I, Hausen HZ. Human papillomavirus type-16-related DNA in genital Bowen's disease and in bowenoid papulosis. *Int J Cancer*. 1983 November 15;32(5):563–565.

14. Tosti A, Morelli R, Fanti PA, Morselli PG, Catrani S, Landi G. Carcinoma cuniculatum of the nail apparatus: Report of three cases. *Dermatology*. 1993;186:217–221.

15. McGrae JD, Greer CE, Manos MM. Multiple Bowen's disease of the fingers associated with human papilloma virus type 16. *Int J Dermatol*. 1993 February;32(2):104–107.

16. Grundmeier N, Hamm H, Weissbrich B, Lang SC, Bröcker E-B, Kerstan A. High-risk human papillomavirus infection in Bowen's disease of the nail unit: Report of three cases and review of the literature. *Dermatology*. 2011;223(4):293–300.

17. Riddel C, Rashid R, Thomas V. Ungual and periungual human papillomavirus–associated squamous cell carcinoma: A review. *J Am Acad Dermatol*. 2011 June;64(6):1147–1153.

18. Rudlinger R, Grob R, Yu Y, Schnyder U. Human papillomavirus-35-positive bowenoid papulosis of the anogenital area and concurrent human papillomavirus-35-positive verruca with bowenoid dysplasia of the periungual area. *Arch Dermatol*. 1989;125(5):655–659.

19. Baran R, Perrin C. Bowen's disease clinically simulating an onychomatricoma. *J Am Acad Dermatol*. 2002 December;47(6):947–949.

20. Baran R, Perrin C. Longitudinal erythronychia with distal subungual keratosis: Onychopapilloma of the nail bed and Bowen's disease. *Br J Dermatol*. 2000 July;143(1):132–135.

21. Zaiac MN, Weiss E. Mohs micrographic surgery of the nail unit and squamous cell carcinoma. *Dermatol Surg*. 2001 March;27(3):246–251.

22. Usmani N, Stables GI, Telfer NR, Stringer MR. Subungual Bowen's disease treated by topical aminolevulinic acid–photodynamic therapy. *J Am Acad Dermatol*. 2005 November;53(5):S273–S276.

23. Gormley RH, Groft CM, Miller CJ, Kovarik CL. Digital squamous cell carcinoma and association with diverse high-risk human papillomavirus types. *J Am Acad Dermatol*. 2011 May;64(5):981–985.

24. Morton CA, Birnie AJ, Eedy DJ. British Association of dermatologists' guidelines for the management of squamous cell carcinoma *in situ* (Bowen's disease) 2014. *Br J Dermatol*. 2014 February;170(2):245–260.

25. Ongenae K, van de Kerckhove M, Naeyaert J-M. Bowen's disease of the nail. *Dermatology*. 2002;204(4):348–350.

26. Guitart J, Bergfeld WF, Tuthill RJ, Tubbs RR, Zienowicz R, Fleegler EJ. Squamous cell carcinoma of the nail bed: A cliniopathological study of 12 cases. *Br J Dermatol*. 1990;123:215–222.

27. Guldbakke K, Brodsky J, Liang M, Schanbacher C. Human papillomavirus type 73 in primary and recurrent periungual squamous cell carcinoma. *Dermatol Surg*. 2008 March;34(3):407–413.

28. Goldminz D, Bennett R. Mohs micrographic surgery of the nail unit. *J Dermatol Surg Oncol*. 1992 August;18(8):721–726.

29. Morton C, Horn M, Leman J et al. Comparison of topical methyl aminolevulinate photodynamic therapy with cryotherapy or fluorouracil for treatment of squamous cell carcinoma in situ: Results of a multicenter randomized trial. *Arch Dermatol*. 2006 June 1;142(6). Available from: http://archderm.jamanetwork.com/article.aspx?doi=10.1001/archderm.142.6.729. Accessed October 14, 2018.

30. Holt PJA. Cryotherapy for skin cancer: Results over a 5-year period using liquid nitrogen spray cryosurgery. *Br J Dermatol*. 1988 August;119(2):231–240.

31. Bath-Hextall FJ, Matin RN, Wilkinson D, Leonardi-Bee J. Interventions for cutaneous Bowen's disease. Cochrane Skin Group, editor. *Cochrane Database Syst Rev*. 2013 June 24; Available from: http://doi.wiley.com/10.1002/14651858.CD007281.pub2. Accessed October 14, 2018.

32. Sau P, McMarlin S, Sperling L, Katz R. Bowen's disease of the nail bed and periungual area a clinicopathologic analysis of seven cases. *Arch Dermatol*. 1994;130(2):204–209.

33. Love WE, Bernhard JD, Bordeaux JS. Topical imiquimod or fluorouracil therapy for basal and squamous cell carcinoma: A systematic review. *Arch Dermatol.* 2009 December 1;145(12). Available from: http://archderm.jamanetwork.com/article.aspx?doi=10.1001/archdermatol.2009.291. Accessed November 19, 2018.

34. Rosen LR, Powell K, Katz SR, Wu HT, Durci M. Subungual squamous cell carcinoma. *Am J Clin Dermatol.* 2010;11(4):285–288.

35. Patel G, Goodwin R, Chawla M et al. Imiquimod 5% cream monotherapy for cutaneous squamous cell carcinoma in situ (Bowen's disease): A randomized, double-blind, placebo-controlled trial. *J Am Acad Dermatol.* 2006 June 1;54(6):1025–1032.

36. Zink BS, Valente L, Ortiz B, Caldas A, Jeunon T, Marques-da-Costa J. Periungual Bowen's disease successfully treated with photodynamic therapy. *Photodiagnosis Photodyn Ther.* 2013 December;10(4):535–537.

37. Calzavara-Pinton PG, Venturini M, Sala R et al. Methylaminolaevulinate-based photodynamic therapy of Bowen's disease and squamous cell carcinoma. *Br J Dermatol.* 2008 July;159(1):137–144.

38. Stender IM, Christian H. Photodynamic therapy with 5-aminolaevulinic acid or placebo for recalcitrant foot and hand warts: Randomised double-blind trial. *Lancet.* 2000 March 18;355(9208):963–966.

39. Jung MY, Lee DY. Successful treatment of periungual pigmented Bowen disease with CO_2 laser. *Br J Dermatol.* 2013 September;169(3):722–723.

40. Sung JM, Kim YC. Photodynamic therapy with epidermal ablation using fractional carbon-dioxide laser in the treatment of Bowen's disease: A case series. *Photodiagnosis Photodyn Ther.* 2017 September;19:84–85.

41. Cai H, Wang Y, Zheng J-C et al. Photodynamic therapy in combination with CO_2 laser for the treatment of Bowen's disease. *Lasers Med Sci.* 2015 July;30(5):1505–1510.

42. Hunt WT, Cameron A, Craig P, de Berker DA. Multiple-digit periungual Bowen's disease: A novel treatment approach with radiotherapy. *Clin Exp Dermatol.* 2013 December;38(8):857–861.

43. Herman JM, Pierce LJ, Sandler HM et al. Radiotherapy using a water bath in the treatment of Bowen's disease of the digit. *Radiother Oncol.* 2008 September;88(3):398–402.

44. VanderSpek LA, Pond GR, Wells W, Tsang RW. Radiation therapy for Bowen's disease of the skin. *Int J Radiat Oncol Biol Phys.* 2005 October;63(2):505–510.

45. Zabawski EJ, Washak RV, Cohen JB, Cockerell JC, Brown SM. Squamous cell carcinoma of the nail bed: Is finger predominance another clue to etiology? A report of 5 cases. *Cutis.* 2001 January;1:59–64.

46. Goodman CR, DeNittis A. Photon irradiation using a water bath technique for treatment of confluent carcinoma in situ of the hand, digits, and nail bed: A case report. *J Med Case Rep.* 2017 December;11(1). Available from: http://jmedicalcasereports.biomedcentral.com/articles/10.1186/s13256-017-1233-3. Accessed November 3, 2018.

47. Arterbery VE, Watson AC. An electronic brachytherapy technique for treating squamous cell carcinoma in situ of the digit: A case report. *BMC Res Notes.* 2013;6(1):147.

3

Brittle Nails

Tatiana Villas Boas Gabbi

3.1 Introduction

Brittle nail syndrome (BNS) is a disorder characterized by increased nail plate fragility, exhibiting surface roughness, raggedness, and peeling. It is a common problem that affects about 20% of the population, with a higher prevalence among the elderly. Women are affected twice as frequently as men.

The nail plate is a coherent arrangement of corneocytes, composed of an intracellular skeleton of keratin fibrils, and an extracellular matrix, formed by keratin-associated proteins. Desmosomes and lipid bilayers are also critical to the coherence of the nail plate. Mechanical properties of hardness and flexibility are related to the organization of keratin filaments as well as nail plate optimal water-binding capacity.

In fact, distinctive clinical features of brittle nail syndrome are onychoschizia and onychorrhexis, and they reflect its pathogenesis. Impaired intercellular adhesive factors of the nail plate are expressed clinically as onychoschizia, showing lamellar splitting of the free edge and distal portion of the nail plate (Figure 3.1). Onychorrhexis reflects matrix involvement and is characterized by longitudinal thinning or ridging of the nail plate with distal splitting (Figure 3.2). Other findings such as horizontal splitting and breaking of the lateral edges have also been described. Granulations in the nail keratin may take place when brittle nail changes are confined to the surface of the nail plate. Patients often complain that their nails are dry, soft, easily breakable, and incapable of growing long.

3.2 How to Confirm the Diagnosis

Brittle nail syndrome can be accessed by dermatological examination and clinical history. Neither a biopsy nor imaging tests are required to establish this diagnosis. Nonetheless, if onychorrhexis is predominant, laboratory tests can be requested to rule out infectious diseases as well as endocrine, metabolic, and nutritional disorders. Depending on clinical history and physical examination, it may also be important to exclude damage to the nail matrix from arsenic poisoning, irradiation, or other factors involving microcirculation and oxygenation.

Differential diagnosis should be made with onychophagia, onychotillomania, lichen planus, and trachyonychia. Van de Kerkhof et al.[1] have proposed a scoring system of key features to better understand therapeutic outcomes.

3.3 Evidence-Based Treatment

Therapeutic approaches for brittle nails depend on whether they are characterized mainly by onychoschizia or onychorrhexis, so that eliciting factors can be investigated, identified, and eliminated.

In cases of onychoschizia, water contact leading to cycles of immersion–desiccation should be avoided or limited by wearing gloves. Protection with rubber gloves worn over light cotton glove liners is advised. In

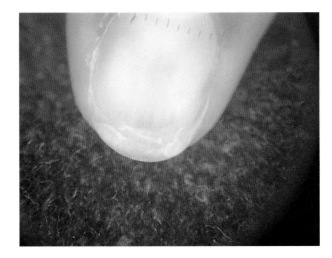

FIGURE 3.1   Onychoschizia. Lamellar splitting of the free edge and distal portion of the nail plate.

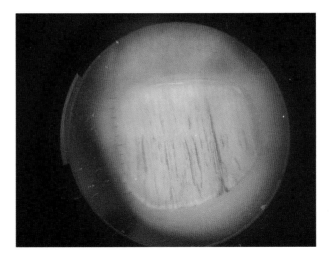

FIGURE 3.2   Onychorrhexis. Longitudinal thinning and ridging of the nail plate.

fact, when occupational exposure to chemicals is involved, gloves are mandatory. Repeated microtraumas to the fingertips due to professional activity or hobbies will benefit from clipping nails short.

For patients with onychorrhexis, investigation should be performed as mentioned earlier in this chapter. Since onychorrhexis can also give rise to onychoschizia, some therapeutic principles are generally advised in BNS aiming to increase water content and to decrease irregularities of the nail plate.

3.3.1 General Measures: Evidence E

- Nail care requires proper and frequent trimming. Cuticles are not to be completely removed. In general, short nails will minimize the microfractures seen on brittle nails.
- Nail lacquers can initially provide a mechanical protection against trauma, as they fill in nail fractures. Depending on their components, they can also improve the nail plate water-binding capacity.
- Nevertheless, nail lacquer removers will eventually be necessary and are likely to increase dehydration substantially.

- Nowadays, there are water-based nail varnish options on the market that are easy to remove and can work both therapeutically and cosmetically.
- Hyperhidrosis should be accessed if present. A study with 500 manual workers showed a positive correlation between this condition and brittle nail syndrome.[2]

3.3.2 Topical Treatment

3.3.2.1 Emollients

Applying emollients, especially those containing phospholipids, urea, and alpha hydroxy acids, significantly improves nail hydration. Humectants, such as glycerin and propylene glycol, and occlusive agents, such as lanoline and petrolatum, can also be recommended (Evidence E).[3]

3.3.2.2 Nail-Hardening Agents

There are two different types of nail-hardening agents available in the market. The first type includes modified nail polishes containing hydrolyzed proteins, artificial or natural fibers (such as nylon or silk), and acrylate resin, among others. They act by creating a protective coat that binds to the nail surface and supports it. They do not alter the nail plate structure. The second type of nail plate–hardening agents acts by promoting keratin cross-linking and can modify the nail plate. They are composed of formaldehyde or hydroxyurea.

Nail-hardening agents containing formaldehyde should be used cautiously, as they can cause dehydration and lead to brittleness, onychoschizia, onycholysis, and subungual hyperkeratosis. They should be reserved for soft nails, for short periods, and always in association with emollients. It is important to avoid formaldehyde in patients who are sensitive to this substance. Hydroxyurea is a safer alternative to formaldehyde (Evidence E).

3.3.2.3 Specific Topical Treatments

Lacquers have been specifically developed to restructure nails affected by dystrophy and fragility. One of them is based on hydroxypropyl chitosan (HPCH), *Equisetum arvense*, and methylsulfonylmethane.[4] Once applied to the nails, HPCH forms an invisible film that adheres to the nail structures and protects them from mechanical trauma. The chitosan polymer backbone bears hydrophilic residues that most likely explain the high affinity of HPCH with keratin. This lacquer is designed to decrease lamellar splitting. There is some data showing its effectiveness on psoriatic nails (Evidence B).[5]

Another lacquer available in the U.S. market is made of 16% polyureaurethane, and when applied to the nails, also adheres tightly to their surface forming a strong but flexible waterproof barrier to environmental hazards.[6] The active penetrates intercellular spaces and nail ridges, also providing mechanical support. It is approved by the U.S. Food and Drug Administration (FDA) for this condition (Evidence E).

3.3.3 Systemic Treatment

3.3.3.1 Biotin: Evidence B

Biotin is a water-soluble vitamin component of the B complex that acts as a coenzyme for several human carboxylases. Biotin deficiency is exceedingly rare and may be inherited or acquired. Acquired forms may occur in cases of severe malnutrition, total parenteral nutrition without biotin supplementation, long-term anticonvulsant or antibiotic therapy, and ingestion of raw egg whites. Inherited conditions include biotinidase deficiency and multiple carboxylase deficiency.

In the early 1990s, investigators began to evaluate the use of biotin in humans as a possible aid in nail health, since biotin had been known for decades to improve hardness and strength in the hoofs of animals.

Two open-label studies with biotin concluded that this vitamin could be an effective treatment for brittle nail syndrome. Floersheim et al.[7] treated 71 patients suffering from brittle nails with oral biotin 2.5 mg daily. By the end of the study, only 45 patients were evaluated. The authors reported an improvement on fingernail firmness and hardness in 41 out of 45 patients (91%), following a 5.5 ± 2.3-month course. Colombo et al.[8] analyzed the fingernail specimens obtained from 22 patients of the previously described study, before and after supplementation with biotin took place, and compared them with samples taken from a group of healthy individuals that did not receive biotin. According to the authors, lamellar splitting improved in all patients and nail thickness was improved by 25%. There is a significant design limitation in this study because 14 subjects had initial and terminal nail specimens obtained, but the removal did not coincide strictly with treatment.

Hochman et al.[9] conducted a small retrospective study that sent a detailed questionnaire to 46 patients suffering from BNS and 2.5 mg of daily biotin as treatment. Responses were obtained from 35 of these patients. The median age was 57 years old (range 21–74) and patients reported that they had the condition for 2 months to 30 years. With treatment duration of 1.5–7 months, 22/35 (63%) had improvement in their nails in 1–4 months (average 2 months).

A double-blind, placebo-controlled study conducted by Gehring[10] documented statistically significant improvement in nail quality, as measured by nail swelling and clinical observation, in biotin-treated patients in comparison with patients receiving placebo.

Published work to date supports the use of 2.5 mg/day of biotin for brittle nails for 6 to 12 months. Side effects reported include gastrointestinal distress. It is important to highlight that biotin intake can potentially interfere with some clinical immunoassay tests such as troponin, serum and urine β-hCG, thyroid function, and some tumor markers. These tests employ the high-affinity interaction between biotin and streptavidin as part of the analyte capture mechanism. The interference can be positive or negative in nature depending on the immunoassay. To address this issue, it is recommended that patients abstain from taking biotin supplements for 48 h.

3.3.3.2 Silicon Supplements: Evidence B

Silicon is the second-most abundant element in nature. Various forms of this mineral can be found, such as silicon dioxide, silica, and orthosilicic acid. There is a growing interest in potential therapeutic effects on human health. Silicon is believed to play an important role in skin, hair, and nail health.

Besides the orthosilicic acid and its stabilized formulations, such as choline chloride-stabilized orthosilicic acid, the most important sources that release orthosilicic acid as a bioavailable form of silicon are colloidal silicic acid (hydrated silica gel), silica gel (amorphous silicon dioxide), and zeolites.

Some authors studied the influence of silicon supplements improving brittle nails. An open study by Lassus in 1993[11] treated 50 patients with 10 mL of colloidal silicic acid for 90 days; brittle nails occurred in 21 patients (mean score 1.9) before treatment and in 10 after treatment (mean score 1.0, P < 0.01).

A randomized, double-blind study analyzed 50 women treated with 10 mg of choline-stabilized orthosilicic acid or placebo for 20 weeks. There was a significant improvement of brittle nails in the group that received the drug, which was not observed in the control group.[12]

3.3.3.3 Bioactive Collagen Peptides: Evidence C

The long-standing belief that ingestion of collagen should be a good option for nail health was lacking scientific evidence until recently. Bioactive collagen peptides (BCP) have been used as a food source and a nutritional supplement for a while now. Even though both gelatin and BCP are obtained from collagen hydrolysis, they have completely different properties. To begin with, collagen peptide obtention requires specific enzymes. These proteases cleave collagen to very low molecular weight peptides, when compared to gelatin. Furthermore, BCP have not only been demonstrated to reach the bloodstream, but also to notably stimulate biosynthesis of extracellular matrix proteins.

In two different prospective randomized placebo-controlled clinical trials, Proksch et al. showed skin improvement in women who ingested, for 8 weeks, 2.5 g/d of Verisol, a specific bioactive collagen peptide. Although nail assessments were not the end point of those studies, an improvement in nail quality was noticed among participants and recorded.[13]

TABLE 3.1

Treatments and Levels of Evidence

Treatment	Level of Evidence
General measures	E[1–3]
Topical emollients	E[2,3]
Topical nail-hardening agents	E[2,3]
Topical hydroxypropyl chitosan (HPCH)	B[4,5]
Topical polyureaurethane 16%	E[6]
Oral biotin	B[7–10]
Oral silicon supplements	B[11,12]
Oral bioactive collagen peptides	C[14]
Oral vitamins and minerals	C[16]

Recently, Hexsel et al. conducted an open study to investigate whether daily ingestion of BCP (2.5 g/day of Verisol) for 6 months could positively influence the symptoms of brittle nails and improve nail growth and strength.[14] They observed that treatment promoted a 12% increase in nail growth rate. A decrease of 42% in the frequency of broken nails was also documented. Additionally, 64% of the participants achieved a global clinical improvement in brittle nails by the end of 24 weeks. After a 4-week washout period, the number of participants showing improvement increased, reaching 88% of them.

3.3.3.4 Vitamins and Minerals Association: Evidence C

In 1999, Bergner[15] treated 1629 patients with an oral supplement for 3–6 months containing L-cystine 60 mg, keratin 60 mg, medicinal yeast 300 mg, calcium pantothenate 180 mg, thiamine nitrate 180 mg, and p-aminobenzoic acid 60 mg. It was an open-label study that evaluated both effluvium and brittle nail syndrome. The mean age of patients was 43.6 years, and 84.6% were female and 15.2% male. Nail alterations were evaluated both by patients and doctors, scoring 87% and 88% of improvement, respectively. Ten patients (0.6%) complained of gastrointestinal disorders that were classified as mild.

In 2007, Lengg et al.[16] performed a double-blind study with this same compound and showed a statistically significant improvement on nails. See further Table 3.1.

REFERENCES

1. Van De Kerkhof PC, Pasch MC, Scher RK, Kerscher M, Gieler U, Haneke E, Fleckman P. Brittle nail syndrome: A pathogenesis-based approach with a proposed grading system. *J Am Acad Dermatol.* 2005;53(4):644–651.
2. Lubach D, Beckers P. Wet working conditions increase brittleness of nails, but do not cause it. *Dermatol.* 1992;185(2):120–122.
3. Iorizzo M, Piraccini BM, Tosti A. Nail cosmetics in nail disorders. *J Cosmet Dermatol.* 2007;1:53–58.
4. Sparavigna A, Caserini M, Tenconi B et al. Effects of a novel nail lacquer based on hydroxypropyl-chitosan (HPCH) in subjects with fingernail onychoschizia. *J Dermatol Clin Res.* 2014;2:1013–1017.
5. Cantoresi F, Sorgi P, Arcese A, Bidoli A, Bruni F, Carnevale C, Calvieri S. Improvement of psoriatic onychodystrophy by a water-soluble nail lacquer. *J Eur Acad Dermatol Venereol.* 2009;23(7):832–834.
6. Iorizzo M. Tips to treat the 5 most common nail disorders: Brittle nails, onycholysis, paronychia, psoriasis, onychomycosis. *Dermatol Clin.* 2015;33(2):175–183.
7. Floersheim GL. Treatment of brittle fingernails with biotin. *Z Hautkr.* 1989;64:41–48.
8. Colombo VE, Gerber F, Bronhofer M et al. Treatment of brittle fingernails and onychoschizia with biotin: Scanning electron microscopy. *J Am Acad Dermatol.* 1990;23:1127–1132.
9. Hochman LG, Scher RK, Meyerson MS. Brittle nails: Response to daily biotin supplementation. *Cutis.* 1993;51:303–330.
10. Gehring W. Biotin: The influence of biotin on nails of reduced quality. *Aktuelle Derm.* 1996;22(1):20–24.

11. Lassus A. Colloidal silicic acid for oral and topical treatment of aged skin, fragile hair and brittle nails in females. *J Int Med Res.* 1993;21(4):209–215.

12. Barel A, Calomme M, Timchenko A, Paepe KD, Demeester N, Rogiers V, … Berghe DV. Effect of oral intake of choline-stabilized orthosilicic acid on skin, nails and hair in women with photodamaged skin. *Arch Dermatol Res.* 2005;297(4):147–153.

13. Proksch E, Schunck M, Zague V, Segger D, Degwert J, Oesser S. Oral intake of specific bioactive collagen peptides reduces skin wrinkles and increases dermal matrix synthesis. *Skin Pharmacol Phys.* 2014;27(3):113–119.

14. Hexsel D, Zague V, Schunck M, Siega C, Camozzato FO, Oesser S. Oral supplementation with specific bioactive collagen peptides improves nail growth and reduces symptoms of brittle nails. *J Cosmet Dermatol.* 2017;16(4):520–526.

15. Bergner T. Diffuse effluvium, damage to hair structure, and disturbances of nail growth treated successfully: Results of a multicenter study. *Dt Derm.* 1999;47:881–884.

16. Lengg N, Heidecker B, Seifert B, Trueb RM. Dietary supplement increases anagen hair rate in women with telogen effluvium: Results of a double-blind, placebo-controlled trial. *Therapy.* 2007;4(1):59–66.

4

Chronic Paronychia

Walter Refkalefsky Loureiro and Hind M. Almohanna

4.1 Introduction

Chronic paronychia is inflammation of the proximal and lateral nail folds that lasted for more than 6 weeks and represents an irritant dermatitis to the breached nail barrier.[1–3] It constitutes approximately 18% of nail dystrophies. Risk factors include persistent exposure to environmental irritants such as wet work;[4] acids, alkalis, and other chemicals used by housekeepers, dishwashers, swimmers, bakers, and florists;[5] and allergens,[6] for example, foods.[7] Furthermore, inflammatory skin diseases, for example, atopic dermatitis and psoriasis, may be associated with chronic paronychia.[8] Also, chronic paronychia develops in some psychiatric disorders with obsessive compulsive traits, such as onychotillomania, nail picking, sucking, or biting.

It is thought that the colonization by fungi and bacteria is a secondary process rather than the primary cause. Although *Candida* spp. is isolated from the nail fold in up to 95% of patients with chronic paronychia, eradication of the yeast does not cure the disease. Therefore, nail fold infection with candida may lead to the persistence of the condition but should not be considered as a causative agent.[2] The main etiologic factor is continuous exposure of the periungual tissues and the matrix to irritants. Also, chronic paronychia is a well-known side effect of systemic medications including taxanes, epidermal growth factor-receptor (EGFR) inhibitors, EGFR tyrosine kinase inhibitors, tyrosine kinase inhibitors, BRAF inhibitors, inhibitors of MEK/ERK, CD20 antagonists, vascular endothelial growth factor inhibitors, and retinoids.[9]

Initially chronic paronychia presents with mild erythema and edema of the proximal and lateral nail folds with loss of the cuticle. After that, the proximal nail fold retracts and becomes hypertrophic along with the lateral nail folds (Figure 4.1).[1,2] Persistent exposure of the nail matrix to irritants disturb the nail plate growth, which manifests as ridging and Beau's lines (Figures 4.2 and 4.3). Moreover, secondary bacterial or fungal infections may lead to discolorations of the nail plate (Figure 4.4). Acute episodes of paronychia on top of chronic may occur, which exacerbate the erythema and swelling.[1,2]

Differential diagnosis includes squamous cell carcinoma (SSC) and SSC in situ (Bowen disease).[10] The clinical features are nonhealing ulceration or persistent eczematous lesion involving the nail folds that does not respond to standard treatments.[10–12] Other mimickers to chronic paronychia are cutaneous leishmaniasis;[13,14] pemphigus vulgaris;[15] pemphigus vegetans;[16] pyodermatitis-pyostomatitis vegetans associated with inflammatory bowel disease, particularly ulcerative colitis;[10] and cutaneous metastases of internal malignancies.[17,18]

4.2 How to Confirm the Diagnosis

The diagnosis of chronic paronychia is usually clinical, based on the characteristic clinical findings, including retraction and hypertrophy of the proximal nail fold, loss of the cuticle, and nail dystrophy. Further support to the clinical diagnosis is the presence of repeated exposure to wet work, chemicals, irritants, or allergens. Fungus investigation (KOH, culture, for PAS [periodic acid–Schiff]) are indicated when there is a suspicion of coexistent onychomycosis. Green discoloration of the nail plate generally

(a)

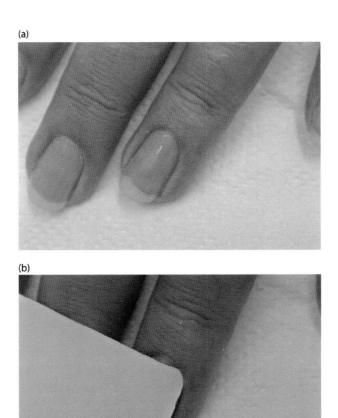

FIGURE 4.1   Swelling and mild erythema of the nail folds (a). Loss of the cuticle and nail plate dystrophy (b).

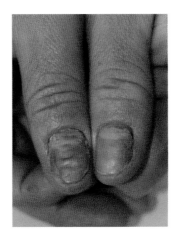

FIGURE 4.2   Persistent exposure to irritants disturbed the nail plate growth causing Beau's lines.

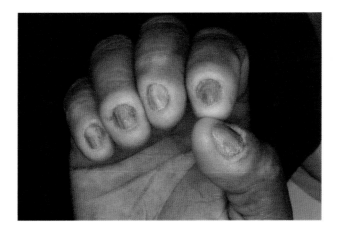

FIGURE 4.3 Hypertrophic proximal and lateral nail folds with cuticle absence and intense nail irregularities: leukonychia, pitting, and discoloration due to melanocytic activation.

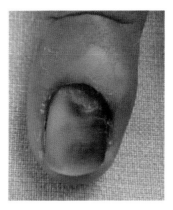

FIGURE 4.4 Discoloration of the nail plate suggesting bacterial colonization by *P. aeruginosa*.

indicates colonization by *Pseudomonas aeruginosa*. If allergic contact dermatitis is suspected, patch testing may be necessary. A "Chronic Paronychia Severity Index Scale" was developed to enable dermatologists to examine all features of this nail disorder.[19]

A skin biopsy is generally not indicated for the diagnosis of chronic paronychia. However, recalcitrant disease and atypical presentations are indications to perform a skin biopsy. Atypical presentations include ulceration, excessive inflammation, or desquamation. In such conditions, histopathologic examination is required to rule out malignancy or other disorders mimicking chronic paronychia.

4.3 Evidence-Based Treatment

4.3.1 General Measures

The mainstay of treatment is avoidance of environmental triggers. Patients have to be instructed to use gloves for all wet work and to keep their hands dry most of the times when possible. In case of contact dermatitis, patients should also avoid exposure to the irritant or allergen. Frequent use of emollients after handwashing and avoiding cuticle removal are essential.

4.3.2 Topical Treatment

We suggest topical corticosteroids rather than antifungals as a first-line treatment for chronic paronychia, in combination with the general measures. A high-potency topical corticosteroid is applied once or twice daily for 2 to 4 weeks or until the lesion is improved. This is supported by the findings of a randomized double-blind placebo-controlled trial comparing topical corticosteroids with systemic antifungal therapy. Topical methylprednisolone aceponate 0.1% cream was associated with a significantly higher cure rate compared with oral antifungal treatment (85% vs. 49% of nails, respectively). Candidal eradication was associated with clinical cure in only 2 patients out of 18 who had positive culture from the proximal nail fold at the beginning of the study.[8]

Topical calcineurin inhibitors can be an alternative treatment option for chronic paronychia in patients who prefer not to use topical corticosteroids. Topical tacrolimus 0.1% ointment was similar in efficacy to betamethasone 17-valerate 0.1% ointment and superior to placebo in one randomized, unblinded study.[20]

Alternative treatment includes a combination of ciclopirox 0.77% topical suspension twice daily and an irritant-avoidance regimen for 6 to 12 weeks.[21]

4.3.3 Surgical Approach

More aggressive techniques may be required to restore the protective nail barrier. Refractory chronic paronychia that failed to respond to medical therapies can be surgically treated. Some surgical procedures have been published.[22] The preferred surgical technique for the author of this chapter is the marsupialization or oblique excision of the eponychium without nail avulsion, as it is simple and very fast to perform (Figures 4.5, 4.7, 4.8).[23] When the patient has a short visible nail plate and wants to increase its area (for cosmetic purposes), then the en bloc surgery is suggested (Figures 4.6 and 4.9). The "en bloc excision"

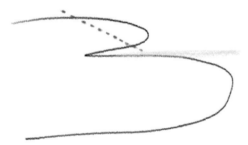

FIGURE 4.5   Schematic for the oblique incision technique: note the inclined orientation of the incision represented by the red dotted line. This incision removes the bulk of the hypertrophic tissue of the eponychium preserving the ventral aspect. There is minimal chance of injuring the nail matrix, thus the use of a protective spatula is not required. The nail matrix and plate are represented by the yellow line.

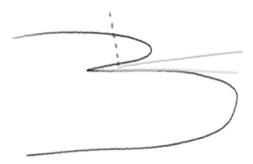

FIGURE 4.6   Schematic of the en bloc excision. The red dotted line represents the gentle slope of the incision; note that the full thickness of the hypertrophic proximal ungual fold is excised. The green line represents a spatula protecting the nail matrix from the scalpel blade, and the yellow line represents the underlying nail matrix and plate.

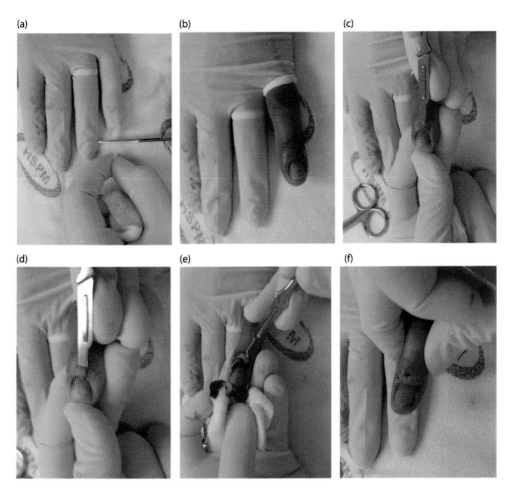

FIGURE 4.7 Step-by-step oblique excision of a crescent-shaped fragment of the hypertrophic proximal nail fold, leaving the ventral part of the eponychium. Open a small hole at the tip of the glove (a). Roll the glove to the base of the finger to exsanguinate and serve as the tourniquet (b). Insert the scalpel blade at approximately 45% angle until the tip os the blade is visible just above the nail plate (c) end (d). Remove the hypertrophic tissue with a crescent shaped incision preserving the roof of the eponychium (e) and (f).

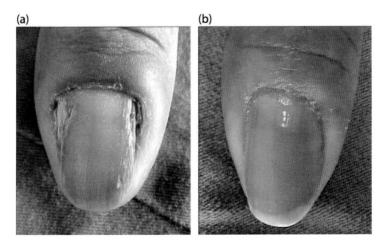

FIGURE 4.8 Before (a) and after (b) 12 months of oblique excision.

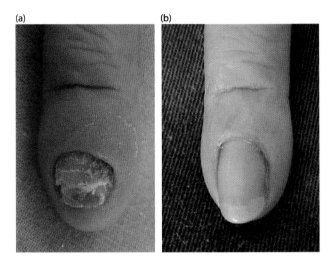

FIGURE 4.9   Before (a) and after (b) 6 months of en bloc excision. Observe the increase of the visible part of the nail plate.

technique includes the removal of the crescent-shaped, full-thickness part of the proximal nail fold with a maximal width of 3 to 6 mm, with or without nail plate avulsion. It was found that 70% of patients who underwent nail plate avulsion with en bloc excision were declared cured compared to 41% without nail plate avulsion after an average follow-up of 16 months (Figure 4.10).[24,25]

The third technique is the "Swiss roll" method that has been considered for paronychia with runaround abscess. In this procedure, the proximal nail fold is lifted, by making an incision on either side, over a nonadherent dressing that is rolled up like a Swiss roll and fixed to the skin with two securing nonabsorbable sutures. Then the nail fold is kept open for 48 hours. After that, if the wound is clean, the sutures can be removed and the proximal nail fold is returned to its anatomical position and left to heal by secondary intention.[26]

The fourth procedure is the "square flap technique," which involves the removal of the fibrotic tissue of the nail folds only, preserving the epidermis and the underlying matrix. In this method, an incision is made on both sides of the proximal nail fold and then a flap is created by making an incision parallel to

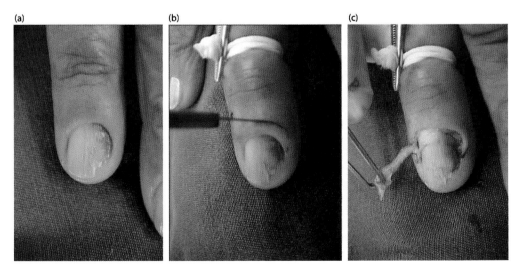

FIGURE 4.10   Perpendicular incision removing en bloc a full-thickness crescent-shape fibrous tissue of the proximal ungual fold, as performed by the authors. Hypertrophyc proximal nail fold (a). Perpendicular incision with approximately 3 mm wide (b). Full thickness removal of the crescent shaped hypertrophic proximal nail fold, including the eponychoum roof (c). (Photos courtesy Dr. Nilton Di Chiacchio.)

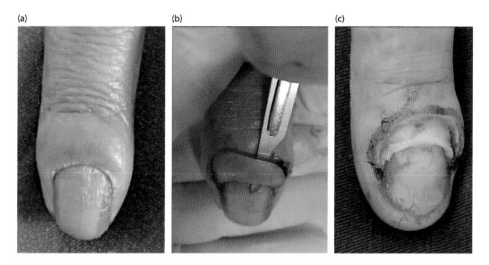

FIGURE 4.11 Oblique incision removing the roof of the proximal nail fold, leaving the ventral part of the eponychium; authors' variation of marsupialization technique. Hypertrophyc proximal nail fold (a). insert the blade tip through the hypertrophic tissue at a 45% angle, until the tip of the blade Is visible just over the nail plate.(b). Remove a crescent shaped hypertrophic preserving the roof of the eponychium (c). (Photos courtesy Dr. Nilton Di Chiacchio.)

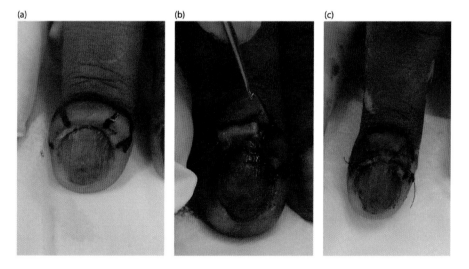

FIGURE 4.12 Square flap technique: (a) Chronic paronychia of the proximal nail fold. The markings show the limits of the hypertrophic fibrous tissue and the location of the incisions. (b) Debulking of the square flap, preserving the epidermis. (c) Square flap sutured in place; note the aspect of the proximal nail fold at the end of the procedure. (Photos courtesy Dr. Robertha Nakamura.)

the epidermis. The flap incision runs underneath the fibrotic tissue but above the nail, to avoid injury to the matrix. Then the flap is flipped and the fibrotic tissue is removed with the scalpel blade. After that, the initial incision is closed primarily with a simple interrupted suture (Figure 4.12).[27]

4.3.4 Comparative Studies of Surgical Interventions

- "Surgical treatment of chronic paronychia: A comparative study of 138 surgeries using two different techniques"[28]—62 patients with a diagnosis of chronic paronychia in 138 nail folds were randomly assigned in equal number to 2 treatment groups with 69 nails each. One group was treated with perpendicular incision and the other with oblique incision. The perpendicular incision is in essence the en bloc excision technique described by Baran,[25] whereas the oblique incision (Figure 4.11) is the eponychium marsupialization described by Keyser and Eaton[23] (the authors considered these terms more graphic and renamed them for descriptive purposes). In none of the procedures was the nail plate was removed. The authors observed clinical cure in 97.1% of the nail folds and improvement in four cases, two of each group. Follow-up was 180 days. They also noted that when perpendicular incision was performed, the resulting visible part of the nail plate was longitudinally bigger; this was not observed with the oblique incision.

- "Eponychial marsupialization and nail removal for surgical treatment of chronic paronychia"[29]— Bednar et al.[29] treated 28 fingers from 25 consecutive patients. The first 7 fingers were treated with marsupialization alone, with recurrence in two patients. The following 18 patients (all with nail dystrophy) were treated with marsupialization and nail plate avulsion; all patients were cured without any case of recurrence ($p < 0.05$) with an average 33-month follow-up. A 3 mm width crescent of skin parallel to the eponychium and extending from the radial to ulnar borders is excised. In contrast to the technique of Keyser and Eaton[23] in which all thickened tissue is removed with the skin, the subcutaneous tissue and fat were left intact in these patients. In 18 patients, marsupialization was associated with partial or total nail plate avulsion. The authors concluded that in patients without dystrophy, the best treatment would be marsupialization alone, while the association of marsupialization and nail avulsion would be reserved for patients with nail irregularities.
- "Surgical cure of chronic paronychia by eponychial marsupialization"[23]
- "Treatment of chronic paronychia: A double-blind comparative clinical trial using singly vaseline, nystatin, and fusidic acid ointment"[30]—A double-blind comparative therapeutic trial divided 80 female patients into three unequal groups: vaseline, nystatin, or fusidic acid. All ointments were effective in clearing chronic paronychia (p < 0.001), without statistic differences between the three groups (p = 0.784).
- "1064 Nd:YAG laser for the treatment of chronic paronychia: A pilot study"[31]—Eleven fingernails in eight patients were treated monthly with long pulsed 1.064 nm Nd:YAG laser for two to five sessions. Patients were also instructed to use gloves and minimize water and detergent exposure. Follow-up consultation was 1 month after the last laser session, with variable improvement of nail folds in 87.5% of patients and 75% showed variable degree of improvement in nail plate.
- "Treatment and prevention of paronychia using a new combination of topicals: Report of 30 cases"[32]
- "Doxycycline for the treatment of paronychia induced by the epidermal growth factor receptor inhibitor cetuximab"[33]

TABLE 4.1

Treatments and Levels of Evidence

Treatment	Level of Evidence
Topical Treatment	
Corticosteroids	A[8]
Tacrolimus	B[20]
Ciclopirox combined	C[21]
Surgical Treatment	
Oblique excision of the eponychium without nail avulsion	B[28] C[24,25]
"En bloc excision"	B[28] C[24,25]
"Swiss roll"	E[26]
"Square flap technique"	D[27]
Eponychial marsupialization and nail removal	C[29]
1064 Nd:YAG laser	D[31]

4.3.5 Patient Education and Preventive Measures

Patient education is paramount to reduce the recurrence of chronic paronychia. In order to prevent chronic paronychia, vigilant skin care of hands is recommended. Patients are advised not to soak their hands in water for prolonged periods of time without wearing protective gloves. They should rather keep their hands and feet dry whenever possible. Extra caution has to be undertaken when trimming the nails. Patients should also avoid any kind of trauma to the nail folds, cuticle, and nail plate. See also Table 4.1.

REFERENCES

1. Rockwell PG. Acute and chronic paronychia. *Am Fam Physician.* 2001;63(6):1113–1116.
2. Shafritz AB, Coppage JM. Acute and chronic paronychia of the hand. *J Am Acad Orthop Surg.* 2014;22(3):165–174.
3. Rigopoulos D, Larios G, Gregoriou S, Alevizos A. Acute and chronic paronychia. *Am Fam Physician.* 2008;77(3):339–346.
4. Daniel CR, 3rd, Daniel MP, Daniel CM, Sullivan S, Ellis G. Chronic paronychia and onycholysis: A thirteen-year experience. *Cutis.* 1996;58(6):397–401.
5. Leggit JC. Acute and chronic paronychia. *Am Fam Physician.* 2017;96(1):44–51.
6. Kanerva L. Occupational protein contact dermatitis and paronychia from natural rubber latex. *J Eur Acad Dermatol Venereol.* 2000;14(6):504–506.
7. Tosti A, Guerra L, Morelli R, Bardazzi F, Fanti PA. Role of foods in the pathogenesis of chronic paronychia. *J Am Acad Dermatol.* 1992;27(5 Pt 1):706–710.
8. Tosti A, Piraccini BM, Ghetti E, Colombo MD. Topical steroids versus systemic antifungals in the treatment of chronic paronychia: An open, randomized double-blind and double dummy study. *J Am Acad Dermatol.* 2002;47(1):73–76.
9. Wollina U. Systemic drug-induced chronic paronychia and periungual pyogenic granuloma. *Indian Dermatol Online J.* 2018;9(5):293–298.
10. Jack C, El Helou T. Non-healing ulcerative paronychia. *Lancet.* 2017;389(10080):1740.
11. Lobato-Berezo A, Fernandez-Valencia-Kettunen CK, Burgos-Lazaro F, Martinez-Perez M, Aguilar-Martinez A, Gallego-Valdes MA. Ungual squamous cell carcinoma mimicking a chronic paronychia: Clinical, pathological and radiological correlation. *Dermatol Online J.* 2015;21(11).
12. Giacomel J, Lallas A, Zalaudek I, Argenziano G. Periungual Bowen disease mimicking chronic paronychia and diagnosed by dermoscopy. *J Am Acad Dermatol.* 2014;71(3):e65–e67.
13. Chaabane H, Turki H. Images in clinical medicine. Cutaneous leishmaniasis with a paronychia-like lesion. *N Engl J Med.* 2014;371(18):1736.
14. Chiheb S, El Machbouh L, Marnissi F. Paronychia-like cutaneous leishmaniasis. *Dermatol Online J.* 2015;21(11).
15. Zawar V, Pawar M, Kumavat S. Recurrent paronychia as a presenting manifestation of pemphigus vulgaris: A case report. *Skin Appendage Disord.* 2017;3(1):28–31.
16. Sukakul T, Varothai S. Chronic paronychia and onychomadesis in pemphigus vegetans: An unusual presentation in a rare autoimmune disease. *Case Rep Med.* 2018;2018:5980937.
17. Ko JH, Young A, Wang KH. Paronychia-like digital cutaneous metastasis. *Br J Dermatol.* 2014;171(3):663–665.
18. Lee CC, Wu YH. Paronychia-like digital metastases of osteosarcoma. *Int J Dermatol.* 2017;56(1):104–105.
19. Atis G, Goktay F, Altan Ferhatoglu Z et al. A proposal for a new severity index for the evaluation of chronic Paronychia. *Skin Appendage Disord.* 2018;5(1):32–37.
20. Rigopoulos D, Gregoriou S, Belyayeva E, Larios G, Kontochristopoulos G, Katsambas A. Efficacy and safety of tacrolimus ointment 0.1% vs. betamethasone 17-valerate 0.1% in the treatment of chronic paronychia: An unblinded randomized study. *Br J Dermatol.* 2009;160(4):858–860.
21. Daniel CR, 3rd, Daniel MP, Daniel J, Sullivan S, Bell FE. Managing simple chronic paronychia and onycholysis with ciclopirox 0.77% and an irritant-avoidance regimen. *Cutis.* 2004;73(1):81–85.
22. Relhan V, Goel K, Bansal S, Garg VK. Management of chronic paronychia. *Indian J Dermatol.* 2014;59(1):15–20.

23. Keyser JJ, Eaton RG. Surgical cure of chronic paronychia by eponychial marsupialization. *Plast Reconstr Surg.* 1976;58(1):66–70.
24. Grover C, Bansal S, Nanda S, Reddy BS, Kumar V. En bloc excision of proximal nail fold for treatment of chronic paronychia. *Dermatol Surg.* 2006;32(3):393–398; discussion 8–9.
25. Baran R, Bureau H. Surgical treatment of recalcitrant chronic paronychias of the fingers. *J Dermatol Surg Oncol.* 1981;7(2):106–107.
26. Pabari A, Iyer S, Khoo CT. Swiss roll technique for treatment of paronychia. *Tech Hand Up Extrem Surg.* 2011;15(2):75–77.
27. Ferreira Vieira d'Almeida L, Papaiordanou F, Araujo Machado E, Loda G, Baran R, Nakamura R. Chronic paronychia treatment: Square flap technique. *J Am Acad Dermatol.* 2016;75(2):398–403.
28. Di Chiacchio N, Debs E, Tassara G. Surgical treatment of chronic paronychia: A comparative study of 138 surgeries using two different techniques. *Surg Cosmetic Derm.* 2009;1(1):21–24.
29. Bednar MS, Lane LB. Eponychial marsupialization and nail removal for surgical treatment of chronic paronychia. *J Hand Surg Am.* 1991;16(2):314–317.
30. Sharquie K, Noaimi A, Galib S. Treatment of chronic paronychia: A double blind comparative clinical trial using singly vaseline, nystatin and fucidic acid ointment. *J Cosmet Dermatol Sci Appl.* 2013;3(4):250–255.
31. El-Komy MH, Samir N. 1064 Nd:YAG laser for the treatment of chronic paronychia: A pilot study. *Lasers Med Sci.* 2015;30(5):1623–1626.
32. Gianni C. Treatment and prevention of paronychia using a new combination of topicals: Report of 30 cases. *G Ital Dermatol Venereol.* 2015;150(4):357–362.
33. Shu KY, Kindler HL, Medenica M, Lacouture M. Doxycycline for the treatment of paronychia induced by the epidermal growth factor receptor inhibitor cetuximab. *Br J Dermatol.* 2006;154(1):191–192.

5

Eczema

Azhar Abbas Ahmed and Antonella Tosti

5.1 Introduction

Nail eczema is usually secondary to hand dermatitis whether the cause of the hand dermatitis is due to endogenous hands/feet eczema, pompholyx, or exogenous factors such as irritant contact dermatitis,[1] or allergic contact dermatitis from acrylate nail products[2] or other allergens.[3] However, in some cases the nail apparatus is the only affected site. All parts of the nail apparatus can be affected, and periungual inflammation can damage the nail matrix function, with development of Beau's line, multiple pits, or trachyonychia.[4,5]

Prevalence of nail changes due to hand eczema varies in different studies from 16%[6] to 32%.[4]

When the nail bed is affected, signs include subungual hyperkeratosis and onycholysis, which can be hemorrhagic. Involvement of the nail folds causes roughness and thickening of the cuticle and with time, loss of the cuticle with chronic paronychia.[7] Nail shining (polished nail) from repeated rubbing of the nail on the itchy skin can be seen in patients with diffuse eczema.[8,9]

Differential diagnosis: Nail psoriasis,[10] onychomycosis, nail lichen planus, and trauma.[11]

5.2 How to Confirm the Diagnosis

In most cases, nail eczema follows the cutaneous eczema or history of acrylate exposure and is therefore easy to diagnose.

A. History including onset, progression, occupation, personal history of atopy.

B. Clinical examination by naked eye may show nail plate surface abnormalities including Beau's lines (Figure 5.1), pitting and trachyonychia, subungual hyperkeratosis, onycholysis, roughness and thickening of the proximal/lateral nail fold, loss of the cuticle, chronic paronychia,[12] and polished nail.[8]

C. Dermoscopy makes the clinical signs more obvious and helps in the diagnosis. Videodermatoscopy allows higher magnifications than the usual handheld dermatoscope. Dermoscopy of the hyponychium allows one to distinguish onycholysis due to eczema from psoriatic onycholysis.

D. Patch testing:[13] Screening test in case of contact dermatitis from acrylic/gel polish nails should include methyl methacrylate (MMA) and 2-hydroxyethyl methacrylate (HEMA).[14]

E. Nail biopsy is usually not necessary as the nail changes normalize after avoiding the precipitating factors.[15]

F. Nail clipping to exclude onychomycosis is usually unnecessary.

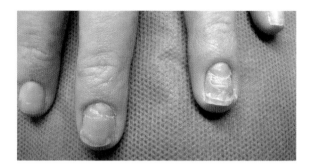

FIGURE 5.1   Irregular Beau's lines in a patient with hand eczema. Not all the nails are affected, and lines are at different levels.

5.3 Treatment of Nail Dermatitis

Treatment is directed toward hand dermatitis if it is the primary cause of nail changes and avoiding the triggering allergen (Figure 5.2). If eczema improves, the nail will gradually return normal with time.

5.3.1 Nonpharmacological Intervention

- Avoid the causative factors.[13,16,17] "Non-touch" techniques should be encouraged in acrylate users.[18]
- Emollient to be applied many times in a day.[13]
- Wear thin cotton gloves under a nonlatex glove when performing wet work or cooking with irritants.[17]
- In case of acrylate contact dermatitis:
  - Clients advised to avoid acrylic and gel polish manicures/pedicures
  - Nail beauticians advised to use a double gloves or nitrile gloves, which will protect from acrylate exposure for up to 6 hours.[19] Wearing a mask and goggles are recommended too[20]
- Avoid cleaning the nail with sharp instruments to lessen further onycholysis.[20]

5.3.2 Topical Treatment

- Topical moderate to high-potency corticosteroids (clobetasol propionate 0.05% cream, betamethasone dipropionate 0.05% cream, etc.) applied for few weeks with or without occlusion.[12,21]

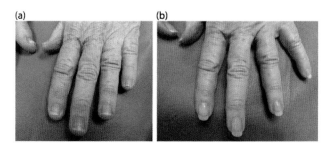

FIGURE 5.2   (a) Psoriasiform contact dermatitis from gel polish manicure. (b) Complete cure after avoiding further exposure and treatment with high-potency topical steroids.

TABLE 5.1

Treatments and Levels of Evidence

Treatment	Level of Evidence
Topical moderate to high-potency corticosteroids	A[12,21]
Topical tacrolimus ointment	A[22]
Intralesional triamcinolone injection	C[23]
Photochemotherapy	C[21]
Alitretinoin	D[24]

- Topical tacrolimus ointment (0.1% or 0.03% ointments) or pimecrolimus 1% cream under occlusion overnight around proximal nail fold;[22] for long-term treatment.[21]
- Topical anti-staphylococcal antibiotics are prescribed for secondary bacterial infection.

5.3.3 Procedures

- Intralesional triamcinolone injection 2.5 mg/mL into the proximal nail fold. Side effects: pain and hematoma, atrophy, whitening may occur.[23]
- Photochemotherapy (NUVB vs. PUVA) as second-line treatment for nail changes associated with hand eczema.[21]

5.3.4 Systemic Treatment

- Short-course systemic steroid rarely required for severe hand eczema with nail changes.
- Alitretinoin 10–30 mg/d[24] (possible side effects: dryness, headache, and occasional report of alitretinoin-induced median nail dystrophy).[25] See further Table 5.1.

REFERENCES

1. Hongal AA, Rajashekhar N, Gejje S. Palmoplantar dermatoses—A clinical study of 300 cases. *J Clin Diagn Res.* 2016;10(8):WC04–WC07.
2. van der Voort EAM, van Neer FJMA, Neumann HAM. Acrylate-induced nail contact allergy. *Int J Dermatol.* 2014;53(9):e390–e392.
3. Mussani F, DeKoven JG. Unilateral hand allergic contact dermatitis due to occupational exposure. *J Cutan Med Surg.* 2014;18(4):283–286.
4. Yu M, Kim SW, Kim MS, Han TY, Lee JH, Son S-J. Clinical study of patients with hand eczema accompanied by nail dystrophy. *J Dermatol.* 2013;40(5):406–407.
5. Crosby DL, Swanson SL, Fleischer AB. Twenty-nail dystrophy of childhood with koilonychia. *Clin Pediatr (Phila).* 1991;30(2):117–119.
6. Simpson EL, Thompson MM, Hanifin JM. Prevalence and morphology of hand eczema in patients with atopic dermatitis. *Dermatitis.* 2006;17(3):123–127.
7. Tosti A, Guerra L, Morelli R, Bardazzi F, Fanti PA. Role of foods in the pathogenesis of chronic paronychia. *J Am Acad Dermatol.* 1992;27(5 Pt 1):706–710.
8. Haneke E. Non-infectious inflammatory disorders of the nail apparatus. *J Dtsch Dermatol Ges.* 2009;7(9):787–797.
9. Wollina U, Nenoff P, Haroske G, Haenssle HA. The diagnosis and treatment of nail disorders. *Dtsch Arztebl Int.* 2016;113(29–30):509–518.
10. DeKoven S, Holness DL. Contact dermatitis caused by methacrylates in nail products. *CMAJ.* 2017;189(37):E1193.
11. Richert B, Caucanas M, André J. Diagnosis using nail matrix. *Dermatol Clin.* 2015;33(2):243–255.

12. Richert B, André J. Nail disorders in children: Diagnosis and management. *Am J Clin Dermatol.* 2011;12(2):101–112.
13. Agarwal US, Besarwal RK, Gupta R, Agarwal P, Napalia S. Hand eczema. *Indian J Dermatol.* 2014;59(3):213–224.
14. Lin Y-T, Tsai S-W, Yang C-W, Tseng Y-H, Chu C-Y. Allergic contact dermatitis caused by acrylates in nail cosmetic products: Case reports and review of the literatures. *Dermatologica Sinica.* 2018;36(4):218–221.
15. Mattos Simoes Mendonca M, LaSenna C, Tosti A. Severe onychodystrophy due to allergic contact dermatitis from acrylic nails. *Skin Appendage Disord.* 2015;1(2):91–94.
16. Takeuchi S, Matsuzaki Y, Ikenaga S et al. Garlic-induced irritant contact dermatitis mimicking nail psoriasis. *J Dermatol.* 2011;38(3):280–282.
17. Militello G. Contact and primary irritant dermatitis of the nail unit diagnosis and treatment. *Dermatol Ther.* 2007;20(1):47–53.
18. Uter W, Geier J. Contact allergy to acrylates and methacrylates in consumers and nail artists—Data of the Information Network of Departments of Dermatology, 2004–2013. *Contact Dermatitis.* 2015;72(4):224–228.
19. Muttardi K, White IR, Banerjee P. The burden of allergic contact dermatitis caused by acrylates. *Contact Dermatitis.* 2016;75(3):180–184.
20. Rieder EA, Tosti A. Cosmetically induced disorders of the nail with update on contemporary nail manicures. *J Clin Aesthet Dermatol.* 2016;9(4):39–44.
21. Diepgen TL, Andersen KE, Chosidow O et al. Guidelines for diagnosis, prevention and treatment of hand eczema—Short version. *J Dtsch Dermatol Ges.* 2015;13(1):77–85.
22. Lee D-Y, Kim W-S, Lee K-J et al. Tacrolimus ointment in onychodystrophy associated with eczema. *J Eur Acad Dermatol Venereol.* 2007;21(8):1137–1138.
23. Grover C, Bansal S, Nanda S, Reddy BSN. Efficacy of triamcinolone acetonide in various acquired nail dystrophies. *J Dermatol.* 2005;32(12):963–968.
24. Milanesi N, D'Erme AM, Gola M. Nail improvement during alitretinoin treatment: Three case reports and review of the literature. *Clin Exp Dermatol.* 2015;40(5):533–536.
25. Winther AH, Bygum A. Can median nail dystrophy be an adverse effect of alitretinoin treatment? *Acta Derm Venereol.* 2014;94(6):719–720.

6

Erythronychia

Cristina Diniz Borges Figueira de Mello

6.1 Introduction

Longitudinal erythronychia is a linear red band that usually extends from the lunula to the distal tip of the nail bed. When limited to one digit, the etiology is usually neoplastic, with onychopapilloma, an idiopathic benign tumor, being the most common diagnosis. The longitudinal red streak results from a localized punctate defect in the distal matrix (due to matrix function loss), inducing a longitudinal ventral groove at the undersurface of the nail, which becomes thinner (Figure 6.2B). In addition, the opposing nail bed swells to fill the concave nail plate, resulting in a vascular congestion that manifests as erythema. The thinned nail plate is more transparent, further enhancing the underlying erythema, and may disintegrate distally, favoring cracks and splits and exposing the nail bed, promoting the formation of multinucleate giant cells and protruding keratosis distally.

Clinically, cases show some or all of the following: longitudinal pink-red nail discoloration, often associated with or composed entirely of splinter hemorrhages, a lucency in the distal matrix, distal V-shaped chipping, splitting, onycholysis of the nail plate at the free edge (Figure 6.1A), and reactive distal nail bed and hyponychial hyperkeratosis (Figure 6.1D). Most individuals with onychopapilloma have no nail-associated symptoms, and seek medical evaluation for cosmetics concerns, distal nail fragility, or because the inconvenience of catching the fragile split's free edge.

Histologic findings characteristic of onychopapilloma include acanthosis, papillomatosis, matrix metaplasia of the nail bed, and distal subungual hyperkeratosis with focal parakeratosis.

The origin of onychopapilloma remains unclear and studies fail to link it to human papillomavirus (HPV) infection. As it occurs mainly on the thumb, one may hypothesize that trauma may be responsible for a reaction pattern.

The differential diagnosis for monodactylous longitudinal erythronychia is broad, including verruca, warty dyskeratoma, glomus tumor, Bowen disease, melanoma, basal cell carcinoma, and other vascular lesions including arteriovenous malformation and traumatic splinter hemorrhages.

6.2 How to Confirm the Diagnosis

Dermatoscopy highlights some clinical alterations, such as splinter hemorrhages (Figure 6.1B) and the keratotic subungual mass (Figure 6.1E) in correspondence to the streak visible at the distal edge of onychopapillomas. Red bands are less visible with contact dermatoscopy as they blanch with lens contact (Figure 6.1B). Onychopapilloma can be diagnosed from a nail clipping. For this purpose, it is very important for the nail clipping to include the entire distal nail plate and not only the affected portion. The diagnosis is suggested by presence of a localized asymmetric keratotic portion underneath the free edge of the nail, composed of layered hyperkeratosis with or without hemorrhage and corresponds to the subungual keratotic mass.

Ultrasound imaging can be used as a noninvasive confirmatory test, revealing in the longitudinal view, a linear hyperechoic structure along the ventral plate and interplate space (Figure 6.1C) and in the transverse view, a round hyperechoic mass below the nail plate (Figure 6.1F).

Surgical exploration and lesion removal results in confirming the diagnosis of the associated condition.

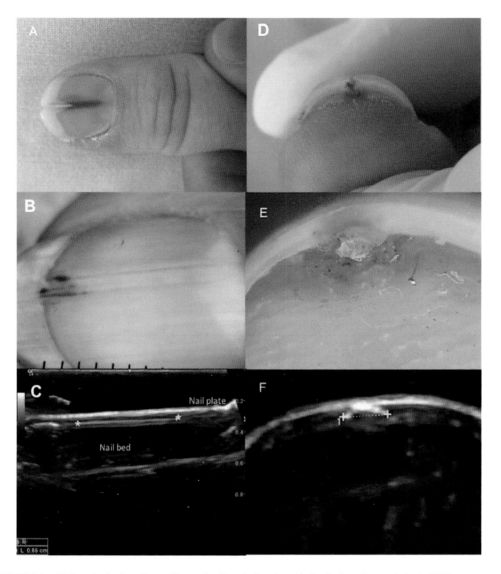

FIGURE 6.1 (A) Longitudinal erythronychia starting from the lunula, with distal triangular onycholysis. (B) Dermatoscopy highlights splinter hemorrhages. (C) Ultrasound in longitudinal view of onychopapilloma (*-*). (D) Clinical, (E) dermatoscopic, and (F) sonographic (+-+) view of the subungual mass under the free margin. (Ultrasound images courtesy Dr. Milena da Rocha e Souza.)

6.3 Evidence-Based Treatment

A static, asymptomatic longitudinal erythronychia does not require treatment. Jellinek has proposed an algorithm to approach patients with longitudinal erythronychia. Stable lesions, where no history or physical examination findings that point to a particular diagnosis, or when the finding is completely incidental, if documented by a good historian or repeated examinations without change, may be followed at regular intervals. It is often reasonable to document and monitor for change carefully over 3–6 months in the first instance. Patients are told to watch the lesion for any change and to return sooner if changes occur.[1]

Where longitudinal erythronychia is broader, with an established split in the nail, atypical in some respect, or in case of changing, evolving, or new lesions, an excisional biopsy (Figure 6.2) should be

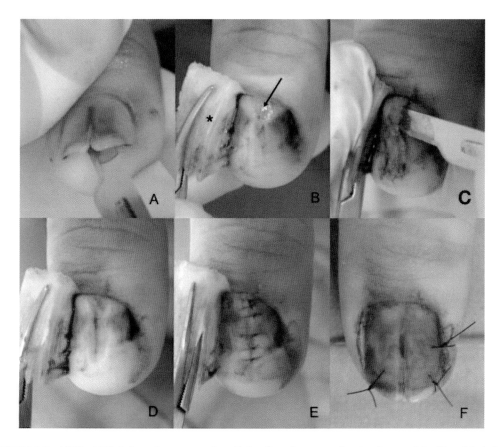

FIGURE 6.2 (A) No. 15 blade is used to separate the nail plate from the tumor, after detachment of the sides of the lesion with an elevator. (B) Lateral curled nail avulsion exposing the tumor (arrow). The defect in the nail can be seen as a groove in the ventral aspect of the nail (*). (C) Deep shave excision of the lesion with No. 15 blade, starting in the mid to distal matrix and carried to the hyponychium. (D) After deeper tangential excision. (E) Reapproximation of the nail bed with 5-0 absorbable sutures. (F) The plate is put back in place and secured to the lateral and distal walls. (Photos courtesy Dr. Nilton Di Chiacchio.)

performed to exclude malignant subungual neoplasm such as a squamous cell carcinoma or a malignant melanoma.[1]

Longitudinal biopsy not only provides adequate tissue for diagnosis, but also usually results in successful treatment of onychopapilloma.[1–6] The procedures start with a delicate lateral avulsion of the nail plate, trying to detach the upper part of the onychopapilloma from the undersurface of the plate, using a surgical No. 15 blade (Figure 6.2A). After lateral curled nail avulsion, the tumor is visualized as subtle pink erythematous swelling in the distal matrix and a longitudinal ridge in the nail bed (Figure 6.2B, arrow). Longitudinal excision is performed starting in the distal matrix and extending up to the digital pulp (Figure 6.2C). Classically, the excision goes down to the bone (Figure 6.3, green dotted line) or is made by tangential longitudinal excision (Figure 6.3, black dotted line). The author of this chapter prefers a deeper tangential excision, halfway between these two procedures (Figure 6.3, blue dotted line; Figure 6.2D). The defect is closed using absorbable stitches (Figure 6.2E), sometimes after generous undermining of the bed, except for the tangential as it only removes a superficial specimen, typically less than 1 mm thick. In all procedures, when possible, the nail plate is put back in place and sutured to the lateral nail folds or distal wall (Figure 6.2F).

In a retrospective analysis of 68 patients with onychopapilloma in which 62 were operated, classical longitudinal excision was compared with tangential longitudinal excision. No statistically significant difference was observed between the two surgical procedures. However, there was a trend in favor of the classical longitudinal excision, which led to fewer recurrences rates.[2] Tosti et al. retrospectively analyzed

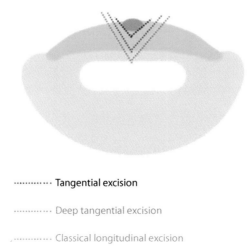

.... Tangential excision

.... Deep tangential excision

.... Classical longitudinal excision

FIGURE 6.3   Scheme illustrating the thickness of the surgical specimens in classical (down to the bone), longitudinal excision (green dotted line), tangential excision (black dotted line), and deep shave excision (halfway) (blue dotted line).

the clinical features of 47 patients with pathologically confirmed onychopapilloma. All cases had a longitudinal excisional biopsy of the tumor. No recurrence was reported, although the surgical procedure performed was not described and the follow-up was only 6 months.[3]

Another retrospective single-center study followed 65 consecutive patients undergoing biopsy of longitudinal erythronychia (either localized or polydactylous). The most common diagnosis was onychopapilloma (41/65, 63%). Longitudinal biopsy was the preferred method of biopsy, with a trapdoor avulsion or lateral plate curl, followed by a longitudinal tangential biopsy of both the distal matrix and nail bed. According to the authors, matrix metaplasia and squamous atypia of the nail bed are readily appreciated with this technique, and scarring is minimized. No recurrence rate was mentioned.[4]

Zaias's procedure is a longitudinal biopsy technique in which a rectangular bloc is excised from the proximal nail fold to the tip of the finger, down to the bone without avulsing the nail plate or either side of it. This includes the hyponychium, the nail bed, and the distal nail matrix. The author recommends that the biopsy should not exceed 3 mm in width within the area of the matrix, in order to avoid a permanent scar.[5]

Recurrence has been observed by de Berker et al. following an isolated excision of distal subungual hyperkeratosis. When distal keratosis is present, longitudinal excision may result in cure as long as it extends all the way back into the involved matrix.[6] See further Table 6.1.

TABLE 6.1

Treatments and Levels of Evidence

Treatment of Onychopapilloma	Level of Evidence
Stable lesions, or when the finding is completely incidental, may be followed at regular intervals.	F[1]
Classical longitudinal excision (CLEx) seems to have a lower recurrence rate than tangential longitudinal excision (TLEx).	C[2]
Longitudinal excisional biopsy of the tumor led to a low rate of recurrence.	C[3]
Minimal scarring results from a 2 mm or smaller longitudinal excisions, including the proximal nail fold, without avulsing the nail plate.	C[5]
Excision of the keratotic focus beneath the distal free edge nick does not result in cure.	D[6]

REFERENCES

1. Jellinek NJ. Longitudinal erythronychia: Suggestions for evaluation and management. *J Am Acad Dermatol.* 2011 January;64(1):167.e1–11.
2. Delvaux C, Richert B, Lecerf P, André J. Onychopapillomas: A 68-case series to determine best surgical procedure and histologic sectioning. *J Eur Acad Dermatol Venereol.* 2018 November;32(11):2025–2030.
3. Tosti A, Schneider SL, Ramirez-Quizon MN, Zaiac M, Miteva M. Clinical, dermoscopic, and pathologic features of onychopapilloma: A review of 47 cases. *J Am Acad Dermatol.* 2016 March;74(3):521–526.
4. Jellinek NJ, Lipner SR. Longitudinal erythronychia: Retrospective single-center study evaluating differential diagnosis and the likelihood of malignancy. *Dermatol Surg.* 2016 March;42(3):310–319.
5. Zaias N. The longitudinal nail biopsy. *J Invest Dermatol.* 1967 October;49(4):406–408.
6. de Berker DA, Perrin C, Baran R. Localized longitudinal erythronychia: Diagnostic significance and physical explanation. *Arch Dermatol.* 2004 October;140(10):1253–1257.

7

Glomus Tumor

Emerson Henrique Padoveze and Suelen Montagner

7.1 Introduction

Glomus tumors (GTs) are rare benign vascular neoplasms arising from the glomus body. This structure is a specialized arteriovenous anastomosis involved in thermoregulation.[1]

Although they can develop anywhere in the body, up to 75% of tumors occur in the hand, most frequently in subungual areas.[2] GTs account for 1.0%–4.5% of all hand tumors, with women being more commonly affected, mainly in their fourth to fifth decade of life.[3] They can be either solitary or multiple.[4] Most typically, they present as a erythronychia (Figure 7.1) or a small, round, bluish nodule visible through the nail plate with a classic triad of symptoms: hypersensitivity to cold, higher pinprick sensitivity, and paroxysmal pain.

The differential diagnosis from other painful tumors—such as leiomyoma, hemangioma, neuroma, gouty arthritis, or eccrine spiradenoma—should be kept in mind while evaluating solitary glomus. Multiple glomus tumors should be carefully differentiated from cavernous hemangioma and blue rubber bleb nevus syndrome, as they can be easily confused with each other.[5]

7.2 How to Confirm the Diagnosis

Glomus tumors, in general, are small and rarely palpable.[6] Diagnosis may be suspected by the clinician and a complementary exam is often required. Dermoscopy of the nail plate and bed is an important diagnostic aid. It may evidence the presence of vascular structures, although not always present.[6]

Imaging studies can be useful in cases of doubtful diagnosis as well as to elicit the anatomical details of the lesion. Radiographs can show cortical thinning or erosive changes in the adjacent bone in some cases. Magnetic resonance imaging (MRI) is an excellent imaging modality for detecting the glomus tumor as small as 2 mm.[4] Ultrasonography is capable of showing the tumor size, site, and shape; however, it is frequently influenced by the surgeon's experience.[7] Ultrasonography can be a better option than MRI when considering the required time, cost, and ability for the test to dynamically enable real-time evaluation of lesions.[8]

The diagnosis can basically be confirmed by the histology that shows a well-circumscribed tumor, composed of conspicuous vasculature surrounded by a mantle of uniformly round glomus cells. The dense fibrous tissue surrounds the mass, forming a pseudocapsule.[9]

7.3 Evidence-Based Treatment

The treatment is surgical. Three different approaches have been discussed: dorsal transungual approach with nail avulsion (Figure 7.2); lateral subperiosteal approach (Figure 7.3); and lateral incision (Figure 7.4). Also see Table 7.1.

The main advantage of the lateral subperiosteal and lateral incision approach is minimum postoperative nail deformity (level of evidence E), with a recurrence rate similar to that of the transungual approach

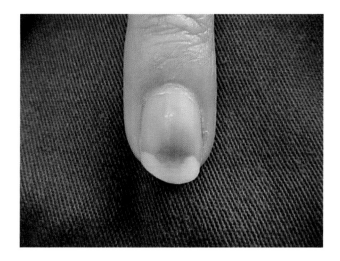

FIGURE 7.1   A small, round, bluish nodule visible through the distal part of the nail plate.

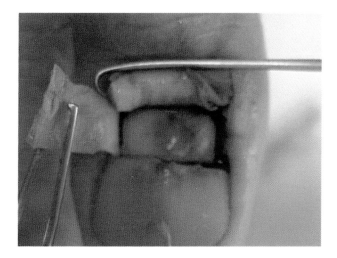

FIGURE 7.2   Dorsal transungual approach with nail avulsion: bluish nodule visible through the nail matrix.

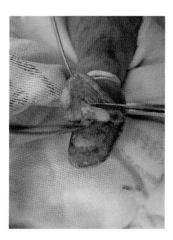

FIGURE 7.3   Subperiosteal approach.

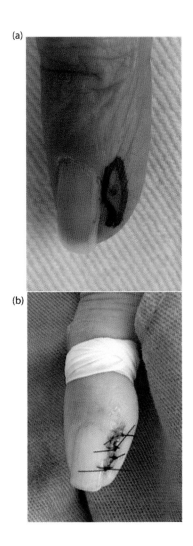

(a)

(b)

FIGURE 7.4   Lateral incision.

TABLE 7.1

Treatments and Levels of Evidence

Surgical Treatments	Level of Evidence
Lateral subperiosteal approach	E[10]
Lateral incision	E[10]
Dorsal transungual approach with nail avulsion	D[11]
Mohs surgery	E[3]

(level of evidence D), but its usefulness is limited to those located on the lateral or pulp finger region.[10] In the transungual approach, the nail plate is carefully lifted and removed for an adequate exposure of the tumor.[11] This approach provides good tumor exposure and helps with its complete removal; however, it may cause nail dystrophy (level of evidence E). Recurrences may be due to an incomplete excision or satellite neoplasms.[10]

Mohs micrographic surgery for glomus tumor is reported. It can reduce the risk of recurrences, thereby avoiding an annoying symptomatology for patients[3] (level of evidence E).

REFERENCES

1. McDermott EM, Weiss AP. Glomus tumors. *J Hand Surg Am.* 2006;31(8):1397–1400.
2. Huang HP, Tsai MC, Hong KT et al. Outcome of microscopic excision of a subungual glomus tumor: A 12-year evaluation. *Dermatol Surg.* 2015;41:487–492.
3. Lambertini M, Piraccini BM, Fanti PA, Dika E. Mohs micrographic surgery for nail unit tumors: An update and a critical review of the literature. *J Eur Acad Dermatol Venereol.* 2018;32:1638–1644.
4. Morey VM, Garg B, Kotwal PP. Glomus tumors of the hand: Review of literature. *J Clin Orthop. Trauma.* 2016;7(4):286–291.
5. Chatterjee JS, Youssef AH, Brown RM, Nishikawa H. Congenital nodular multiple glomangioma: A case report. *J Clin Pathol.* 2005;58:102–103.
6. Maehara LSN, Yamada S, Michalany NS et al. Diagnosis of glomus tumor by nail bed and matrix dermoscopy An. *Bras. Dermatol. An Bras Dermatol.* 2010;85(1):236–238.
7. Baek HJ, Lee SJ, Cho KH et al. Subungual tumors: Clinicopathologic correlation with US and MR imaging findings. *Radiographics.* 2010;30:1621–1636.
8. Moon ES, Choi MS, Kim MS et al. Distribution of glomus tumors in fingers. *J Korean Soc Surg Hand.* 2009;14:138–143.
9. Kim SH, Suh HS, Choi JH et al. Glomus tumor: A clinical and histopathologic analysis of 17 cases. *Ann Dermatol.* 2000;12:95–101.
10. Lee SH, Roh MR, Chung KY. Subungual glomus tumors: Surgical approach and outcome based on tumor location. *Dermatol Surg.* 2013;39:1017–1022.
11. Moon SE, Won JH, Kwon OS, Kim JA. Subungual glomus tumor: Clinical manifestations and outcome of surgical treatment. *J Dermatol.* 2004;31:993–997.

8

Hematomas

Shari R. Lipner

8.1 Introduction

Subungual hematoma, or subungual hemorrhage, is defined as a blood collection between the nail bed or matrix and the nail plate. It may arise from an acute trauma or from repetitive minor trauma to the nail unit. It is a very common chief complaint or incidental finding in dermatologic practice. Patients or referring physicians are often concerned about subungual melanomas especially when the pigmented area is present for some time. Less often patients present because the subungual hematoma is causing pain.

8.2 How to Confirm the Diagnosis

A full medical history is performed in evaluating nail hematomas. All comorbidities are elicited in the history, specifically asking about bleeding or clotting disorders. Past and present medications are reviewed including blood thinners. If a patient is taking a blood thinner, such as aspirin, hematomas are more likely.[1] If there is an acute trauma, such as a heavy object falling on the toenail, the patient will likely recall the time of injury. However, if there is chronic trauma from tight or high-heeled shoes, the patient is unlikely to recollect.

A complete dermatological examination is necessary in evaluating nail hematomas. The physical examination requires removal of nail cosmetics and artificial nails followed by an examination of the skin, hair, mucosa, and all 20 nails. Violaceous patches on the skin may indicate senile purpura, a bleeding disorder, or medication use such as prednisone or warfarin. The nails should be examined on a flat surface with the fingers and toes spread apart. A complete examination requires an evaluation of the patient while standing, as well as the gait to check for toe overlap, pressure on particular toes, or favoring one side of the body with weight. The nails, nail folds, and hyponychium are examined, as well as the degree of onycholysis when present. The digit is also examined for motor function, sensation, and circulation. Pressure is applied to the dorsal digit and strength of extension is evaluated. Capillary refill is employed to test circulation.

Subungual hematomas present as well-circumscribed spots or patches seen through the nail plate (Figure 8.1). The hallux is most often affected and up to a third of patients will have more than one nail involved. The color is more likely to be pink to purple if the trauma occurred 1–5 weeks before presentation and brown-black at 16 weeks or more.[2] It may affect the proximal or distal parts of the nail plate or the entire nail. Typically, the proximal border of the hematoma follows the shape of the lunula. If enough blood accumulates under the nail, onycholysis may ensue. In acute cases, there may be an area of leukonychia overlying the heme.

Dermoscopy is a helpful tool in evaluating subungual hematomas. Because the nail plate has a convex surface, contact dermoscopy with ultrasound gel is preferred. The most common pattern is the homogeneous pattern, which can be seen in 92% of cases.[2] Other patterns in descending order of frequency are peripheral fading, globular pattern, streaks, periungual hemorrhages, and nail plate dystrophy.[2] Subungual hematomas can be distinguished dermoscopically from subungual melanomas,

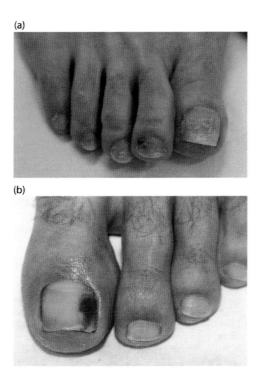

FIGURE 8.1 Subungual hematoma, clinical presentation. (a) Right second toenail with well-circumscribed dark brown patch involving the proximal and lateral nail plate. Note the overlap of the second and third toe, likely contributing to chronic microtrauma. (b) Left great toenail with well-circumscribed dark brown patch involving the lateral and mid-distal nail plate.

with longitudinal irregular bands or lines, ulcerations, triangular-shaped bands, and vascular pattern in the latter but not the former.[2]

Nail hematoma has a broad differential diagnosis and includes etiologies of melanonychia. Recognition of characteristic features from the history and physical examination are helpful in ruling in/out other nail disorders. For example, a history of significant wet work, onycholysis, and green-black discoloration of the nail plate may be a sign of green nail syndrome due to *Pseudomonas aeruginosa* nail infection. An expanding black band involving the hallux, with pigment involving the proximal nail fold (Hutchinson's sign) warrants a nail matrix biopsy to rule out subungual melanoma.[3] Table 8.1 summarizes the differential diagnosis of subungual hematoma.

Most cases of subungual hematoma can be diagnosed with history, physical examination, dermoscopy, and high-quality interval digital photography (Figure 8.2). A careful history may elicit a history of trauma consistent with nail hematoma, but it is important to keep in mind that trauma is also a risk factor for nail unit melanoma.[4] A recent history of silver nitrate application, henna, tar, or tobacco use may imply exogenous pigment, and these pigments can easily be wiped off with an alcohol pad or scraped off with a curette or 15 blade. In cases of onychomycosis, there is often accompanying onycholysis, yellowing, and subungual hyperkeratosis, as well as interdigital scale and multiple nails affected.[5] A clipping with histopathology, or potassium hydroxide with microscopy, fungal culture, or polymerase chain reaction on subungual debris can be used to confirm the presence or absence of a fungal infection.[6–8] While nail hematomas can present as longitudinal melanonychia, this presentation is an exception rather the rule. If there are features concerning for a nail unit melanoma, even in the presence of clinical or dermoscopic features suggestive of a hematoma, a nail unit biopsy should be performed to rule out malignancy.[9]

It is important to employ high quality standardized digital photography at each visit to monitor outgrowth of the hematoma with nail growth. A baseline measurement of the distance between the cuticle and most proximal border of the hematoma with subsequent interval measurements is helpful to document improvement. After reassuring the patient of the diagnosis, counseling on normal nail growth

TABLE 8.1

Differential Diagnosis of Subungual Hematoma (Melanonychia)

Condition	Clinical Findings
Subungual hematoma	Brown-black spot or patch seen through the nail plate; melanonychia may follow shape of lunula; dermoscopy show homogeneous areas, globules, streaks, peripheral fading; grows out with nail plate growth
Exogenous pigment	Jet-black discoloration of nail plate or nail folds; melanonychia follows shape of proximal nail fold; wipes off with alcohol pad or scrapes off with curette
Fungal melanonychia	Longitudinal brown-black band that is often wider distally and narrower proximally; onycholysis and subungual hyperkeratosis; dermoscopy shows scales of varying colors (yellow, orange, brown, black)
Pseudomonas aeruginosa nail infection	Green-black patch seen through nail plate; may be accompanying onycholysis; dermoscopy shows medial fading of the pigment
Melanotic macule (melanocytic activation)	Longitudinal gray-brown band that often involves multiple nails; dermoscopy shows gray background with regular gray lines in terms of color, thickness, and spacing
Nail matrix nevus	Longitudinal brown band; dermoscopy shows brown background with regular brown lines in terms of color, thickness, and spacing
Nail unit melanoma	Longitudinal brown-black band that is often 3 mm or more in width; Hutchinson's sign may be present; dermoscopy shows brown background with irregular gray lines in terms of color, thickness, and spacing, and there may be loss of parallelism; up to one-third of nail unit melanomas are amelanotic

rates (2–3 mm month/fingernails, 1 mm/month toenails), gives the patient realistic expectations on resolution of the hematoma. Patient-initiated photographs using smartphones are also helpful to monitor improvement or lack thereof.[10]

Clippings can be useful in diagnosing nail hematomas in select cases. If the pigment is distal or localized to an onycholytic part of the nail plate, the nail plate can be painlessly clipped. The sample is then placed into a formalin bottle, processed, and evaluated by the dermatopathologist. Diaminobenzidine staining will highlight the area of hemorrhage.[11] The presence of blood in the clipping, however, does not rule out other etiologies of melanonychia including nail unit melanoma. A quick and easy way to diagnose subungual hemorrhage is to perform distal clippings from the area of hematoma, place the clippings on a urinalysis strip, and add a drop of water with a syringe. Green color formation after 60 seconds is indicative of blood.[12]

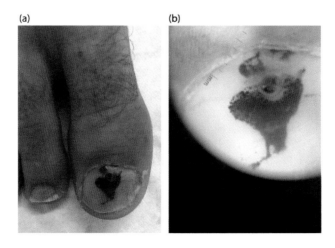

FIGURE 8.2 Subungual hematoma, clinical presentation and dermoscopy. (a) Left great toenail with well-circumscribed dark brown patch involving the proximal and central nail plate. Note a prior punch biopsy was performed through the nail plate. (b) Dermoscopy of panel A, showing homogeneous areas, peripheral fading, globules, and streaks.

TABLE 8.2

Treatments and Levels of Evidence

Treatment	Level of Evidence
Conservative – "wait and see"	E[10]
"Hematoma selfies"	
Evacuation of the hematoma	E[13–16]

Imaging is necessary in some cases of subungual hematoma. Involvement of the entire nail plate, significant distal onycholysis or proximal nail plate detachment, pain, or limited range of motion of the digit or toe requires x-ray examination. With significant trauma, there may be an underlying bone fracture of the toe or digit. Advanced imaging techniques such as ultrasound or MRI are rarely required. Presence of a fracture should prompt referral to an orthopedist.

8.3 Evidence-Based Treatment

In almost all cases, suspected subungual hematomas can be managed expectantly. After baseline standardized digital photography, the patient can be followed every 2–3 months in the office with physical examination and interval photography until the heme grows out completely. An alternative is for the patient to send "hematoma selfies" through a secure patient portal.[10] If onycholysis is present, the detached portion is clipped back. If there is any sensitivity in the nail, a Band-Aid or gauze with paper tape can be applied to afford some protection. In cases where a malignancy is in the differential diagnosis, a nail unit biopsy is performed.

Evacuation of the hematoma is rarely required. Some authors have advocated for evacuation when 60% of the nail plate is involved, but this is only required when there is significant pain in the nail unit.[13] Anesthesia is usually not required, but a digital block can be performed if needed. Informed consent is obtained after discussing risks and benefits including loss of the nail, recurrence of hematoma, and infection. After cleansing the nail unit with chlorhexidine or betadine, an electrocautery tip is held perpendicular to the nail plate to produce a small hole through the nail plate over the central area of hematoma. An alternative is a flamed paper clip. The blood will drain on its own or a capillary tube can be used to facilitate drainage.[14,15] A contraindication to using electrocautery or a paper clip is acrylic nails since they are flammable. Alternatively, an 18-gauge needle or 2 mm punch biopsy can be inserted and gently twisted into the nail plate over the central area of hematoma.[14–16] These techniques should resolve the majority of the hematoma and related pain, but at times a second trephination is needed for relief. Vaseline and a pressure dressing are applied to the wound and the patient is instructed to keep the bandage clean and dry for 48 hours. There is no evidence for use of prophylactic antibiotics for evacuation of subungual hematoma.[17] See further Table 8.2.

REFERENCES

1. Braun RP, Baran R, Le Gal FA et al. Diagnosis and management of nail pigmentations. *J Am Acad Dermatol*. 2007;56(5):835–847.
2. Mun JH, Kim GW, Jwa SW et al. Dermoscopy of subungual haemorrhage: Its usefulness in differential diagnosis from nail-unit melanoma. *Br J Dermatol*. 2013;168(6):1224–1229.
3. Lipner SR, Scher RK. Evaluation of nail lines: Color and shape hold clues. *Cleve Clin J Med*. 2016;83(5):385–391.
4. Bormann G, Marsch WC, Haerting J, Helmbold P. Concomitant traumas influence prognosis in melanomas of the nail apparatus. *Br J Dermatol*. 2006;155(1):76–80.
5. Lipner SR, Scher RK. Long-standing onychodystrophy in a young woman. *JAMA*. 2016;316(18):1915–1916.
6. Lipner SR, Scher RK. Part I: Onychomycosis: Clinical overview and diagnosis. *J Am Acad Dermatol*. 2018;80(4):835–851.

7. Lipner SR, Scher RK. Onychomycosis: A small step for quality of care. *Curr Med Res Opin.* 2016;32(5):865–867.
8. Lipner SR, Scher RK. Confirmatory testing for onychomycosis. *JAMA Dermatol.* 2016;152(7):847.
9. Daniel CR, 3rd, Jellinek NJ. Subungual blood is not always a reassuring sign. *J Am Acad Dermatol* 2007;57(1):176.
10. Chelidze K, Ko D, Lipner SR. The nail hematoma selfie. *J Am Acad Dermatol.* 2018;78(6):e137–e138.
11. Stephen S, Tosti A, Rubin AI. Diagnostic applications of nail clippings. *Dermatol Clin.* 2015;33(2):289–301.
12. Huang YH, Ohara K. Medical pearl: Subungual hematoma: A simple and quick method for diagnosis. *J Am Acad Dermatol.* 2006;54(5):877–878.
13. Fehrenbacher V, Blackburn E. Nail bed injury. *J Hand Surg Am.* 2015;40(3):581–582.
14. Dean B, Becker G, Little C. The management of the acute traumatic subungual haematoma: A systematic review. *Hand Surg.* 2012;17(1):151–154.
15. Patel L. Management of simple nail bed lacerations and subungual hematomas in the emergency department. *Pediatr Emerg Care.* 2014;30(10):742–745; quiz 746–748.
16. Khan MA, West E, Tyler M. Two millimetre biopsy punch: A painless and practical instrument for evacuation of subungual haematomas in adults and children. *J Hand Surg Eur Vol.* 2011;36(7):615–617.
17. Costello J, Howes M. Best evidence topic report. Prophylactic antibiotics for subungual haematoma. *Emerg Med J.* 2004;21(4):503.

9

Herpes Simplex

Matilde Iorizzo

9.1 Introduction

Herpes simplex virus (HSV) infection of the nail unit may be caused by HSV type 1 or HSV type 2. HSV type 1 is generally responsible for gingivostomatitis, herpes labialis, and keratitis. HSV type 2 is generally responsible for genital lesions, but they can be caused by HSV type 1 as well.

Worldwide, the prevalence of HSV type 1 infections is greater than HSV type 2 infections: according to a recently released report by the Centers for Disease Control, in fact, the prevalence of HSV type 1 and HSV type 2 is 47.8% and 11.9%, respectively, among individuals aged 14–49 years.[1] Nail unit infections result from a contagion by another affected area (autogenous inoculation) or from a close contact with a person actively shedding the virus (exogenous inoculation). Healthy skin is not a transmission route for HSV; therefore disrupted epidermis is necessary to get the infection. HSV remains viable on surfaces for a very short period, but short enough for transmission. Clinically, the two viruses give an identical picture, so it is impossible to establish the responsible agent without a diagnostic test. Defining the agent is important in order to identify the presumed source of contagion.[2]

After a prodromal period (20 days, but less than 6 hours in recurrent infections) of local tenderness, erythema, and swelling, clusters of small and tense vesicles appear around the perionychium (Figure 9.1).[3] More rarely the vesicles develop within the nail bed producing onycholysis (Figure 9.2). Lymphangitis, axillary/inguinal adenopathy, and flu-like symptoms may also be observed, even if they are rare. This period is extremely contagious due to viral shedding. In the next days the vesicles increase in size and sometimes also coalesce in a large bulla. Vesicular liquid, clear at the beginning, becomes turbid and in rare cases purulent or hemorrhagic (Figure 9.3). After the acute phase, there is a rupture of the vesicles that dry, forming crusts. Healing generally occurs in 15–20 days in primary infection, less in recurrences. It is rare to have periungual skin scars or permanent nail dystrophies.

HSV may affect the periungual skin of the terminal phalanx with the typical vesicles but also start as an acute, extremely painful paronychia often confused with bacterial paronychia. For this last reason, HSV of the nail unit is also miscalled herpetic whitlow (or felon):[4] this term is incorrect because, by definition, there is no pus discharge.

After the first infection and replication in the epidermal cells, HSV is sequestered from the host immune surveillance and remains dormant in the dorsal root ganglia. HSV typically persists throughout the host's lifetime. Due to an immune system imbalance, HSV can reactivate and reach the skin through the peripheral nervous fibers. Reactivation does not necessarily imply clinical symptoms.

However, the clinical presentation of recurrences is generally less severe and less lasting than the first infection.

Any finger may be involved, even more than one at the same time.[5] Fingernails, especially the index finger, are more frequently affected than toenails. Compared with males, females have a higher prevalence of both HSV types. The same is true for children, especially finger suckers and nail biters.[6] Medical and dental personnel are the adult group most hit by this disease.[7,8] The degree of host immune competence is responsible for the severity of clinical manifestations and, for this reason, in immunocompromised patients, HSV infections are more severe, more persistent, and recur more frequently. In this group of

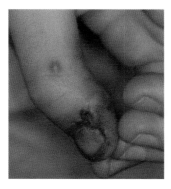

FIGURE 9.1   Clusters of small and tense vesicles around the perionychium. (Courtesy of Prof. A. Tosti.)

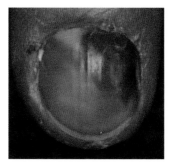

FIGURE 9.2   Presence of vesicles within the nail bed producing hemorrhagic onycholysis. (Courtesy of Prof. A. Tosti.)

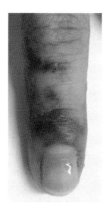

FIGURE 9.3   Vesicular liquid in rare cases becomes hemorrhagic.

patients, in fact, viral shedding is more frequent.[9,10] Ulcerated and necrotic bullae can be observed, which can often lead the clinician to a misdiagnosis.

The most common disorders from which HSV should be differentiated is acute bacterial paronychia. This last one gives usually a purulent discharge not present in HSV infections. A diagnostic test is, however, always advisable to make a prompt and correct diagnosis. If there is no possibility of doing the test and when there is no response to topical/systemic antibiotics, an HSV infection should always be suspected. Contrary to HSV, herpes zoster virus infections are very rare around the nail unit and Coxsackievirus infections are responsible for more disseminated vesicles even if they may lead to a misdiagnosis due to a very frequent concomitant gingivostomatitis. Many other dermatological disorders can present with pustular lesions around the nail unit, such as pustular psoriasis, parakeratosis pustulosa, blistering distal dactylitis, dyshidrotic eczema, pemphigus, and pemphigoid. When the clinical picture is doubtful, a Tzanck test or polymerase chain reaction (PCR) needs to be performed.

9.2 How to Confirm the Diagnosis

The diagnosis of HSV infection is generally clinical; a biopsy is never required.

In doubtful cases or simply to confirm the clinical diagnosis, a Tzanck smear, a culture, a PCR, or a serum analysis can be performed.

The Tzanck test (a superficial scraping from the base of a freshly incised vesicle, stained with Wright-Giemsa, and then evaluated under a light microscope) reveals characteristic acantholytic and multinucleate giant cells ("balloon" giant cells). This test is very fast and cheap, but it does not permit distinguishing between type 1 and type 2 HSV.[11] It does not even permit distinguishing between HSV and herpes zoster virus.

For this reason, culture and PCR are then necessary. Material for culture and PCR is a vesicular liquid, obtained by swabbing the base of a freshly ulcerated vesicle and moved to a viral media. Culture is the gold standard test, but PCR is faster and more sensitive, but also more expensive.[2] The problem of culture is that it takes 3–7 days to provide results and, in some cases, treatment should be started earlier. Vesicles contain the highest concentration of HSV within the first 24–48 hours after their appearance. After this time the test could be negative.

Serum analysis for HSV antibodies is also helpful to differentiate between type 1 and type 2 HSV, but it is generally performed to establish the history of prior infections. High levels of IgG are in fact consistent with a nonactive lesion. Serum analysis is also helpful when the vesicles are localized in difficult-to-access areas like the nail bed.

9.3 Evidence-Based Treatment

Treatment of HSV infections is primarily aimed at symptomatic relief: to reduce pain and to accelerate healing. There is currently no cure, in fact, for HSV outbreaks. Treating the primary infection, even if done early (within 24–48 hours of symptom onset), does not prevent recurrences but could reduce their number per year and their severity.[12,13] It is very important, contrary to acute bacterial paronychia, not to incise herpetic vesicles to avoid spreading of the infection and bacterial superinfection, even if it may reduce tension-related pain.[14]

Since HSV type 2 is the most common causative agent of HSV infections in the nail unit,[2] treatment guidelines for this specific virus are generally followed:[15]

- Adult patients and children older than 12 years—Oral acyclovir 200 mg, five times a day (every 4 hours with a night pause of 8 hours, due to the very short elimination half-life of 2.5 hours, but 400 mg three times a day is another option) for 10 days as the first option. As a second option, valacyclovir 500 mg, two times a day for 10 days and famciclovir 250 mg, three times a day for 10 days. Five days of treatment are enough in recurrences. To prevent recurrences, a chronic course, 6 months of acyclovir 400 mg two times a day, valacyclovir 500 mg/day or famciclovir 250 mg twice a day should be taken into account.

    There is not a specific number of recurrences per year that justify the chronic use of systemic antivirals: From two on they could be used.

- Immunocompromised adult patients and children older than 12 years—Oral acyclovir 400 mg three times a day until the risk of infection passes.

- Patients younger than 12 years of age—Oral acyclovir 400 mg suspension (2.5 mL every 4 hours) or the 250 mg intravenous infusion (5–20 mg/kg every 8 hours) are generally utilized for a variable period (5–20 days) depending on the severity of the infection.

Although widely used, clinical studies have demonstrated that topical 5% acyclovir cream and ointment provide a small benefit in reducing the duration of symptoms. Moreover, the topical application will not get the drug to the site of reactivation and does not influence the host immune response.[16] Penciclovir 1% cream and docosanal 10% cream are two other available options. This last one is only approved for orolabial HSV and the use for another location should be considered *off-label*. Compared to oral treatments that are available only by medical prescription, topicals are OTC (over-the-counter) products and are more accessible to patients.

No specific guidelines of care are available for HSV of the nail unit, and in the literature all the available papers reporting treatment outcomes are limited case series (level of evidence D) or individual case reports (level of evidence E).

REFERENCES

1. McQuillan G, Kruszon-Moran D, Flagg EW, Poulose-Ram R. *Prevalence of Herpes Simplex Virus Type 1 and Type 2 in Persons Aged 14–49: United States, 2015–2016*. Atlanta, GA: Centers for Disease Control and Prevention. Published online February 7, 2018.
2. Fatahzadeh M, Schwartz RA. Human herpes simplex virus infections: Epidemiology, pathogenesis, symptomatology, diagnosis and management. *J Am Acad Dermatol*. 2007;57:737–763.
3. Gill MJ, Arlette J, Buchan KA. Herpes simplex virus infection of the hand. *J Am Acad Dermatol*. 1990;22:111–116.
4. Stern H, Elek SD, Millar DM, Anderson HF. Herpetic whitlow, a form of cross-infections in hospitals. *Lancet*. 1959;2:871–874.
5. Péchère M, Friedli A, Krisher J. Multiple herpes simplex type 1 whitlow lesions. *Annales de Dermatologie et Vénéréologie*. 1999;126:646.
6. Muller SA, Hermann EC Jr. Association of stomatitis and paronychias due to herpes simplex. *Archives of Dermatology*. 1970;101:396–402.
7. Rosato FE, Rosato EF, Plotkin SA. Herpetic paronychia—An occupational hazard in the medical personnel. *New Engl J Med*. 1970;283:804–805.
8. Herbert AM, Bagg J, Walker DM et al. Seroepidemiology of herpes virus infections among dental personnel. *J Dent*. 1995;23:339–342.
9. Garcia-Plata MD, Moreno-Gimenez JC, Vexez-Garcia A et al. Herpetic whitlow in an AIDS patient. *J Eur Acad Dermatol Venereol*. 1999;12:241–242.
10. Camasmie HR, Leda SB, Lupi O et al. Chronic herpetic whitlow as the first manifestation of HIV infection. *AIDS*. 2016;30:2254–2256.
11. Durdu M, Ruocco V. Clinical and cytologic features of antibiotic-resistant acute paronychia. *J Am Acad Dermatol*. 2014;70:120–126.
12. Cernik C, Gallina K, Brodell RT. The treatment of herpes simplex virus infections: An evidence-based review. *Arch Intern Med*. 2008;168:1137–1344.
13. Nikkels AF, Pierard GE. Treatment of mucocutaneous presentations of herpes simplex virus infections. *Am J Clin Dermatol*. 2002;3:475–487.
14. Feder HM Jr, Long SS. Herpetic whitlow. Epidemiology, clinical characteristics, diagnosis, and treatment. *Am J Dis Child*. 1983;137:861–863.
15. World Health Organization (WHO). *WHO Guidelines for the Treatment of Genital Herpes Simplex Virus*. Geneva: WHO; 2016.
16. Cunningham A, Griffiths P, Leone P et al. Current management and recommendations for access to antiviral therapy of herpes labialis. *J Clin Virol*. 2012;53:6–11.

10

Ingrowing Nail

Azzam Alkhalifah, Florence Dehavay, and Bertrand Richert

10.1 Introduction

An ingrowing nail, or onychocryptosis, is the impingement of the nail plate into the surrounding soft tissue leading to a foreign-body reaction. This is the result of an imbalance between the width of the nail bed and plate and nail folds. One should understand that the problem could be the nail itself, the periungual tissues, or both, which guides the therapeutic approach.

Although it can be seen in all age groups, its incidence peaks in teenagers. Ingrowing toenails represent 20% of all foot problems encountered by general practitioners, and about 10,000 new cases are registered in the United Kingdom each year. The big toe is affected in the vast majority of cases.[1,2]

Among the different types of ingrowing nails, the most common type is distal lateral ingrowing. The condition is very painful and alters the patient's daily activities. In addition to redness, swelling, and tenderness, the presence of granulation tissue, oozing, and sometimes secondary infection can be present. In chronic stages, fibrosis and hyperkeratosis of the surrounding skin without signs of acute inflammation can be seen.

Many severity classification indexes have been published in the literature. The Heifetz Index (Table 10.1) remains the most commonly used as it is simple, easy, fast, and guides the management.

10.2 Diagnosis

The diagnosis is clinical; no investigations are needed. Swabs should be performed when infection is suspected. Nevertheless, in atypical cases with chronic, oozing subungual lesions, the clinician should think of other differential diagnoses, especially squamous cell carcinoma and amelanotic melanoma. For this reason, the granulation tissue accompanying ingrown nails should always be sent for histopathological analysis.

10.3 Treatment

Conservative treatments, requiring high patient compliance, could be effective in mild or sometimes moderate cases, but they are associated with high recurrence rate.

Surgical treatment is indicated either when conservative treatments have failed or when the condition is painful or recurrent and the patient asks for a radical solution.

10.3.1 Topical Treatments

The acute inflammation seen in ingrowing nails is mostly a foreign-body reaction rather than a secondary infection, although both can be associated.

The use of topical corticosteroids alone or mixed with topical antibiotics to treat inflammatory and infected ingrown nails is of common practice, but studies are still needed to confirm their efficacy.

TABLE 10.1

Heifetz Index

Stage	Clinical Signs
I	Inflammatory: Slight erythema and swelling of the nail grooves
II	Suppuration and acute infection
III	Severe with granulation tissue in the nail grooves (acute) or hypertrophy of the surrounding tissues (chronic)

Daily soaking in warm soapy water, or a mix of water and Epsom salts, have been described to reduce inflammation,[3] but confirmatory studies are missing.

As for systemic treatments, oral antibiotics did not prove their effectiveness to reduce healing time or postoperative morbidity after phenol matricectomy.[4] Level of evidence B.

10.3.2 Conservative Treatments

The aim of nonsurgical approaches is to stop the nail plate/soft tissue conflict. For that several techniques have been developed: traction, separation techniques, restoring a normal shape to the nail, or reduction of the transverse curvature of the nail with a device.

They are usually successful in treating the acute episode, but recurrence is usual.

The best indication is when the mild to moderate ingrowing results from a transitory cause (e.g., too tight shoes, onychoptosis, improper trimming in the corners). They are summarized in Table 10.2 along with their evidence-based level.

10.3.2.1 Fold Traction Technique

Taping is the easiest and the least aggressive treatment.

Taping has been reported to have a success rate of 44.5% after a 2-month follow-up of 750 affected toenails.[5] It consists of applying a 4 cm long adhesive tape on the edge of the affected fold and pulling it continuously away from the nail edge by turning the tape around the toe (Figure 10.1). It must be adherent and should be changed at least once daily to keep the traction continuous. A modified "slit-tape strap" procedure was effective in treating 140 ingrown toenails with a recurrence rate of 13%. However, most of these patients received combined conservative treatments.[6] Level of evidence C.

Limitation is allergy to the colophony contained in the adhesive tape and sweating that impairs the adherence to the skin.

10.3.2.2 Separation Techniques

10.3.2.2.1 Cotton Insertion

Applying a piece of cotton wool under the corner of the nail can provide good results with variable recurrence rates. It elevates the offending plate from the lateral sulcus. This can be done with normal sterile cotton wool,[7] collodion-coated wisp of cotton,[8] cotton pladgets soaked in chlorhixidine after

TABLE 10.2

Conservative Treatments and Levels of Evidence

Conservative Treatment	Level of Evidence
Orthonyxia is effective, more comfortable, but not more successful than wedge resection in treating ingrown toenails	B[20]
Taping alone is helpful in treating more than a third of nonpreviously treated ingrown nails	C[5]
Cotton insertion techniques can treat mild, noninfected ingrown nails	C[7–11]
Gutter treatment is more successful than avulsion alone	C[12]
Gutter is more effective when fixed with cyanoacrylate	C[13]

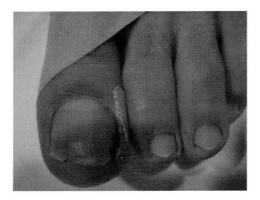

FIGURE 10.1   Fold traction technique: Taping.

a surgical cleaning of the fold,[9] "cotton nail cast" when fixed with cyanoacrylate,[10] or "rolled cotton padding."[11] These procedures may require local anesthesia, as the insertion of the cotton under the lateral nail plate might be painful. Level of evidence C.

10.3.2.2.2 Gutter Splinting

The aim of the procedure is similar to that of the cotton methods. It definitely requires a distal block. In a prospective randomized comparative trial, a plastic gutter (made from an infusion tube) inserted around the lateral edge of the nail, after surgical debridement, showed a cure rate of 56% at a one-year follow-up compared to 84% with wedge resection of the matrix. When compared to simple avulsion, higher rates of failure were seen in the avulsion group.[12] The gutter can be fixed with an adhesive tape, a stitch to the nail, with formable acrylics.[13,14] Level of evidence C.

A Cochrane systematic review found that surgical treatment of ingrown nails was significantly more effective in preventing the recurrence than gutter treatment (RR 0.63, 95% CI 0.47–0.85),[1] although one trial had shown that both were equally effective.[15] Level of evidence B.

10.3.2.2.3 Dental Floss

Dental floss to separate the plate from the fold has been used successfully to treat ingrown toenails.[16] Level of evidence C.

10.3.2.3 Acrylic Nail

The procedure is aimed to restore a normal shape to the plate with subsequent counterpressure onto the distal pulp. The best indication is a too short nail in the corner or a missing part of the nail.[13] The acrylic resin can also be used to fix a gutter. In a technique that uses the acrylic resin to combine splinting and orthonyxia, it can reach a success rate of up to 91.8%.[17] Level of evidence C.

10.3.2.4 Orthonyxia (Nail Brace)

Orthonyxia is a technique that aims to lift up the lateral sides of the plate. It was first created by E. E. Stedman in 1872 and appeared in Europe and Australia in the 1980s.[18] It can be a helpful, but usually not a permanent, solution for ingrown nails secondary to an increased transverse curvature of the plate. Two types of braces are available: adhesive ones (memory alloy), with a thin composite strip; and hooked ones. A prospective study in 2005 found comparable results between brace treatment and Emmert's wedge excision with less pain and rest days in the brace group (level of evidence B).[19] Another prospective randomized blinded study showed less recurrences in the wedge excision group compared to brace treatment (nonsignificant), although complete recovery time and postoperative morbidity significantly favored the brace treatment (level of evidence B).[20] Several retrospective studies have reported the effectiveness of nail braces.[21–23]

10.3.3 Surgical Treatment

Surgical procedures are the first choice approach for moderate-to-severe ingrowing, failure of a conservative treatment, or when the cause of ingrowing cannot be definitively corrected with conservative methods (due to too wide nail, overcurvature of the plate). According to the type of ingrowing, there are two main surgical approaches: narrowing the nail plate or debulking the soft tissues. Each approach can be done by different procedures with good results, as long as they are performed in appropriate cases. Partial or complete nail avulsion alone to treat ingrown nails should be avoided, as it provides only temporary relief with recurrence in most patients.[24]

10.3.3.1 Nail Plate Narrowing

The aim of the various procedures is to remove the offending lateral part of the plate and to radically remove or destroy the corresponding part of the matrix, to prevent any recurrence. The matrix can be removed surgically or destroyed with a laser device, by electrocoagulation, or chemically.

The main limitation of these procedures is that they are operator-dependent, which explains why different studies on the same procedure may report different success rates. The difficulty of all of these procedures, chemical ones excluded, is the anatomical variation of the lateral horn of the matrix. They are summarized in Table 10.3 along with their evidence-based level.

10.3.3.1.1 Wedge Excision

Wedge excision was first described by Winograd in 1929 and developed since then under different names with some slight modifications to the procedure. They all involve surgically removing the ingrown part of the nail along with the corresponding matrix (Figure 10.2). When done with expertise, it gives a low

TABLE 10.3
Narrowing Treatments and Their Levels of Evidence

Nail Narrowing	Level of Evidence
Post-phenolization curettage reduces healing time, increases postoperative bleeding, leads to lower rates of infection, and increases postoperative pain (all significant)	A[47]
NaOH matricectomy has faster tissue normalization than phenol	A[51]
Both 88% phenol and 100% TCA are effective in treating ingrown nails	A[59]
100% TCA produce more oozing and inflammation than 88% phenol	A[59]
Oral antibiotics are not effective in reducing postoperative morbidity or healing time after phenol matrixectomy	B[4]
Topical gentamycin doesn't decrease infection nor recurrence rates after wedge resection or phenolization	B[28]
Phenolization is more successful than wedge resection in treating ingrown nails	B[28,35–37]
Phenolization is less painful than wedge resection	B[35,37]
Post-phenol application of 20% ferric chloride reduces oozing time	B[46]
Wedge resection is more successful than gutter treatment	B[12]
Total nail avulsion doesn't add benefit to the wedge resection	C[26]
Wedge resection with electrocoagulation has fewer recurrences than wedge resection alone	C[27]
Wedge resection with phenol has fewer recurrences than wedge resection alone	C[29,32,33]
Wedge resection with phenol has fewer recurrences than phenol alone	C[33]
The addition of phenol after wedge resection decreases the postoperative pain	C[33]
Phenol is effective and safe for diabetics	C[53,54]
Phenol is effective and safe for children	C[29,55]
10% NaOH matricectomy is effective and safe for diabetics	B[56]
10% NaOH matricectomy is effective and safe for children	C[57]
Er:YAG laser is more effective than Emmet's operation to treat ingrown nails	B[65]
CO_2 laser is effective in treating ingrown nails	C[61–64]

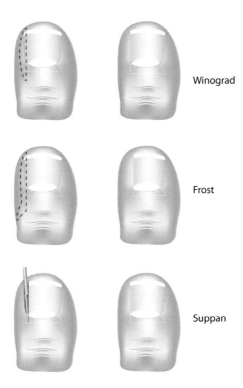

Winograd

Frost

Suppan

FIGURE 10.2 Various types of wedge excisions.

recurrence rate. The best reported results[25–27] reach the success rates observed in chemical ones. In some other series, the recurrence rate was high, up to half of treated patients.[28–30] The recurrences and spicules grow from missed parts of the matrix, due to the individual variations in the length and the curvature of the matrix horns. Some surgeons rise the success rate of the wedge resection by adding phenolization[31] or electrocoagulation[27] right after. The addition of phenol gave significantly lower recurrence rates than wedge resection alone[29,32] and phenolization alone,[33] although it was more invasive and nonsignificantly more painful than phenolization alone. Surgical matricectomy using an operative microscope has been shown in a retrospective study to provide 100% success rate, although no other studies have been published about this method since 2010.[34]

10.3.3.1.2 Chemical Techniques

Partial matricectomy can be obtained with chemical cautery. It has the advantage of being less invasive, less painful, and less operator-dependent than the surgical wedge resection, with very high success rates. After applying a tourniquet, the lateral part of the nail (3–5 mm width) is avulsed to its most proximal end, to unveil the matrix. Then the chemical cauterant, which can be phenol (80%–90%), sodium hydroxide (10%), or trichloroacetic acid (100%), is applied for a determined time (Figure 10.3).

Several prospective, comparative studies demonstrated that *phenolization* was more successful[28,33,35–38] and less painful[35,37] than the various techniques of wedge excision. In skilled hands, phenol matricectomy ensures a very low recurrence or spicule rates of less than 3%.[39–44] An application time of 4 minutes is necessary to destroy the full thickness of the nail bed epithelium as shown by a study on fresh cadavers.[45]

Oozing for 2–6 weeks is the main drawback of the procedure. Patients should perform daily home care to avoid a secondary infection. However, 20% ferric chloride[46] and post-phenol curettage[47] of the necrotized tissues may help to reduce oozing and shorten healing time. In addition to its cauterizing effect, phenol has bactericidal[48] and demyelination[49] effects, which gives the molecule the advantages of being antiseptic and anesthetic. The latter effect offers a very comfortable postop for patients.

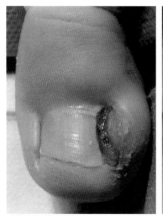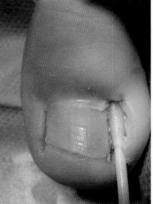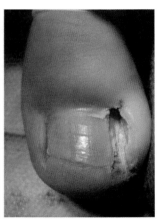

FIGURE 10.3   Chemical cautery procedure.

Sodium hydroxide 10% has shown similar success rates when applied for 1 minute, with shorter period of oozing and complete healing.[50–52] Both phenol[29,53–55] and sodium hydroxide[56,57] are effective and safe for diabetics and children.

Trichloroacetic acid (TCA) 100% matricectomy showed a comparable success rate[58] with a shorter healing time. However, this could not be verified on a prospective, randomized, double-blind study. It showed that phenol and TCA are both effective with an overall success rates in both groups of 100%, but oozing and inflammation was observed to be less with phenol treatment. Postop pain was very low for both cauterants. TCA did not offer any advantage in terms of postoperative morbidity compared with phenol. It is an excellent alternative when phenol is not available.[59]

Recently, 90% *bichloracetic acid* has been used in a case series with a success rate of 98%.[60]

The literature is very rich in prospective and retrospective studies showing the very high success rates of chemical cauteries. In addition, these procedures are easy to perform and have a low cost. They are considered the gold standard to treat moderate-to-severe ingrowing without permanent tissue hypertrophy.[1,2]

10.3.3.1.3 Laser Matricectomy

Lasers, mainly CO_2 lasers, can be used to treat ingrown nails by vaporizing the lateral matrix. Its advantage is being hemostatic by the direct coagulation effect of the laser. Similar to the wedge resection, laser is operator-dependent and recurrence happen when the most proximal and lateral parts of the matrix are not reached by the laser beam. To ensure success rates, an incision is always needed in the lateral-proximal folds junction to expose the lateral horn of the matrix, but recurrence may however happen. In some studies, CO_2 laser[61–64] and erbium YAG laser[65] gave high cure rates comparable to those seen with the phenolization.

10.3.3.1.4 Other Techniques

Acceptable results have been reported with electrocautery matricectomy,[66–68] which remains inferior to phenolization with longer healing time in electrocautery.[69] Nail matrix destruction with cryotherapy after a partial nail avulsion has also been reported.[70] These techniques are no longer recommended.

10.3.3.2 Debulking Techniques

Another surgical approach is to focus not on the plate itself but on the adjacent soft tissues. The role of the soft tissue was interestingly suggested by the Pearson et al. prospective study that failed to find any significant difference in toenail shape between ingrown toenails and controls.[71]

The surgical procedures involving only the soft tissues, also called "debulking," are especially useful when facing hypertrophic nail folds. The nail is not narrowed and retains its natural dimensions, and

TABLE 10.4

Debulking Treatments and Levels of Evidence

Debulking Techniques	Level of Evidence
Knot technique has less relapse rate and number of additional surgeries required than the Winograd technique	A
Vandenbos procedure is effective with low rate of recurrence and good cosmetic outcomes	B
Noël procedure is effective with low rate of recurrence	B
Monaldi technique is effective with low rate of recurrence but nonoptimal cosmetic results	B
Cologlu technique is superior to wedge resection	B
Howard-Dubois procedure is effective in treating ingrown nails	C
Super-U procedure is effective with good cosmetic outcomes	C
Knot technique is effective with low rate of recurrence	C
Other techniques with excision of the lateral fold and flap are effective	C

the cosmetic outcome is excellent. The recurrence rates are low but the downtime is long and in some instances, a loss of skin sensitivity is reported.

Many surgical techniques, with small variations between each of them, have been described. The vast majority are retrospective studies with grade C recommendation.

Well-designed randomized controlled studies are definitely needed to determine the best indication of each technique.[72]

Debulking procedures are summarized in Table 10.4 along with their evidence-based level.

10.3.3.2.1 Howard-Dubois Procedure

The Howard-Dubois procedure was first described by Howard at the end of the 19th century,[73] then reintroduced more than half a century later by Dubois who made it quite popular in France.[74]

Surgical technique: The aim is to remove a crescent of soft tissue at the tip of the toe, parallel to the hyponychium to allow lowering of the distal pulp. A fish-mouth incision is performed about 5 mm below the level of the distal lateral grooves, running from the medial to the lateral aspect of the distal interphalangeal joint. A second incision is performed to create a wedge reaching about 3–5 mm at its maximum width at the distal tip of the phalanx. All incisions are carried down to the bone. The crescent is removed using sharp-pointed scissors and suturing may be performed with simple interrupted stitches or running lock stitches to avoid bleeding. Removal of an adequate amount of soft tissue and suturing the defect will pull down the distal wall, thus freeing the nail (Figure 10.4).

Indications: Technique of choice for distal embedding and a good approach for moderate hypertrophic lateral folds.

Advantages: Excellent cosmetic outcomes.

Disadvantages: Wound margin necrosis may happen if too much traction is exerted onto the distal wall during suture. This is a painful procedure from traction on the soft tissues.

Studies: Murray et al. described a series of 20 patients with procedures on 25 toes. All the patients had previously undergone another surgery and a cure rate of 60% was achieved with a follow-up of 9 months.[75] Level of evidence C.

10.3.3.2.2 Vandenbos Procedure

The Vandenbos procedure was first described in 1959 by Vandenbos and Bowers[76] and recently brought back in vogue by Chapeskie who slightly modified the initial procedure.[77]

Surgical technique: A wide excision removing a big bite of the lateral fold starting in the proximal nail fold and reaching the tip of the toe is performed, leaving the most distal part of the pulp. At anytime the procedure involves the nail bed or the matrix. The debulking is generous with a

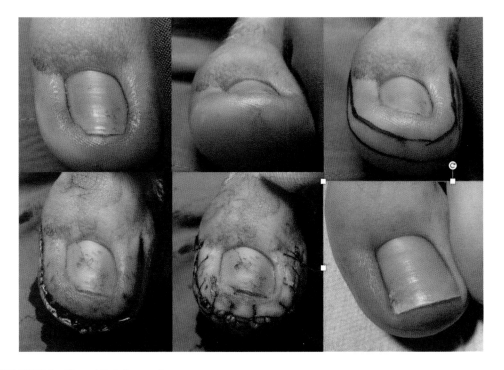

FIGURE 10.4   Howard-Dubois procedure.

defect of approximately 1.5 by 3 cm and occasionally exposing of a portion of the bony phalanx. Hemostasis can be obtained by gentle electrocautery, and the wound is left for secondary intention healing (Figure 10.5).

Indications: Severe hypertrophy of the lateral nail folds.

Advantages: Very easy procedure, even for the beginner. Moderate pain as there is no traction from stitching.

Disadvantages: Heavy bleeding may occur. Long healing time (up to 8 weeks). Soakings three times daily until healed.

Studies: Vandenbos and Bowers performed a retrospective case series with 55 patients. No recurrence was observed, but the follow-up time was not indicated.[76] Level of evidence C.

Chapeskie and Kovac performed a retrospective study in a mixed adult–pediatric population with 124 patients and 212 surgical sites with a median follow-up time of 8 years. No recurrence was observed,

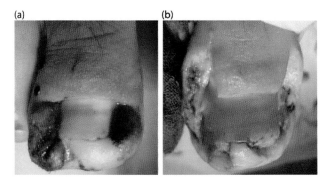

FIGURE 10.5   Vandenbos procedure.

meaning a cure rate of 100% with excellent cosmetic outcomes and high rates of patient satisfaction.[78] Level of evidence C.

Haricharan et al. performed a prospective study in a pediatric population of 50 patients with 67 procedures and a median follow-up time of 14 months. They reported a cure rate of 100% with no recurrence and excellent cosmetic results with very high patient satisfaction.[79] Level of evidence B.

Livingston et al. performed a prospective study, which they name "NAILTEST," in a young population (children, adolescents, and young adults) of 39 patients with 59 procedures under general anesthesia and a median follow-up time of 6 months. They acknowledged no recurrence rate, and 95% of participants and 100% of parents would recommend this procedure.[80] Level of evidence B.

10.3.3.2.3 Super-U Procedure

The Super-U debulking technique, very similar to the Vandenbos technique, was developed in 1989 by Peres Rosa, a Brazilian dermatologist.[81,82]

> *Surgical technique:* All hypertrophic tissues are generously removed in a U-shaped manner around the distal tip of the toe. In contrast to the Vandenbos procedure, the proximal nail fold is not involved and the median part of the toe tip is excised. Hemostasis is obtained by a running lock suture around the wound followed by secondary intention healing (Figure 10.6).
>
> *Indications:* Severe hypertrophy of the lateral or distal nail folds.
>
> *Advantages:* Excellent cosmetic outcomes. Very easy procedure, even for the beginner. Moderate pain as there is no traction from stitching.
>
> *Disadvantages:* Heavy bleeding may occur. Long healing time (up to 8 weeks). Soakings two times daily until healed.
>
> *Studies:* Correa et al. performed a retrospective study on 10 patients with 11 procedures and a median follow-up time of 1 year. They observed two (18%) recurrences, and the majority (9/10) of the patients were satisfied.[83] Level of evidence C.

10.3.3.2.4 Noël's Procedure

This technique was described in 2008 by Noël, a Swiss dermatologist.[84]

> *Surgical technique:* A wedge-shaped ellipse of soft tissue, including the fibrotic and granulation tissue, is vertically removed, on one or both sides of the nail, without touching the plate or the matrix. The incision lines strictly follow the lateral sides of the nail, skimming the lateral aspect of the bony phalanx, down to the lower-third of the toe, to remove a large amount of soft tissues between the bone and the skin. The defect is closed by simple interrupted sutures (Figure 10.7).

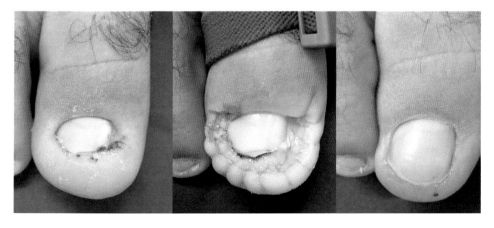

FIGURE 10.6 Super U procedure. (Courtesy Nilton di Chiacchio.)

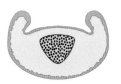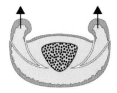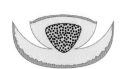

FIGURE 10.7   Noël's procedure.

Indications: Moderate-to-severe hypertrophy of the lateral nail folds.

Advantages: Quick downtime healing. Limited bleeding.

Disadvantages: Moderate pain. Advanced surgery for skilled surgeons.

Studies: Only the original paper reports a prospective study with 23 adult patients with a minimum follow-up of one year. Complete cure was achieved in all cases with no recurrence and an excellent cosmetic outcome.[84] Level of evidence B.

10.3.3.2.5 Other Procedures

Besides the most popular debulking techniques described earlier, the literature offers a plethora of surgical procedures. Some of them were selected.

10.3.3.2.5.1 Knot Technique   In 2015, Ince et al. proposed a new surgical technique named the "knot technique."[85]

Surgical technique: The aim of this technique is to raise the lateral part of the ingrown nail. After a wedge excision of the lateral soft tissues, the wound margins are sutured with 8–10 knots. The latter are placed under the nail and after passing the needle through the plate, the last knot is secured on the nail surface. These successive knots are used to depress the soft tissue and elevate the lateral part of the nail. Stitches are removed after 3–5 weeks.

Indications: Moderate-to-severe hypertrophy of the lateral nail folds.

Advantages: Easy procedure, even for the beginner. Short downtime.

Disadvantages: Stitches to be kept for 3 to up to 5 weeks. The procedure could be painful from the traction on the lateral soft tissues.

Studies: Ince et al. performed a case series of 30 patients with stage 2 or 3 ingrown nails. They included 34 toenails and reported only one (3%) recurrence in the median follow-up of 20 months.[85] Level of evidence C.

Ince and coworkers also carried out a prospective randomized study comparing the Winograd procedure and his technique (knot technique). Seventy-five patients were enrolled with a total of 90 ingrown nails in stage 2 or 3. Thirty-five patients with 45 ingrown nails were treated with the knot technique and 40 patients with 45 ingrown nails were treated with the Winograd procedure. After a median follow-up time of 13 months, the relapse rate and number of additional surgeries required were significantly greater ($p < 0.05$) in the Winograd group.[86] Level of evidence A.

10.3.3.2.5.2 Monaldi Technique   The peculiarity of the Monaldi technique relies in the plantar approach. It was described by Gualdi and his coworkers in 2014.[87]

Surgical technique: A fusiform resection of hallux healthy plantar pulp, starting 1 cm below the hyponychium and extending proximally up to the interphalangeal joint is performed. The incision should be deep to remove enough soft tissue to close the defect. The wound is closed with a running suture or simple interrupted sutures.

Indications: Hypertrophy of the lateral nail folds.

Advantages: Very easy procedure. Scar hidden on the plantar aspect of the toe. Short downtime.

Disadvantages: Scar on the plantar aspect of the toe may impair gait. Nonoptimal cosmetic results. Loss of skin sensitivity.

Study: The only study is the one from Gualdi et al. It was a prospective study on 20 patients with 24 nail surgeries and a follow-up of 16 months. The authors reported a 4% rate of recurrence, all patients complained about the cosmetic results, and 20% observed a reduction in skin sensitivity.[87] Level of evidence B.

10.4 Unilateral Excision of Lateral Fold

Multiple techniques are described in the literature with different shapes of excision (triangular, elliptical, semielliptical, crescent, or radical), with or without nail avulsion (with or without nail matricectomy), and with or without suture. Most of them are variants of the previously described surgical techniques. The following summarizes the most relevant ones.

Bose performed a radical excision of the lateral nail folds (adjacent to the nail border) followed by secondary healing (Figure 10.8). It may be considered as a unilateral variant of the Vandenbos procedure.[88] Level of evidence C.

Persichetti et al. proposed a technique, without matricectomy, where the nail is removed first then bilateral elliptical excisions (not adjacent to the nail border) are performed and the defect sutured to evert the nail fold. It may be considered as a variant of the Howard-Dubois procedure completed with a total nail avulsion. On a series of 120, they reported a rate of recurrence of 5.5% in the 6–12-month follow-up period.[89] Level of evidence C.

Aksakal et al. developed a technique very similar to Persichetti's, with only avulsion of the lateral third of the plate. Thirty surgeries on 22 patients were performed with 5 (17%) recurrences during the 8–10-month follow-up.[90] Level of evidence C.

Sarifakioglu and Sarifakioglu reported a series with a similar technique as Aksakal's. It may be considered as a hemi–Howard-Dubois with partial nail avulsion.[91] Level of evidence C.

Zhu et al. proposed a modified technique combining a bilateral wedge resection removing the lateral matrix horns, as described by Winograd, with only closure of the most proximal and distal parts of the defect. They retrospectively reviewed 131 patients treated with the technique. They observed 10 recurrences with 6 patients requiring new surgery.[92] Level of evidence C.

10.5 Flaps

Tweedie and Ranger used a transposition flap after preliminary removal of granulation tissue. The flap is elevated, parallel to the lateral nail fold with a proximal pedicle. The lower part of the flap is trimmed

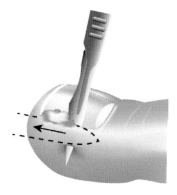

FIGURE 10.8 Bose procedure.

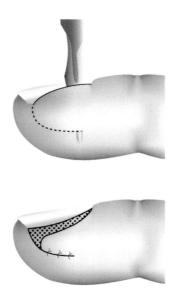

FIGURE 10.9   Tweedie and Ranger flap.

to allow a lower transposition of the flap. After suturing the flap, a small upper defect is then left to heal by secondary intention (Figure 10.9). The treatment is not technically difficult and is effective with a 90% success rate but pain may be observed.[93] Level of evidence C.

Cologlu et al. showed in a comparative study that a partial matricectomy with a lateral fold advancement flap was superior to wedge resection in terms of recurrence ($p \leq 0.05$), spicules ($p \leq 0.05$), reoperation ($p \leq 0.05$), and patients' satisfaction (p $\leq$ 0.05).[94] Level of evidence B.

El-Shaer proposed a variant of the Winograd technique where the closure is obtained by freeing a flap from the lateral aspect of the toe.[95] Level of evidence C.

Aksoy et al. developed a procedure that they named "lateral foldplasty." This complex technique combines, after curettage of the granulation tissue, two flaps: first a rectangular skin flap on the lateral fold and a second triangular flap on the adjacent lateral part of the tip of the toe. After trimming, the two flaps are sutured, which results in the lowering of the distal part of the lateral nail fold. This flap can be associated with a small lateral surgical matrix excision if necessary. They retrospectively analyzed the procedure in 32 patients with 52 ingrown toenails. They reported 4% of recurrence, 1 partial flap necrosis, and good cosmetic outcomes.[96] Level of evidence C.

In conclusion, there is no cure-all technique for ingrowing toenails. After careful examination of each individual case, the surgeon should decide which technique would be the most accurate to the type of ingrown nail, the patient's desire, the downtime, and the surgeon's own skills. More well-conducted comparative trials are definitely needed to evaluate each technique in precise conditions.

REFERENCES

1. Eekhof JA, Van Wijk B, Knuistingh Neven A, van der Wouden JC. Interventions for ingrowing toenails. *Cochrane Database Syst Rev.* 2012;4:CD001541.
2. Rounding C, Bloomfield S. Surgical treatments for ingrowing toenails. *Cochrane Database Syst Rev.* 2005;2:CD001541.
3. Daniel CR, 3rd, Iorizzo M, Tosti A, Piraccini BM. Ingrown toenails. *Cutis.* 2006;78(6):407–408.
4. Reyzelman AM, Trombello KA, Vayser DJ, Armstrong DG, Harkless LB. Are antibiotics necessary in the treatment of locally infected ingrown toenails? *Arch Fam Med.* 2000;9(9):930–932.
5. Tsunoda M, Tsunoda K. Patient-controlled taping for the treatment of ingrown toenails. *Ann Fam Med.* 2014;12(6):553–555.
6. Watabe A, Yamasaki K, Hashimoto A, Aiba S. Retrospective evaluation of conservative treatment for 140 ingrown toenails with a novel taping procedure. *Acta Derm Venereol.* 2015;95(7):822–825.

7. Senapati A. Conservative outpatient management of ingrowing toenails. *J R Soc Med*. 1986;79(6):339–340.
8. Ilfeld FW. Ingrown toenail treated with cotton collodion insert. *Foot Ankle*. 1991;11(5):312–313.
9. Connolly B, Fitzgerald RJ. Pledgets in ingrowing toenails. *Arch Dis Child*. 1988;63(1):71–72.
10. Gutierrez-Mendoza D, De Anda Juarez M, Avalos VF, Martinez GR, Dominguez-Cherit J. "Cotton nail cast": A simple solution for mild and painful lateral and distal nail embedding. *Dermatol Surg*. 2015;41(3):411–414.
11. d'Almeida LF, Nakamura R. Onychocryptosis treatment pearls: The "rolled cotton padding" maneuver and the "artificial resin nail" technique. *Dermatol Surg*. 2016;42(3):434–436.
12. Wallace WA, Milne DD, Andrew T. Gutter treatment for ingrowing toenails. *Br Med J*. 1979;2(6183):168–171.
13. Arai H, Arai T, Nakajima H, Haneke E. Formable acrylic treatment for ingrowing nail with gutter splint and sculptured nail. *Int J Dermatol*. 2004;43(10):759–765.
14. Taheri A, Mansoori P, Alinia H, Lewallen R, Feldman SR. A conservative method to gutter splint ingrown toenails. *JAMA Dermatol*. 2014;150(12):1359–1360.
15. Peyvandi H, Robati RM, Yegane RA et al. Comparison of two surgical methods (Winograd and sleeve method) in the treatment of ingrown toenail. *Dermatol Surg*. 2011;37(3):331–335.
16. Woo SH, Kim IH. Surgical pearl: Nail edge separation with dental floss for ingrown toenails. *J Am Acad Dermatol*. 2004;50(6):939–940.
17. Matsumoto K, Hashimoto I, Nakanishi H, Kubo Y, Murao K, Arase S. Resin splint as a new conservative treatment for ingrown toenails. *J Med Invest*. 2010;57(3–4):321–325.
18. Chiriac A, Solovan C, Brzezinski P. Ingrown toenails (unguis incarnatus): Nail braces/bracing treatment. *Proc (Bayl Univ Med Cent)*. 2014;27(2):145.
19. Harrer J, Schoffl V, Hohenberger W, Schneider I. Treatment of ingrown toenails using a new conservative method: A prospective study comparing brace treatment with Emmert's procedure. *J Am Podiatr Med Assoc*. 2005;95(6):542–549.
20. Kruijff S, van Det RJ, van der Meer GT, van den Berg IC, van der Palen J, Geelkerken RH. Partial matrix excision or orthonyxia for ingrowing toenails. *J Am Coll Surg*. 2008;206(1):148–153.
21. Liu CW, Huang YC. Efficacy of a new nail brace for the treatment of ingrown toenails. *J Dtsch Dermatol Ges*. 2018;16(4):417–423.
22. Shih YH, Huang CY, Lee CC, Lee WR. Nail brace application: A noninvasive treatment for ingrown nails in pediatric patients. *Dermatol Surg*. 2019;45(2):323–326.
23. Guler O, Tuna H, Mahirogullari M, Erdil M, Mutlu S, Isyar M. Nail braces as an alternative treatment for ingrown toenails: Results from a comparison with the Winograd technique. *J Foot Ankle Surg*. 2015;54(4):620–624.
24. Grieg JD, Anderson JH, Ireland AJ, Anderson JR. The surgical treatment of ingrowing toenails. *J Bone Joint Surg Br*. 1991;73(1):131–133.
25. Gabriel SS, Dallos V, Stevenson DL. The ingrowing toenail: A modified segmental matrix excision operation. *Br J Surg*. 1979;66(4):285–286.
26. Huang JZ, Zhang YJ, Ma X, Wang X, Zhang C, Chen L. Comparison of wedge resection (Winograd procedure) and wedge resection plus complete nail plate avulsion in the treatment of ingrown toenails. *J Foot Ankle Surg*. 2015;54(3):395–398.
27. Acar E. Winograd method versus Winograd method with electrocoagulation in the treatment of ingrown toenails. *J Foot Ankle Surg*. 2017;56(3):474–477.
28. Bos AM, van Tilburg MW, van Sorge AA, Klinkenbijl JH. Randomized clinical trial of surgical technique and local antibiotics for ingrowing toenail. *Br J Surg*. 2007;94(3):292–296.
29. Islam S, Lin EM, Drongowski R et al. The effect of phenol on ingrown toenail excision in children. *J Pediatr Surg*. 2005;40(1):290–292.
30. Anderson JH, Greig JD, Ireland AJ, Anderson JR. Randomized, prospective study of nail bed ablation for recurrent ingrowing toenails. *J R Coll Surg Edinb*. 1990;35(4):240–242.
31. Karaca N, Dereli T. Treatment of ingrown toenail with proximolateral matrix partial excision and matrix phenolization. *Ann Fam Med*. 2012;10(6):556–559.
32. Fulton GJ, O'Donohoe MK, Reynolds JV, Keane FB, Tanner WA. Wedge resection alone or combined with segmental phenolization for the treatment of ingrowing toenail. *Br J Surg*. 1994;81(7):1074–1075.
33. Issa MM, Tanner WA. Approach to ingrowing toenails: The wedge resection/segmental phenolization combination treatment. *Br J Surg*. 1988;75(2):181–183.

34. Yabe T, Takahashi M. A minimally invasive surgical approach for ingrown toenails: Partial germinal matrix excision using operative microscope. *J Plast Reconstr Aesthet Surg.* 2010;63(1):170–173.

35. van der Ham AC, Hackeng CA, Yo TI. The treatment of ingrowing toenails. A randomised comparison of wedge excision and phenol cauterisation. *J Bone Joint Surg Br.* 1990;72(3):507–509.

36. Morkane AJ, Robertson RW, Inglis GS. Segmental phenolization of ingrowing toenails: A randomized controlled study. *Br J Surg.* 1984;71(7):526–527.

37. Herold N, Houshian S, Riegels-Nielsen P. A prospective comparison of wedge matrix resection with nail matrix phenolization for the treatment of ingrown toenail. *J Foot Ankle Surg.* 2001;40(6):390–395.

38. Caronia V, Battistioli M, Gualandi O, Marchese M, Bonotto G. [Treatment of the ingrown toenail by phenol cauterization (ASLUF)]. *Minerva Chir.* 2001;56(2):199–203.

39. Bostanci S, Ekmekci P, Gurgey E. Chemical matricectomy with phenol for the treatment of ingrowing toenail: A review of the literature and follow-up of 172 treated patients. *Acta Derm Venereol.* 2001;81(3):181–183.

40. Di Chiacchio N, Belda W, Jr., Di Chiacchio NG, Kezam Gabriel FV, de Farias DC. Nail matrix phenolization for treatment of ingrowing nail: Technique report and recurrence rate of 267 surgeries. *Dermatol Surg.* 2010;36(4):534–537.

41. Vaccari S, Dika E, Balestri R, Rech G, Piraccini BM, Fanti PA. Partial excision of matrix and phenolic ablation for the treatment of ingrowing toenail: A 36-month follow-up of 197 treated patients. *Dermatol Surg.* 2010;36(8):1288–1293.

42. Kimata Y, Uetake M, Tsukada S, Harii K. Follow-up study of patients treated for ingrown nails with the nail matrix phenolization method. *Plast Reconstr Surg.* 1995;95(4):719–724.

43. Zaraa I, Dorbani I, Hawilo A, Mokni M, Ben Osman A. Segmental phenolization for the treatment of ingrown toenails: Technique report, follow up of 146 patients, and review of the literature. *Dermatol Online J.* 2013;19(6):18560.

44. Ramsay G, Caldwell D. Phenol cauterization for ingrown toenails. *Arch Emerg Med.* 1986;3(4):243–246.

45. Becerro de Bengoa Vallejo R, Losa Iglesias ME, Viejo Tirado F, Serrano Pardo R. Cauterization of the germinal nail matrix using phenol applications of differing durations: A histologic study. *J Am Acad Dermatol.* 2012;67(4):706–711.

46. Aksakal AB, Atahan C, Oztas P, Oruk S. Minimizing postoperative drainage with 20% ferric chloride after chemical matricectomy with phenol. *Dermatol Surg.* 2001;27(2):158–160.

47. Alvarez-Jimenez J, Cordoba-Fernandez A, Munuera PV. Effect of curettage after segmental phenolization in the treatment of onychocryptosis: A randomized double-blind clinical trial. *Dermatol Surg.* 2012;38(3):454–461.

48. Marcos-Tejedor F, Aldana-Caballero A, Martinez-Nova A. Effect of phenol and sodium hydroxide in the bacterial load at nail fold after partial matricectomy. *Dermatol Surg.* 2017;43(2):316–317.

49. Boberg JS, Frederiksen MS, Harton FM. Scientific analysis of phenol nail surgery. *J Am Podiatr Med Assoc.* 2002;92(10):575–579.

50. Tatlican S, Eren C, Yamangokturk B, Eskioglu F. Letter: Retrospective comparison of experiences with phenol and sodium hydroxide in the treatment of ingrown nail. *Dermatol Surg.* 2010;36(3):432–434.

51. Grover C, Khurana A, Bhattacharya SN, Sharma A. Controlled trial comparing the efficacy of 88 phenol versus 10 sodium hydroxide for chemical matricectomy in the management of ingrown toenail. *Indian J Dermatol Venereol Leprol.* 2015;81(5):472–477.

52. Bostanci S, Kocyigit P, Gurgey E. Comparison of phenol and sodium hydroxide chemical matricectomies for the treatment of ingrowing toenails. *Dermatol Surg.* 2007;33(6):680–685.

53. Felton PM, Weaver TD. Phenol and alcohol chemical matrixectomy in diabetic versus nondiabetic patients. *A retrospective study. J Am Podiatr Med Assoc.* 1999;89(8):410–412.

54. Giacalone VF. Phenol matricectomy in patients with diabetes. *J Foot Ankle Surg.* 1997;36(4):264–267; discussion 328.

55. Mitchell S, Jackson CR, Wilson-Storey D. Surgical treatment of ingrown toenails in children: What is best practice? *Ann R Coll Surg Engl.* 2011;93(2):99–102.

56. Tatlican S, Eren C, Yamangokturk B, Eskioglu F, Bostanci S. Chemical matricectomy with 10% sodium hydroxide for the treatment of ingrown toenails in people with diabetes. *Dermatol Surg.* 2010;36(2):219–222.

57. Yang G, Yanchar NL, Lo AY, Jones SA. Treatment of ingrown toenails in the pediatric population. *J Pediatr Surg.* 2008;43(5):931–935.

58. Kim SH, Ko HC, Oh CK, Kwon KS, Kim MB. Trichloroacetic acid matricectomy in the treatment of ingrowing toenails. *Dermatol Surg.* 2009;35(6):973–979.
59. Andre MS, Caucanas M, Andre J, Richert B. Treatment of ingrowing toenails with phenol 88 or trichloroacetic acid 100: A comparative, prospective, randomized, double-blind study. *Dermatol Surg.* 2018;44(5):645–650.
60. Terzi E, Guvenc U, Tursen B, Tursen U, Kaya TI. The effectiveness of matrix cauterization with bichloracetic acid in the treatment of ingrown toenails. *Dermatol Surg.* 2017;43(5):728–733.
61. Takahashi M, Narisawa Y. Radical surgery for ingrown nails by partial resection of the nail plate and matrix using a carbon dioxide laser. *J Cutan Laser Ther.* 2000;2(1):21–25.
62. Lin YC, Su HY. A surgical approach to ingrown nail: Partial matricectomy using CO_2 laser. *Dermatol Surg.* 2002;28(7):578–580.
63. Andre P. Ingrowing nails and carbon dioxide laser surgery. *J Eur Acad Dermatol Venereol.* 2003;17(3):288–290.
64. Serour F. Recurrent ingrown big toenails are efficiently treated by CO_2 laser. *Dermatol Surg.* 2002;28(6):509–512.
65. Wollina U. Modified Emmet's operation for ingrown nails using the Er:YAG laser. *J Cosmet Laser Ther.* 2004;6(1):38–40.
66. Kim M, Song IG, Kim HJ. Partial removal of nail matrix in the treatment of ingrown nails: Prospective randomized control study between curettage and electrocauterization. *Int J Low Extrem Wounds.* 2015;14(2):192–195.
67. Ozan F, Dogar F, Altay T, Ugur SG, Koyuncu S. Partial matricectomy with curettage and electrocautery: A comparison of two surgical methods in the treatment of ingrown toenails. *Dermatol Surg.* 2014;40(10):1132–1139.
68. Farrelly PJ, Minford J, Jones MO. Simple operative management of ingrown toenail using bipolar diathermy. *Eur J Pediatr Surg.* 2009;19(5):304–306.
69. Misiak P, Terlecki A, Rzepkowska-Misiak B, Wcislo S, Brocki M. Comparison of effectiveness of electrocautery and phenol application in partial matricectomy after partial nail extraction in the treatment of ingrown nails. *Pol Przegl Chir.* 2014;86(2):89–93.
70. Yilmaz A, Cenesizoglu E. Partial matricectomy with cryotherapy in treatment of ingrown toenails. *Acta Orthop Traumatol Turc.* 2016;50(3):262–268.
71. Pearson HJ, Bury RN, Wapples J, Watkin DF. Ingrowing toenails: Is there a nail abnormality? A prospective study. *J Bone Joint Surg Br.* 1987;69(5):840–842.
72. DeBrule MB. Operative treatment of ingrown toenail by nail fold resection without matricectomy. *J Am Podiatr Med Assoc.* 2015;105(4):295–301.
73. Howard WR. Ingrown toenail; its surgical treatment. *N Y Med J.* 1893(57):579.
74. Dubois JP. [Treatment of ingrown nails]. *Nouv Presse Med.* 1974;3(31):1938–1940.
75. Murray WR, Robb JE. Soft-tissue resection for ingrowing toenails. *J Dermatol Surg Oncol.* 1981;7(2):157–158.
76. Vandenbos KQ BW. Ingrown toenail: A result of weight bearing on soft tissue. *US Armed Forces Med J.* 1959;10(10):1168–1173.
77. Chapeskie H. Ingrown toenail or overgrown toe skin?: Alternative treatment for onychocryptosis. *Can Fam Physician.* 2008;54(11):1561–1562.
78. Chapeskie H, Kovac JR. Case series: Soft-tissue nail-fold excision: A definitive treatment for ingrown toenails. *Can J Surg.* 2010;53(4):282–286.
79. Haricharan RN, Masquijo J, Bettolli M. Nail-fold excision for the treatment of ingrown toenail in children. *J Pediatr.* 2013;162(2):398–402.
80. Livingston MH, Coriolano K, Jones SA. Nonrandomized assessment of ingrown toenails treated with excision of skinfold rather than toenail (NAILTEST): An observational study of the Vandenbos procedure. *J Pediatr Surg.* 2017;52(5):832–836.
81. Rosa IP GM, Mosca FZ. Tratamento cirúrgico da hipercurvatura do leito ungueal. *An Bras Dermatol.* 1989;64(2):115–117.
82. Rosa IP, Di Chiacchio N, Di Chiacchio NG, Caetano L. "Super U"—A technique for the treatment of ingrown nail. *Dermatol Surg.* 2015;41(5):652–653.
83. Correa J, Magliano J, Agorio C, Bazzano C. Super U technique for ingrown nails. *Actas Dermosifiliogr.* 2017;108(5):438–444.

84. Noël B. Surgical treatment of ingrown toenail without matricectomy. *Dermatol Surg.* 2008;34(1):79–83.
85. Ince B, Dadaci M, Altuntas Z. Knot technique: A new treatment of ingrown nails. *Dermatol Surg.* 2015;41(2):250–254.
86. Ince B, Dadaci M, Bilgen F, Yarar S. Comparison between knot and Winograd techniques on ingrown nail treatment. *Acta Orthop Traumatol Turc.* 2015;49(5):539–543.
87. Gualdi G, Monari P, Crotti S, Calzavara-Pinton PG. Surgical treatment of ingrown toe nail: The Monaldi technique, a new simple proposal. *Dermatol Surg.* 2014;40(2):208–210.
88. Bose B. A technique for excision of nail fold for ingrowing toenail. *Surg Gynecol Obstet.* 1971;132(3):511–512.
89. Persichetti P, Simone P, Li Vecchi G, Di Lella F, Cagli B, Marangi GF. Wedge excision of the nail fold in the treatment of ingrown toenail. *Ann Plast Surg.* 2004;52(6):617–620.
90. Aksakal AB, Oztas P, Atahan C, Gurer MA. Decompression for the management of onychocryptosis. *J Dermatolog Treat.* 2004;15(2):108–111.
91. Sarifakioglu E, Sarifakioglu N. Crescent excision of the nail fold with partial nail avulsion does work with ingrown toenails. *Eur J Dermatol.* 2010;20(6):822–823.
92. Zhu X, Shi H, Zhang L, Gu Y. Lateral fold and partial nail bed excision for the treatment of recurrent ingrown toenails. *Int J Clin Exp Med.* 2012;5(3):257–261.
93. Tweedie JH, Ranger I. A simple procedure with nail preservation for ingrowing toe-nails. *Arch Emerg Med.* 1985;2(3):149–154.
94. Cologlu H, Kocer U, Sungur N, Uysal A, Kankaya Y, Oruc M. A new anatomical repair method for the treatment of ingrown nail: Prospective comparison of wedge resection of the matrix and partial matricectomy followed by lateral fold advancement flap. *Ann Plast Surg.* 2005;5(54):306–311; discussion 12.
95. El-Shaer WM. Lateral fold rotational flap technique for treatment of ingrown nail. *Plast Reconstr Surg.* 2007;120(7):2131–2133.
96. Aksoy B, Aksoy HM, Civas E, Oc B, Atakan N. Lateral foldplasty with or without partial matricectomy for the management of ingrown toenails. *Dermatol Surg.* 2009;35(3):462–468.

11

Lichen Planus

Bianca Maria Piraccini, Aurora Alessandrini, and Michela Starace

11.1 Introduction

Nail lichen planus (LP) is not rare. Nail abnormalities are seen in approximately 10% of adult patients with cutaneous lichen planus, but without skin involvement can also occur, making the diagnosis more difficult; moreover, a mild oral LP being detected in less than one-fourth of the patients only after examination. Association with scalp LP (lichen planopilaris or frontal fibrosing alopecia) is exceptional.[1] Nail LP shares with lichen planopilaris the aggressive behavior that may lead to a scarring outcome.[2] LP of the nail apparatus considerably affects the quality of life, due to the impaired manual activity produced, the cosmetic discomfort, the chronic nature, the scarce response to treatment, and the numerous recurrences.

Evidence suggests LP to be autoimmune in nature and that abnormalities are caused by basal keratinocytes in a process mediated by T cells that express autoantigen on their surface.[3] For this reason, nail lichen planus may be associated with skin and systemic autoimmune disorders, especially in children, or with disorders characterized by altered immune response, including alopecia areata, vitiligo, autoimmune thyroid disease, celiac disease, chronic inflammatory liver diseases, psoriasis, atopic dermatitis, localized scleroderma, polymyalgia, and Sjögren syndrome.[2,4,5] Stress was an evident triggering factor in 20% of patients in a study of 20 cases.[6]

The prevalence of nail LP is equally distributed among both sexes and occurs most commonly around the fifth or sixth decades of life,[7] but recently a study reported a higher prevalence in males,[8] even if onset in childhood may occasionally occur.[5] A recent article reported nail involvement in about 14% of children with skin LP.[4]

Usually, LP involves several to all nails, with various degrees of severity and with the thumbs showing the most severe signs. Fingernails are more often affected than toenails. Toenails have less specific signs, as nail thinning is less evident. The longitudinal shape of the signs is the typical feature. The inflammatory infiltrate of LP may localize to all the different components of the nail apparatus, alone or in combination, producing symptoms due to altered function or to destruction of the involved area. Most commonly, nail LP affects the nail matrix.

Depending on severity of the inflammatory damage and the localization of the pathological process, nail LP may clinically be presented in five different variants:

- "Typical" nail lichen planus (of matrix, of nail bed, or of matrix + nail bed): Accounting for about 80% of the cases
- Trachyonychia: Responsible for about 8% of the cases
- Idiopathic atrophy of the nails: Accounting for less than 5% of patients
- Yellow nail syndrome (YNS)–like LP: Rare
- Bullous-erosive LP: Extremely rare

Nail matrix LP is the most common type and is presented by nail thinning with longitudinal ridging and fissuring (onychorrhexis).[2,7,8] The longitudinal pattern of the nail damage is quite characteristic. The nails are thinned and show deep longitudinal fissures that reach the distal margin, which is irregular and

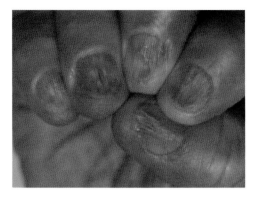

FIGURE 11.1   Clinical picture of nail matrix lichen planus: nail thinning with longitudinal ridging and fissuring (onychorrhexis) are evident in most of the nails.

short (Figure 11.1). A spotty nail matrix inflammation results in different degrees of thinning and ridging within the nail plate. Severity of inflammatory signs varies from nail to nail. In severe cases, the nail plate is severely thinned and appears as scales on the nail bed. An irregular punctate or diffuse redness of the lunula area, named mottled lunula, which is not specific for nail LP, is seen in approximately 25% of the patients, especially in the thumbs.[7,9] This sign indicates an inflammation of the nail matrix. Where the longitudinal fissuring is absent, there are present longitudinal red streaks on the nail plate (longitudinal erythronychia) that are a sign of inflammation but without destruction of the nail plate. Another possible sign of inflammation is the presence of longitudinal melanonychia due to a melanocytic activation[10] (Figure 11.2). All the clinical features of nail matrix lichen planus are most evident in the fingernails, while in the toenails longitudinal ridging and fissuring are present as isolated signs only rarely, as they are most commonly associated with nail plate thickening, which makes the clinical diagnosis difficult.

(a)

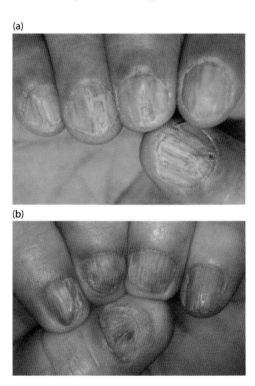

(b)

FIGURE 11.2   Atypical types of nail LP: (a) Longitudinal erythronychia and (b) longitudinal melanonychia.

Dorsal pterygium is a possible outcome of nail matrix LP, and indicates a pathognomonic focal scarring of the nail matrix. Destruction of a part of the matrix, with absent production of the nail plate, leads to adhesion of the dorsal skin to the nail bed. This clinically appears as a V-shaped extension of the proximal nail fold that splits the nail plate in two portions with a fusion of the two splitting parts, usually in the center but possibly also in the lateral part as a fissure. Development of dorsal pterygium is uncommon and does not correlate with duration of the nail LP. Dorsal pterygium may remain stable or become wider, indicating progression of matrix scarring and the overlying proximal nail fold.

Nail bed LP causes onycholysis, which is not specific of nail LP and is usually associated with nail matrix involvement. The nails show proximal onycholysis with or without subungual hyperkeratosis. When the onycholysis is complete, a possible nail plate shedding can occur and permanent atrophy may result. Diagnosis of nail LP is difficult when onycholysis is the prevalent symptom and requires pathological examination. LP of the nail bed may rarely cause hypertrophic LP, characterized by diffuse nail thickening due to homogeneous nail bed hyperkeratosis. A characteristic finding in nail bed lichen planus is the "pup tent" sign, in which the nail plate splits, elevates longitudinally, and the lateral edges angle downward.[11]

When LP involves the nail matrix in a mild diffuse way, it produces trachyonychia.[12] One or several/all nails are presented by an opaque nail plate due to fine longitudinal striations covered by minute scales, often with mild nail thinning. In these cases, the diagnosis of nail LP is only possible with a pathological study of the nail matrix after a biopsy (Figure 11.3). Trachyonychia due to LP is uncommon and mostly seen in children.[13] Even when caused by nail LP, trachyonychia is always a benign condition and does not produce pterygium. Psoriasis, alopecia areata, and atopic dermatitis can be other possible causes.

Idiopathic atrophy of the nails is a rare variety of lichen planus, almost exclusively observed in Asians, and may sometimes be hereditary.[14,15] It is characterized by onset in childhood with acute and rapid development of pterygium of several nails with progressive atrophy, in the absence of subjective symptoms or other cutaneous signs. The involved digits show total or subtotal absence of the nail plate with dorsal pterygium. The proximal nail fold may show atrophy and telangiectasia.

In the toenails, clinical signs of LP are associated with marked nail thickening, and fissuring is rarely evident and this form recalls an aspect such as yellow nail syndrome (YNS)–LP. The nails are often yellow in color with similar features of YNS.[16] Only the evaluation of fingernails may suggest the diagnosis.

Bullous LP of the nails is an uncommon and extreme variant of LP where bullous or ulcerative lesions develop in the matrix and nail bed resulting in complete shedding of the nail plate and nail scarring combine with bullae and erosions on the soles and occasionally on the palms.[17] It can affect fingernails or toenails: absence of the nail plates, nail bed erosions, and marked inflammation of the periungual skin lead to total nail loss with anonychia (Figure 11.4).

Uncommon clinical presentations of nail LP include nail degloving, which describes partial or total avulsion of the nail and surrounding tissue that has been reported in a case of nail LP[18] and nail LP with involvement of the periungual tissues, which appears with pruriginous erythematous scaly or

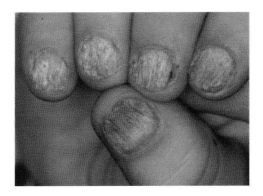

FIGURE 11.3 Trachyonychia due to nail LP, histologically proven.

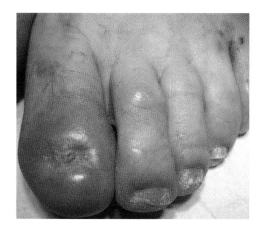

FIGURE 11.4   Bullous LP of the nails, characterized by nail scarring with bullae and erosions on the soles.

violaceous hyperkeratotic plaques with well-defined edges in the proximal nail fold and the distal pulp.[19] The proximal nail fold may also show a diffuse bluish-red discoloration with or without swelling, with evident Wickham striae.[20]

Nail LP in children is rarer than in adults, and usually induces milder nail changes. In most cases, nail LP in children are presented by the clinical features that characterize typical nail LP of adults of one or several/all nails with nail thinning and longitudinal ridging, fissuring, and distal splitting, due to nail matrix involvement or with onycholysis due to nail bed involvement. The development of dorsal pterygium is rare in children; trachyonychia and idiopathic atrophy of the nails are more frequent.[13]

Moreover, dorsal pterygium may result as a scarring from causes such as bullous diseases, digital ischemia, traumatic damage to the nail, accidental, or surgical. Due to the nail thickening of LP, onychomycosis with yellow discoloration, onycholysis and subungual hyperkeratosis, and yellow nail syndrome with green-yellow discoloration and nail plate hypercurvature are to be excluded.

11.2 How to Confirm the Diagnosis

The diagnosis of nail LP may be easy in a patient with LP of the skin, but it is difficult when the disease is limited to the nails. The different signs of nail LP can in fact resemble those seen in other nail disorders and a prompt diagnosis is crucial before having a scarring outcome.

Other possible nail diseases that can mimic nail lichen planus due to the presence of nail thinning and longitudinal ridging are nail ageing due to the fragility of the nail plate; nail psoriasis, especially in the nail bed involvement and sometimes it requires a biopsy for definitive diagnosis; and systemic amyloidosis that may produce uniformly thinned, brittle, longitudinally ridged (onychorrhexis) nails that are split distally.[21,22] A longitudinal nail biopsy with Congo red staining is needed to demonstrate amyloid deposits in the nail matrix and bed. Graft-versus-host disease (GVHD), where dorsal pterygium, longitudinal ridging, and distal splitting of the fingernails are the typical features, is typically associated with skin lesions.[23]

Bullous LP must be differentiated from inflammatory and neoplastic diseases able to cause nail plate loss and bleeding, and the pathology is mandatory for the diagnosis. Unless the patient has clinical signs of LP of the skin mucosae, diagnosis of nail LP requires a biopsy. First, many diseases that can mimic lichen planus must be excluded. Second, as treatment of nail LP requires systemic or intralesional drugs, in order to avoid permanent scarring, having a pathological confirmation of the diagnosis helps to increase patient's acceptance of therapy.

Onychoscopy enhances visualization of the longitudinal fissures of the nail plate due to lichen planus reaching the distal nail and partial absence of the nail plate (Figure 11.5). In the early stages of disease, the signs are represented by pitting and may progress to trachyonychia, then in the advanced stage appear as lamellar fragmentation, onycholysis, and subungual hyperkeratosis, especially when the affected area is

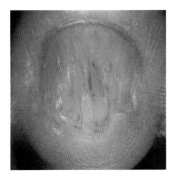

FIGURE 11.5   Onychoscopy of nail LP. This instrument permits a better visualization of the longitudinal fissures of the nail plate and of dorsal pterygium (10× magnification).

the nail bed, culminating in the classical signs of the lichen of the nail matrix. Dermoscopic observation of the proximal nail plate, where it emerges from the nail fold, permits evaluating the disease's course in a short time, since it shows the newly formed nail plate. These signs are typical when the disease involves the nail matrix and are mainly seen in the fingernails.[2,24]

Histological aspects of typical nail lichen planus are characterized by a dense band-like lymphocytic infiltrate of the nail matrix or nail bed dermis, associated with hyperkeratosis, hypergranulosis, and acanthosis of the nail matrix epithelium. Diffuse granulosis, a linear pattern at the dermo-epithelial junction, or irregular epithelial hyperplasia of the epithelium are detected as well. Nail matrix atrophy and granulosis in the epithelium, and melanophages in the superficial dermis in old lesions are observed in longstanding cases and in idiopathic atrophy of the nails.[7]

11.3 Evidence-Based Treatment

Therapy on the basis of the level of evidence is reviewed in Table 11.1.

Treatment of nail LP is direct to stopping the inflammatory response, but it is difficult, as not all patients respond to therapy. Mild forms of lichen planus may resolve spontaneously, and so, often, no treatment is necessary. However, more severe inflammation and potentially scarring disease should be treated more aggressively to prevent permanent dystrophy.

Optimal therapy is still lacking, and systemic or intralesional steroids are the treatment of choice.

TABLE 11.1

Treatments and Levels of Evidence

Treatment	Level of Evidence
Intramuscular triamcinolone acetonide	A[7]
Intradermal triamcinolone injections in the proximal nail matrix (PNM)	B[29]
Topical steroids	B[30]
Azathioprine	E[28]
Tacrolimus 0.1% cream	C[30]
Prednisone	C[7,13]
Cyclosporine A	E[33]
Etretinate	E[31,32,33]
Fumaric acid esters	E[32]
Alitretinoin	E[25,27]
Etanercept	E[34]

11.3.1 Systemic Treatment

11.3.1.1 Systemic Steroids

Treatment with steroids is effective in two-thirds of patients, producing total or subtotal regression of nail symptoms, independently of age and severity of disease.[2] Fingernails respond more often and quickly than toenails. Patients who do not respond to systemic steroids are unlikely to benefit from other therapies.

The modality of steroids therapy is on the basis of the number nails involved and the degree of inflammation, which can be locally injected if one to three nails are involved, or are prescribed systemically.

Systemic steroids include intramuscular triamcinolone acetonide (0.5–1.0 mg/kg per month for 2–6 months, then tapered), which can be utilized both in adults (Figure 11.6) and in children with nail LP with optimal tolerability and oral prednisone, at a dose up to 60 mg per day, or 0–5 mg/kg on alternate days for an average of 3–6 months, resulting in total resolution of the nail changes.[7,13]

11.3.1.2 Alitretinoin

Oral alitretinoin has recently been shown to be effective in patients with nail lichen planus over a period of 6–9 months. An initial dose of 30 mg daily can be used for the first 3 months and then be reduced to 10 mg daily to maintain long-term efficacy.[25–27]

11.3.1.3 Azathioprine

Azathioprine 100 mg daily may be used in association with systemic steroids in nonresponder patients in order to increased response to therapy,[2] but it is reported as successful therapy in only two cases of erosive lichen planus.[28]

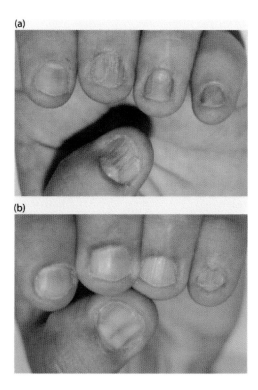

FIGURE 11.6   Clinical picture of nail LP (a) before and (b) after 3 months of intramuscular triamcinolone acetonide.

11.3.1.4 Intralesional Steroids Injections

Intralesional steroids can be used with LP involving a maximum four nails. Diluted triamcinolone acetonide at the dosage of 3–5 mg/mL is injected into each of four periungual sites monthly (Figure 11.7). Injection sites should be at the lateral distal digit at the sites of the matrix and nail bed so that the solution can diffuse to the center of the digit to bathe the undersurface of these structures. Five to six injections are necessary to achieve visible improvement.[29]

11.3.2 Topical Treatment

11.3.2.1 Topical Steroids

Potent fluorinated corticosteroids can be used topically under occlusion. In addition to topical corticosteroids, other topical medications have been used in nail lichen planus. Topical tacrolimus has been used with success in five cases.[30]

11.3.2.2 Other Treatments

Many studies are reported of the use of other systemic treatments, but the efficacy has been tested only in a single case, such as etretinate 0.3–0.4 mg/kg/day, which can be used in patients nonrespondent to systemic steroids, alone[2] or associated with topical steroids applied on the nail fold,[31] fumaric acid esters,[32] or ciclosporin.[33]

(a)

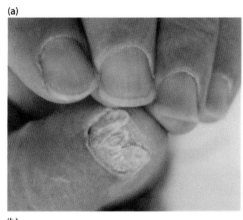

(b)

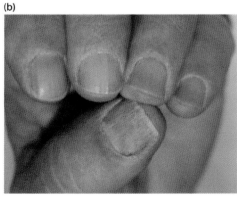

FIGURE 11.7 Clinical improvement of nail LP of fingernails after intralesional steroids injections (a) before treatment and (b) after three sessions of injections.

11.3.2.3 Biologics

In the end, only one case of nail lichen planus has been treated with a biological therapy and specifically etanercept, which led to a marked improvement of relapsing toenail lichen planus.[34]

11.4 Prognosis

Surely a bad prognosis is reported in cicatricial and severe forms of nail LP, such as idiopathic atrophy or bullous variant, where the therapy is indicated to stop the progression and avoid scarring and total nail loss. In other forms, the answer is dependent upon the degree of the inflammation and the starting of atrophy. If the matrix and nail bed are completely involved with an exuberant destructive inflammatory process, a total loss of the nail plate and permanent atrophy with scarring will result. Nail LP has a negative long-term prognosis in a considerably high percentage of patients, if we consider patients who do not respond to the initial steroid treatment (20% of cases) and those with nonresponsive relapses (about 30% of the cured patients). Cicatricial outcome with the formation of dorsal pterygium is, however, rare and does not appear to be related to duration of the disease.

About 20% of patients with nail LP treated with systemic steroids developed distal subungual onychomycosis of fingernails or toenails in the long-term follow-up.[2]

11.5 Conclusion

In summary, one-third of the patients do not respond to therapy. Also 10% of the patients who respond to therapy do not heal completely, but maintain mild nail lesions, consisting of small superficial fissures of the nail plate distal margin and longitudinal bands of leukonychia. Relapse of nail LP occurs in about 60% of the cured patients and is not always responsive to a further treatment with steroids.

REFERENCES

1. Macpherson M, Hohendorf-Ansari P, Trüeb RM. Nail involvement in frontal fibrosing alopecia. *Int J Trichol.* 2015;7:64–66.
2. Piraccini BM, Saccani E, Starace M et al. Nail lichen planus: Response to treatment and long term follow-up. *Eur J Dermatol.* 2010;20:489–496.
3. Shiohara T, Mizukawa Y, Takahashi R, Kano Y. Pathomechanisms of lichen planus autoimmunity elicited by cross-reactive T cells. *Curr Dir Autoimmun.* 2008;10:206–226.
4. Pandhi D, Singal A, Bhattacharya SN. Lichen planus in childhood: A series of 316 patients. *Pediatr Dermatol.* 2014;31:59–67.
5. Tosti A, Piraccini BM, Cambiaghi S, Jorizzo M. Nail lichen planus in children: Clinical features, response to treatment, and long-term follow-up. *Arch Dermatol.* 2001;137:1027–1032.
6. Chiheb S, Haim H, Ouakkadi A et al. Clinical characteristics of nail lichen planus and follow-up: A descriptive study of 20 patients. *Ann Dermatol Venereol.* 2015;142:21–25.
7. Tosti A, Peluso AM, Fanti PA et al. Nail lichen planus. Clinical and pathological study of 24 patients. *J Am Acad Dermatol.* 1993;28:724–730.
8. Goettmann S, Zaraa I, Moulonguet I. Nail lichen planus: Epidemiological, clinical, pathological, therapeutic and prognosis study of 67 cases. *J Eur Acad Dermatol Venereol.* 2012;26:1304–1313.
9. Baran R. The red nail—Always benign? *Actas Dermosifiliogr.* 2009;100(Suppl. L):106–113.
10. Baran R, Jancovici E, Sayag J et al. Longitudinal melanonychia in lichen planus. *Br J Dermatol.* 1985;113:369–370.
11. Boyd AS, Neldner KH. Lichen planus. *J Am Acad Dermatol.* 199;25:593–619.
12. Scher RK, Fischbein R, Ackerman AB. Twenty-nail dystrophy: A variant of lichen planus. *Arch Dermatol.* 1978;114:612–613.
13. Peluso AM, Tosti A, Piraccini BM et al. Lichen planus limited to the nails in childhood: Case report and literature review. *Pediatr Dermatol.* 1993;10:36–39.

14. Suarez SM, Scher RK. Idiopathic atrophy of the nails. A possible hereditary association. *Pediatr Dermatol.* 1990;7:39–41.

15. Tosti A, Piraccini BM, Fanti PA et al. Idiopathic atrophy of the nails: Clinical and pathological study of 2 cases. *Dermatology.* 1995;190:116–118.

16. Tosti A, Piraccini BM, Cameli N. Nail changes in lichen planus may resemble those of yellow nail syndrome. *Br J Dermatol.* 2000;142:848–849.

17. Isogai Z, Koashi Y, Sunohara A et al. Ulcerative lichen planus: A rare variant of lichen planus. *J Dermatol.* 1997;24 (4):270–272.

18. Baran R, Perrin C. Nail degloving, a polyetiologic condition with 3 main patterns: A new syndrome. *J Am Acad Dermatol.* 2008;58:232–237.

19. Tosti A, Ghetti E, Piraccini BM, Fanti PA. Lichen planus of the nails and fingertips. *Eur J Dermatol.* 1998;8:447–448.

20. Lallas A, Kyrgidis A, Tzellos TG et al. Accuracy of dermoscopic criteria for the diagnosis of psoriasis, dermatitis, lichen planus and pityriasis rosea. *Br J Dermatol.* 2012 Jun;166(6):1198–1205.

21. Fanti PA, Tosti A, Morelli R et al. Nail changes as the first sign of a systemic amyloidosis. *Dermatologica* 1991;183:44–46.

22. Renker T, Haneke E, Röcken C, Borradori L. Systemic light-chain amyloidosis revealed by progressive nail involvement, diffuse alopecia and sicca syndrome: Report of an unusual case with a review of the literature. *Dermatology.* 2014;228:97–102.

23. Sanli H, Arat M, Oskay T, Gürman G. Evaluation of nail involvement in patients with chronic cutaneous graft versus host disease: A single-center study from Turkey. *Int J Dermatol.* 2004;43:176–80.

24. Nakamura R, Broce AA, Palencia DP, Ortiz NI, Leverone A. Dermatoscopy of nail lichen planus. *Int J Dermatol.* 2013;52:684–687.

25. Pinter A, Pätzold S, Kaufmann R. Lichen planus of nails—Successful treatment with alitretinoin. *J Dtsch Dermatol Ges.* 2011;9:1033–1034.

26. Alsenaid A, Eder I, Ruzicka T et al. Successful treatment of nail lichen planus with alitretinoin: Report of 2 cases and review of the literature. *Dermatology.* 2014;229:293–296.

27. Iorizzo M. Nail lichen planus—A possible new indication for oral alitretinoin. *J Eur Acad Dermatol Venereol.* 2016;30:509–510.

28. Lear JT, English JS. Erosive and generalized lichen planus responsive to azathioprine. *Clin Exp Dermatol.* 1996;21:56–57.

29. De Berker D, Lawrence CM. 1998. A simplified protocol of nail steroid injection for psoriatic nail dystrophy. *Br J Dermatol.* 1998;138:90–95.

30. Ujiie H, Shibaki A, Akiyama M et al. Successful treatment of nail lichen planus with topical tacrolimus. *Acta Derm Venereol.* 2010;90:218–219.

31. Kato N, Ueno H. Isolated lichen planus of the nails treated with etretinate. *J Dermatol.* 1993;20:577–580.

32. Schulze-Dirks A. Nail involvement in lichen planus—Effective treatment with fumaric acid esters. *J Eur Acad Dermatol Venereol.* 2002;16(Suppl. 1):76–79.

33. Florian B, Angelika J, Ernst SR. Successful treatment of palmoplantar nail lichen planus with cyclosporine. *J Dtsch Dermatol Ges.* 2014;12:724–725.

34. Irla N, Schneiter T, Haneke E et al. Nail lichen planus: Successful treatment with etanercept. *Case Rep Dermatol.* 2010;2:173–176.

12

Melanoma

Eckart Haneke

12.1 Introduction

Although nail melanomas are usually quoted as being particularly rare, this is not true when calculating the small surface of all nails taken together—roughly 0.6% of the body surface—and their proportion of 1.5%–2.5% of all melanomas in Caucasians.[1] When looking further at the matrix origin of approximately 75% of the nail melanomas, then the matrix making up for only one-third of the nail field rather appears to be a hot spot of melanoma development.

Most nail melanoma patients are over 35 years old with a peak age of 50–70 years. Ungual melanomas in children are exceptional[2] (Figure 12.1).

Ungual melanomas occur in all skin types with roughly equal frequency; however, the percentage of nail melanomas is higher in those who develop cutaneous melanomas at a much lower percentage. The nails of the big toes, thumb, index, and middle fingers are most frequently affected. Ultraviolet exposure is not an etiological factor in nail melanomas.

About two-thirds to three-quarters of all nail melanomas are pigmented and produce a longitudinal melanonychia. This is the diagnostic hallmark for nail melanomas; however, amelanotic melanomas do occur (Figure 12.2) and are clinically nonspecific, most of them originating from the nail bed.

Another strong hint at the diagnosis of an ungual melanoma is periungual pigmentation, called the Hutchinson sign. This may be very subtle and require dermatoscopy to be seen, which is called the micro-Hutchinson. In early cases, the brown streak in the nail cannot clinically be attributed to a benign or malignant melanocytic process. It often takes many months or years until the brown band reaches a certain width or occupies more than one-third of the nail.

Criteria for possible malignancy are asymmetry, different shades of brown to black, irregular striation within the band, width over 5 mm or occupying more than a third of the nail, a streak wider proximally than distally, and nail dystrophy even when this is very subtle; race is not a particular risk factor.[3]

Really specific dermatoscopic features allowing the diagnosis of nail melanoma to be made with certainty do not (yet) exist.[4] A bleeding tumor with nail dystrophy in association with a longitudinal melanonychia is usually a far-advanced deep melanoma and associated with a poor prognosis.

The differential diagnosis includes all longitudinal brown and black nail pigmentations, particularly bacterial and fungal melanonychias. Subungual hematoma very rarely produces a longitudinal band and usually shows small peripheral dark brown to red globules in the periphery under the dermatoscope.[5]

12.2 How to Confirm the Diagnosis

The management of any lesion suspicious of nail melanoma has to face the problem of underdiagnosis with the potential of delaying the treatment or overdiagnosis with overtreatment in case of a benign melanocytic or even nonmelanocytic lesion. In case of any doubt, a stepwise approach is recommended:

1. Clinical diagnosis
2. Dermatoscopy

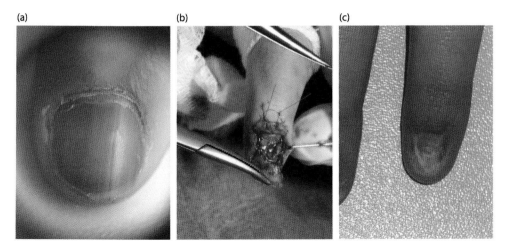

FIGURE 12.1 Subungual melanoma in an 11-year-old girl. (a) Before operation. (b) Virtually the entire matrix is tangentially excised. (c) After 4 months, most of the nail has regrown.

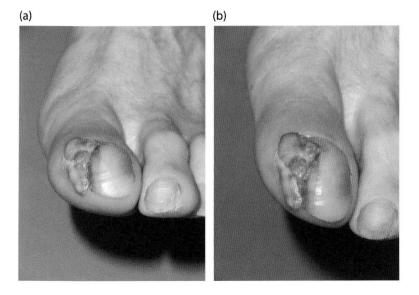

FIGURE 12.2 (a, b) Advanced neglected amelanotic melanoma of the big toe nail.

3. Histopathology of a nail clipping
4. Tangential biopsy of the lesion with/without intraoperative dermatoscopy of the pigment spot in the matrix; if available immediate postexcisional confocal laser scanning microscopy may be used

Unfortunately, there are no laboratory examinations and further imaging techniques that can help in the case of an early melanonychia.

It is often said that the prognosis of nail melanoma is—compared to that of other acral lentiginous melanomas— particularly poor. Although this appears to be the case in many patients, this is not due to a particularly high malignancy of this special localization but due to late diagnosis and treatment as well as often year- and even decade-long neglect and misdiagnosis (see Figures 12.2 and 12.3).

With the advent of the horizontal tangential matrix and nail bed biopsy with a very low postbiopsy nail dystrophy potential, there is no excuse not to biopsy an acquired longitudinal melanonychia in an adult over 30 years.[5,6]

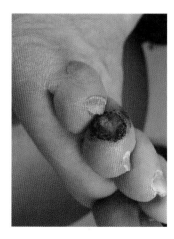

FIGURE 12.3   Ulcerated melanoma of the fourth right toe.

12.3 Evidence-Based Treatment

The mainstay of nail melanoma treatment is surgery. The history of ungual melanoma surgery from high amputation to metacarpal/metatarsal phalangeal to proximal and finally distal interphalangeal amputation with no worsening of the prognosis has given strong evidence that it is not the degree of amputation but the time of surgery that is crucial for the prognosis.[1] (See Figures 12.4 and 12.5.)

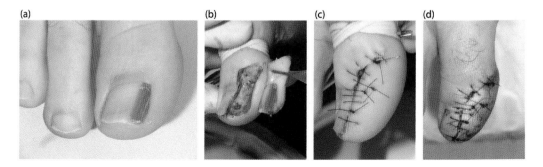

FIGURE 12.4   Atypical melanocytic hyperplasia (= in situ melanoma) of the big toe nail matrix. (a) Before surgery. (b) Segmental excision of the involved portion of the nail. (c) End of surgery. (d) Two days after surgery.

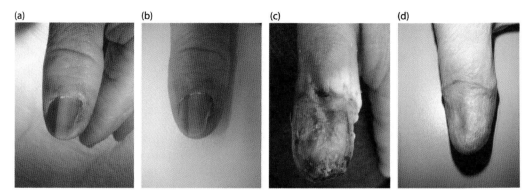

FIGURE 12.5   A 65-year-old female patient with subungual melanoma in situ of her thumb. (a, b) Clinical aspect before surgery. (c) Seven days after total removal of the dorsal half of the distal phalanx and full-thickness skin graft. (d) Six months after surgery.

Since 1978, we have adopted a functional nonamputational approach for in situ and early invasive melanoma,[7] which has been confirmed 25 years later in a large series comparing wide local excision ("functional surgery") with amputation: The prognosis of the patients with functional surgery was better than that of the patients who underwent amputation.[8,9] In the more than 40 years after the first report of functional surgery for nail melanoma, this approach has gained international acceptance, particularly among dermatosurgeons. At present, in situ and thin subungual melanomas are treated by local surgery,[10,11] thick melanomas with a Breslow Index over 2.5 mm by amputation.[12]

Technically, an adequate anesthesia of the involved digit is performed: proximal digital block for fingers 1 and 5 and all toes, transthecal anesthesia for fingers 2–4. Ropivaine 0.5%–1% is preferred as it has a rapid onset of action and a very long duration of 12 to 18 hours. A tourniquet is applied: for fingers a sterile surgical glove tourniquet is the easiest, for toes a Penrose drain may be used. A 2 cm wide metal band with a screw to tighten it can be used for all digits. For functional surgery, an excision is carried around the nail apparatus approximately 6 mm around its anatomical borders. In case of a positive Hutchinson sign, a 10 mm wide margin around it is recommended[13] as occult intraepithelial tumor cells were detected by molecular genetic techniques up to 9 mm around the Hutchinson sign.[14] Then the entire nail unit is dissected from the bone of the distal phalanx paying particular attention not to leave any epithelial remnants of the lateral matrix horns behind; if this is the case a spicule and a recurrence from the residual matrix epithelium may develop. Another challenging area is the firm connection of the distal nail bed with the distal dorsal tuft (tuberositas unguicularis); sometimes a pointed nail clipper aids in superficially removing it with the overlying nail bed. Visible arteries and veins are ligated at the proximal wound margin and electrocautery of more bleeders may be performed after releasing the tourniquet. Some dermatosurgeons perform a running locked suture all around the wound to stop excessive postoperative bleeding. Tulle gras with plenty of Vaseline-based ointment and a thick padded dressing with slight compression are applied and left for 24–48 h. The extremity is elevated for 48 hours. Pain medication is given according to the pain threshold of the patient. We change the dressing, which is usually blood-stained, after 1 or at latest 2 days before the clotted blood is hard like concrete; this renders the dressing change relatively comfortable.

Experience has shown that immediate wound coverage with a free skin graft shortens the wound healing period, but better functional and esthetic results are obtained with guided second intention healing and delayed grafting or even spontaneous reepidermization. The final result is a functionally perfect and cosmetically acceptable digit.

In case of a nail melanoma thicker than 2.5 mm, amputation is generally recommended. This should be done as a distal amputation leaving as much of the digit as possible.[15] The skin of the digital pad can usually be preserved and used as a flap to cover the tip and dorsal aspect of the wound.

A case of successful treatment with imiquimod of a recurrent in situ melanoma after conservative surgery was recently described.[16]

There is no general consensus concerning sentinel lymph node biopsy and postoperative lymphonodectomy in thick nail melanomas. Metastasizing nail melanomas are treated according to the guidelines of cutaneous melanomas. See further Table 12.1.

TABLE 12.1

Treatments and Levels of Evidence

Treatment of Ungual Melanomas	Level of Evidence
Functional surgery is superior in in situ and early advanced nail melanoma	A[1,6–11]
Defect repair by full-thickness skin grafts is not superior to second intention healing after complete resection of the nail apparatus	C[11]
Level of amputation, if necessary, does not influence survival	C[1,9]
Generally accepted guidelines for nail melanoma surgery do not yet exist	E[1]
Experience with targeted melanoma treatments in nail melanoma is lacking	F[1]
Safety margin around anatomical borders of the nail unit should be 5–6 mm, 10 mm Hutchinson sign	F[13,14]

REFERENCES

1. Haneke E. Ungual melanoma—Controversies in diagnosis and treatment. *Dermatol Ther.* 2012;25:510–524.
2. Tosti A, Piraccini BM, Cagalli A, Haneke E. In situ melanoma of the nail unit in children: Report of two cases in fair-skinned Caucasian children. *Pediatr Dermatol.* 2012;29:79–83.
3. Thai KE, Young R, Sinclair RD. Nail apparatus melanoma. *Australas J Dermatol.* 2001;42:71–81; quiz 82–83.
4. Di Chiacchio N, Farias DC, Piraccini BM et al. Consensus on melanonychia nail plate dermoscopy. *An Bras Dermatol.* 2013;88:309–313.
5. Haneke E, Baran R. Melanonychia. *Dermatol Surg.* 2001;27:580–584.
6. Haneke E. Operative Therapie akraler und subungualer Melanome. In: Rompel R, Petres J (eds), *Operative und onkologische Dermatologie. Fortschritte der operativen und onkologischen Dermatologie.* Berlin: Springer; 1999, pp. 210–214.
7. Haneke E, Binder D. [Subungual melanoma with linear nail pigmentation]. *Hautarzt.* 1978;29:389–391.
8. Moehrle M, Metzger S, Schippert W, Garbe C, Rassner G, Breuninger H. "Functional" surgery in subungual melanoma. *Dermatol Surg.* 2003;29:366–374.
9. Slingluff CL Jr, Vollmer R, Seigler HF. Acral melanoma: A review of 185 patients with identification of prognostic variables. *J Surg Oncol.* 1990;45:91–98.
10. Nakamura Y, Ohara K, Kishi A et al. Effects of non-amputative wide local excision on the local control and prognosis of in situ and invasive subungual melanoma. *J Dermatol.* 2015;42:861–866.
11. Duarte AF, Correia O, Barros AM, Ventura F, Haneke E. Nail melanoma in situ: Clinical, dermoscopic, pathologic clues, and steps for minimally invasive treatment. *Dermatol Surg.* 2015;41:59–68.
12. Park KG, Blessing K, Kernohan NM. Surgical aspects of subungual malignant melanomas. The Scottish Melanoma Grou[. *Ann Surg.* 1992;216:692–695.
13. Haneke E. *Histopathology of the Nail: Onychopathology.* Boca Raton, FL: CRC Press; 2017.
14. North JP, Kageshita T, Pinkel D, LeBoit PE, Bastian BC. Distribution and significance of occult intraepidermal tumor cells surrounding primary melanoma. *J Invest Dermatol.* 2008;128:2024–2030.
15. Montagner S, Belfort FA, Belda W Jr, DiChiacchio N. Descriptive survival study of nail melanoma patients treated with functional surgery versus distal amputation. *J Am Acad Dermatol.* 2018;79:147–149.
16. Ocampo-Garza J, Gioia Di Chiacchio N, Haneke E, le Voci F, Paschoal FM. Subungual melanoma in situ treated with imiquimod 5% cream after conservative surgery recurrence. *J Drugs Dermatol.* 2017;16:268–270.

13

Melanonychias

Nilton Di Chiacchio and Nilton Gioia Di Chiacchio

13.1 Introduction

Longitudinal melanonychia is defined as a brown or black longitudinal streak in the nail plate from the matrix to the distal part of the nail plate, due to increased activity of melanocytes or melanocytic hyperplasia of the nail matrix.

Hypermelanosis (melanocytc activation) can appear in dark-skinned individuals, and can be caused by chronic traumas, drugs, infections, dermatologic disorders, pregnancy, endocrine disorders, Peutz-Jeghers syndrome, or Laugier-Hunziker syndrome, among others.

Melanocytic hyperplasia can be observed in cases of nevus, lentigo, and melanoma of the nail matrix.[1]

The importance of knowledge of the longitudinal melanonychias is the early diagnosis of melanoma.[2]

13.2 How to Confirm the Diagnosis

A longitudinal melanocytic band of the nail plate indicates the diagnosis of longitudinal melanonychia, but some clinical features,[3] and patterns of the dermoscopy of nail plate, nail matrix, and nail bed support the diagnosis of nail melanoma.[4,5]

Biopsy or tangential excision is indicated in suspicious cases, and histopathological examination is considered the gold standard for the diagnosis of melanonychia.

13.2.1 Clinical Features

In adults, some clinical features are considered worrisome, such as involvement of a single digit, pigment variegation, darkening and spreading of the pigmentation, proximal widening of the pigmented band (melanonychia with triangular shape), nail plate dystrophy, the medial part of the lesion is dark and its lateral part clearer and blurred, and involvement of the nail folds and the hyponychium (Hutchinson sign). In children, these signs may appear in benign cases and are not considered worrying.[3]

13.2.2 Dermoscopy of Nail Plate

Dermoscopy patterns of nail plate pigmentation, described in 2002,[4] suggest that

- Gray color means melanocytic activation (hypermelanosis)
- Brown color means melanocytic hyperplasia, and the regularity of lines, according to parallelism, spacing, color, and thickness, suggest a benign pole (regular) or a malignant pole (irregular)

A consensus of experts[6] concluded that dermoscopy of the nail plate is not always so easy to interpret, and some concepts should be taken into account:

- It is difficult to distinguish a light brown from a gray background.
- A regular pattern is not often observed, even in benign lesions.
- Color homogeneity and width of each individual longitudinal line are important and should be considered.
- Background with areas of different hue of pigmentation is suggestive of melanoma, even in the absence of irregular lines.
- Melanoma in adults often shows a diffuse dark background with barely visible lines.
- In children, dark background with barely visible lines, and brown bands with lines irregular in color, width, and spacing are not indicative of nail melanoma.

13.2.3 Dermoscopy of Nail Matrix and Bed (Intraoperative Dermoscopy)

Dermoscopy of the nail matrix and bed is considered better than dermoscopy of nail plate, because it allows a direct and fine visualization of pigmentation, revealing aspects not observed when the nail plate is interposed, and it is indicated just in suspicious cases, when biopsy or excision of pigmented lesion is mandatory.[5]

Four different patterns were described:

- Regular gray with discreet lines and absence of globules observed in cases of hypermelanosis
- Regular brown lines, frequently seen in cases of lentigo
- Regular brown with globules or blotches in the major part of nevi
- Irregular and disorganized with irregular globules in cases of melanoma

13.2.4 Biopsy with Punch, "S" Excision (Lateral Longitudinal Excision), and Tangential Excision (Shaving Biopsy)

Sufficient specimens for histopathological diagnosis are obtained by a number of techniques, however, the tangential excision avoids a permanent nail dystrophy sometimes observed when biopsy with punch is performed and also allows a complete removal of pigmented lesion (Figure 13.1).

"S" excision is well-indicated in cases of lateral melanonychias. This technique allows a complete removal of the lesion (en bloc) (Figure 13.2).[7]

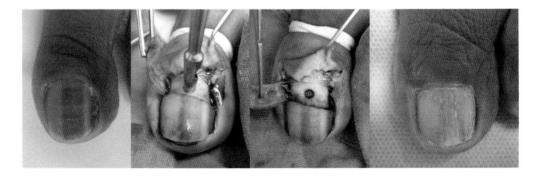

FIGURE 13.1 Biopsy of pigmented lesion of the nail matrix, with a 3 mm punch. After 2 years, a longitudinal thickness of the nail plate can be observed.

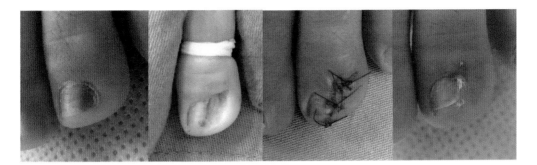

FIGURE 13.2   Longitudinal lateral excision, "S" excision. After 7 months there is no nail dystrophy.

13.3 Evidence-Based Treatment

The treatment of longitudinal melanonychias can be conservative (wait and see) or surgical (removing the pigmented lesion of the matrix).

13.3.1 Conservative Treatment (Wait and See)

Conservative treatment is indicated when

- The doctor is convinced that clinical and dermoscopy features obviously indicates a benign lesion
- In the pediatric population
- The parent or even the patient agrees with the treatment and undertakes the periodic review

Melanonychia striata is almost always associated with benign melanocytic proliferations in childhood, despite some cases when nail melanomas have been described.[8–10] Numerous reports show that in cases with worrisome clinical and dermoscopy features, histopathological findings reveal benign lesions—lentigo or nevus.[11–13] Furthermore, in children, biopsy or surgical removal are generally avoided unless necessary (Figures 13.3 and 13.4).[14]

Just a few reports show the regression of longitudinal melanonychia in children.[15,16]

13.3.2 Surgical Treatment: Tangential Excision

Tangential excision was first described by Haneke in 1999.[17] Others techniques have been described, with the same goal—thin and complete removal of the pigmented lesion, avoiding nail plate dystrophy.[18,19]

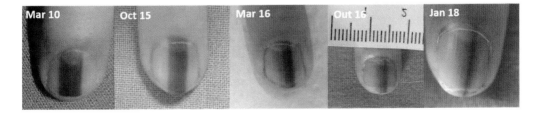

FIGURE 13.3   Wait and see. Eight-year follow-up: Melanonychia decreases.

(a)

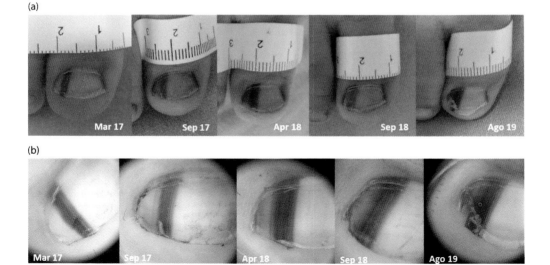

(b)

FIGURE 13.4   Wait and see. Two-year follow-up: (a) Clinical; (b) on dermoscopy. Note the worsening melanonychia with widening the width of the pigmented band and distal dystrophy of the nail plate.

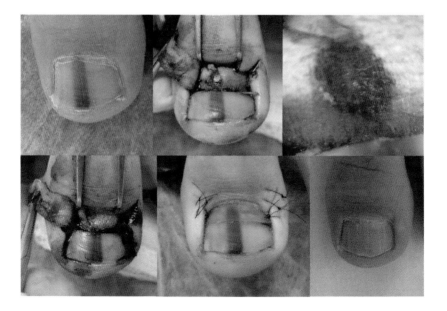

FIGURE 13.5   Tangential excision. Direct view of the nail matrix pigmented lesion. Intraoperative dermoscopy reveals regular linear brown pattern with dots and blotches. After 2 years, no nail dystrophy is observed. Histopathological examination confirmed a nevus.

After block anesthesia, the proximal nail fold is reclined back, the proximal half of the nail plate is detached of the nail bed, and also reclined laterally, allowing a direct view of the lesion. A delicate incision is performed around the pigmented lesion and removed like a thin graft. The nail plate and proximal nail fold are replaced and sutured. The specimen is placed and flattened on filter paper to be sent to the pathologist (Figure 13.5).[20]

The recurrence of melanonychia occurs in a few cases, when the lesion is not completely removed or in cases of hypermelanosis.[21,22] See further Table 13.1.

TABLE 13.1

Conservative/Surgical Treatments and Levels of Evidence

Treatment	Level of Evidence
Conservative	
Wait and see	E[20]
Surgical	
Excisional biopsy with punch	NA
Lateral longitudinal excision	NA
Tangential excision	B[15,16]

REFERENCES

1. Leung AKC, Lam JM, Leong KF, Sergi CM. Melanonychia striata: Clarifying behind the Black Curtain. A review on clinical evaluation and management of the 21st century. *Int J Dermatol*. 2019 April 21 [Epub].
2. Di Chiacchio N, Hirata SH, Enokihara MY, Michalany NS, Fabbrocini G, Tosti A. Dermatologists' accuracy in early diagnosis of melanoma of the nail matrix. *Arch Dermatol*. 2010 April;146(4):382–387.
3. Haneke E, Baran R. Longitudinal melanonychia. *Dermatol Surg*. 2001 June;27(6):580–584.
4. Ronger S, Touzet S, Ligeron C, Balme B, Viallard AM, Barrut D, Colin C, Thomas L. Dermoscopic examination of nail pigmentation. *Arch Dermatol*. 2002 October;138:1327–1333.
5. Hirata SH, Yamada S, Enokihara MY, Di Chiacchio N, de Almeida FA, Enokihara MMSS, Michalany NS, Zaiac M, Tosti A. Patterns of nail matrix and bed of longitudinal melanonychia by intraoperative dermatoscopy. *J Am Acad Dermatol*. 2011 August;65(2):297–303.
6. Di Chiacchio ND, Farias DC, Piraccini BM et al. Consensus on melanonychia nail plate dermoscopy. *An Bras Dermatol*. 2013 March–April;88(2):309–313.
7. Jellinek N. Nail matrix biopsy of longitudinal melanonychia: Diagnostic algorithm including the matrix shave biopsy. *J Am Acad Dermatol*. 2007 May;56(5):803–810.
8. Bonamonte D, Arpaia N, Cimmino A, Vestita M. In situ melanoma of the nail unit presenting as a rapid growing longitudinal melanonychia in a 9-year-old white boy. *Dermatol Surg*. 2014 October;40(10):1154–1157.
9. Tosti A, Piraccini BM, Cagalli A, Haneke E. In situ melanoma of the nail nit in children: Report of two cases in fair-skinned Caucasian children. *Pediatr Dermatol*. 2012;29:79–83.
10. Iorizzo M, Tosti A, Di Chiacchio N, Hirata SH, Misciali C, Michalany N, Domiguez J, Toussaint S. Nail melanoma in children: Differential diagnosis and management. *Dermatol Surg*. 2008 July;34(7):974–978.
11. Cooper C, Arva NC, Lee C, Yélamos O, Obregon R, Sholl LM, Wagner A, Shen L, Guitart J, Gerami P. A clinical, histopathologic, and outcome study of melanonychia striata in childhood. *J Am Acad Dermatol*. 2015 May;72(5):773–779.
12. Tseng YT, Liang CW, Liau JY, Chang K, Tseng YH, Chen JS, Liao YH. Longitudinal melanonychia: Differences in etiology are associated with patient age at diagnosis. *Dermatology*. 2017;233(6):446–455.
13. Goettmann-Bonvallot S, Andre J, Belaich S. Longitudinal melanonychia in children: A clinical and histopathologic study of 40 cases. *J Am Acad Dermatol*. 1999;41:17–22.
14. Tasia M, Lecerf P, Richert B, André J. Paediatric nail consultation in an academic centre in Belgium: A 10-year retrospective study. *J Eur Acad Dermatol Venereol*. 2019 March 5 [Epub].
15. Maddy AJ, Tosti A. Spontaneous regression of a nail matrix melanocytic nevus in a child. *Pediatr Dermatol*. 2017 September;34(5):e254–e256.
16. Taniguchi K, Kaku Y, Fukuda M, Fujisawa A, Tanioka M, Dainichi T, Miyachi Y, Otsuka A, Honda T, Kabashima K. Ten-year follow up of longitudinal melanonychia in childhood: A case report. *J Dermatol*. 2019 March;46(3):e89–e90.
17. Haneke E. Surgical therapy of acral und subungual melanomas. In: Rompel R, Petres J (eds), *Surgical and Oncological Dermatology. Proceedings of Surgical and Oncological Dermatology*, Berlin: Springer; 1999; vol. 15, pp. 210–214.

18. Zhou Y, Chen W, Liu ZR, Liu J, Huang FR, Wang DG. Modified shave surgery combined with nail window technique for the treatment of longitudinal melanonychia: Evaluation of the method on a series of 67 cases. *J Am Acad Dermatol.* 2019 March 28 [Epub].
19. Zaiac MN, Ocampo-Garza J. Modified tangential excision of the nail matrix. *J Am Acad Dermatol.* 2018 August 3 [Epub].
20. Ocampo-Garza J, Di Chiacchio NG, Dominguez-Cherit J, Fonseca Noriega L, Di Chiacchio N. Submitting tangential nail-matrix specimens. *J Am Acad Dermatol.* 2017 November; 77(5):e133–e134.
21. Richert B, Theunis A, Norrenberg S, André J. Tangential excision of pigmented nail matrix lesions responsible for longitudinal melanonychia: Evaluation of the technique on a series of 30 patients. *J Am Acad Dermatol.* 2013 July;69(1):96–104.
22. Samie FH. Tangential excision of pigmented nail matrix lesions responsible for longitudinal melanonychia: Evaluation of the technique on a series of 30 patients. *J Am Acad Dermatol.* 2019 May 23 [Epub].

14

Myxoid Cysts

Nilton Gioia Di Chiacchio and Nilton Di Chiacchio

14.1 Introduction

Myxoid cysts were first described in 1883 by Hyde as synovial lesions of the skin.[1] Known by many different names (the synonyms reflect the different opinions as to their etiology and pathogenesis), they are considered one of the most common pseudotumors of the nail apparatus, occur in a variety of clinical forms, and have a wide range of treatments.[2] Clinically, they appear as a 3–10 mm skin-colored to dome-shaped papules on the proximal nail fold of the fingers (occasionally on the toes) on people between the ages of 40–70 years, and more commonly in women than in men.[3] Mostly the lesions are solitary, but in some cases more than one digit is affected, and rarely two lesions can be found on the same finger (Figure 14.1).[2] They are often asymptomatic, but they sometimes can be painful and cause a reduction in motility, as well as weakness and deformity in the nails.[4] Some authors claim that "myxoid pseudocyst" would be a more appropriate name, since histological examination shows that an epithelial lining does not surround the collection of mucinous fluid.[2,5,6]

The exact mechanism of formation of these cysts is still unknown. Basically they can be merely a focal mucinosis of the distal phalanx (proximal nail fold), also known as the myxomatous type, or they can have a connection to the distal interphalangeal joint (ganglion type), where a herniation of synovial linings or tendon sheaths is observed.[2,6] The connection with the joint can be seen in about 85% of the lesions, by injecting 0.05–0.1 mL of sterile methylene blue solution.[2] The degenerative nature of myxoid cysts is often associated with distal interphalangeal joint osteoarthritis, specially the ganglion type.[2] Nail dystrophy is

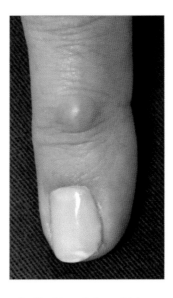

FIGURE 14.1 Dome-shaped papule above the distal interphalangeal joint.

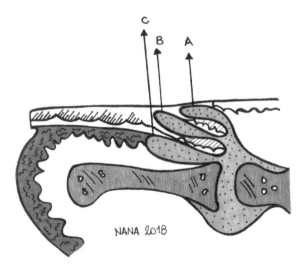

FIGURE 14.2   (A) Within the proximal nail fold, (B) beneath the proximal nail fold and above the nail plate, and (C) beneath the nail matrix. (Adapted from De Berker DA, Lawrence CM, *Dermatol Surg*, 2001 March;27(3):296–299.)

often noticed about 6 months before the cyst is clinically seen and can occur in the nail matrix or in the nail bed, depending to the location of the cyst and the pressure exerted by it.[6,7]

Clinically, the cyst can be classified into three different types according to its location (Figure 14.2). In type A, the cyst is located between the crease of the distal interphalangeal joint and the cuticle, can be superficial or deep, and deeper and distal lesions can produce a longitudinal groove in the nail plate (Figure 14.3a,b). In type B, the cyst is located beneath the proximal nail fold, and it arises from the most proximal recess of the nail fold as it reflects anteriorly to make the beginning of the matrix, resulting in a longitudinal groove in the nail plate (deeper than that arising from the dorsum of the proximal nail fold). It can produce a steplike series of fluctuations within the groove, reflecting the changing volume of the cyst, helping in the differential diagnosis with fibroma, which can also produce a small keratotic tip (Figures 14.4 and 14.5). Finally, type C presents as a tumor beneath the nail matrix, clinically seen as a hemiovercurvature of the nail plate, with violaceous swelling under the nail. Atrophic nail dystrophy may be observed in cases when there is too much pressure from beneath the nail matrix, and rarely is there a history of discharge of mucoid content (Figure 14.6).[8]

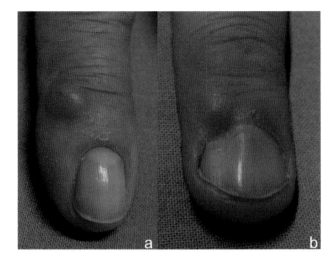

FIGURE 14.3   (a) Cyst type A—proximal and superficial. (b) Cyst type A—distal and deeper, producing a longitudinal groove.

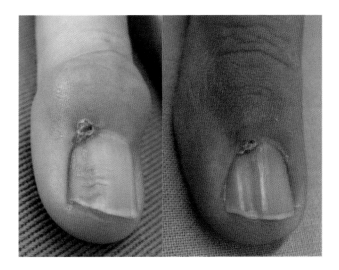

FIGURE 14.4   Cyst type B with and without the transversal lines.

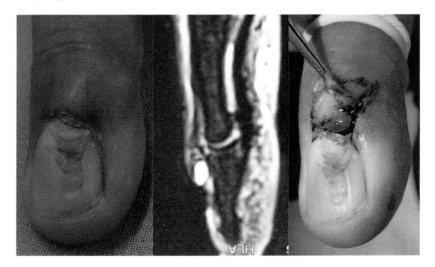

FIGURE 14.5   Cyst type B. Clinical and intraoperative aspects, including an MRI image.

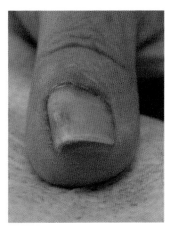

FIGURE 14.6   Cyst type C. Under the nail matrix.

14.2 How to Confirm the Diagnosis

The diagnosis of a myxoid cyst is mostly clinically, however, in difficult lesions or before surgery, transillumination, dermoscopy, ultrasound, and magnetic resonance imaging are helpful tools.[3,9,10]

Transillumination is based on the transmission of light through the body to distinguish between cystic and solid masses. When used to confirm the diagnosis of a myxoid cyst, the light will pass by the cyst easily, resulting in lucent-filling defects.[11]

Dermoscopy can be used as a helpful adjuvant and noninvasive tool in the diagnosis of myxoid cysts, showing a particular lattice pattern, serpiginous spots to be identified when no pressure is applied on the cysts. Some authors demonstrated that these cysts have an atypical vascular pattern that disappears after vitro pressure, leaving a translucent pattern with bright white areas.[6,9,10]

For cysts located beneath the nail matrix, ultrasound and MRI are indicated to confirm the fluid-filled nature of the lesion before surgery. MRI can identify the communication of the cyst with the distal interphalangeal joint; as can ultrasound if operated by an experienced doctor.[3,12] A myxoid cyst appears as an anechoic area of the ultrasound picture; no vascularity is normally seen inside the cyst, which can help differentiate it from glomus tumors.[12]

Histopathology confirms the diagnosis, showing a myxomatous area in the wall of the pseudocyst in more than 90% of the cases. The epidermis is thinned and there is a large area of myxoid tissue without any cyst lining. Myxoid areas are positive with Alcian blue and Hale's colloidal iron stain. Cells are positive for vimentin and actin, and negative for desmin (immunohistochemistry).[2]

14.3 Evidence-Based Treatment

Before treatment it is important to remember to clarify some important aspects of the disease to the patient. The first is the fact that it is a benign disease, and the patient should know that before the decision to be treated or not. The second is recurrence can happen, especially due to the etiology of the cyst. The patient should be advised that conservative and surgical treatment options are available, and conservative options are more prone to have recurrences when compared to surgical options.

Many treatment options for myxoid cysts are described in the literature, including "wait and see" as an option, since spontaneous regressions are cited in a few reports.[13] In most cases, treatment is needed due to the comorbidities that these lesions can cause.

Basically, the treatment options aim for the removal of the cyst and creating a fibrosis on the connection of the cyst with the distal interphalangeal joint in order to avoid recurrence.[3,14]

Intra-articular methylene blue solution can be used to identify the connection (or connections) of the cyst with the interphalangeal joint, which would decrease the recurrence rates.[3,15] When osteophytes are associated with the distal interphalangeal joint, they should be treated with another technique.[16]

The most common conservative or nonsurgical options and their cure rates are sclerotherapy, 77%; cryotherapy, 72%; corticosteroid injection, 62%; expression of the cyst content, 39%; CO_2 laser, 88%; and infrared coagulation, 76%. The total cure rate for these modalities is 69%.[14]

Surgical techniques and their cure rates are simple cyst excision, 90%; destruction of cyst pedicle, 92%; skin, cyst, and osteophyte excision with primary closure, 93%; skin and cyst excision with local flap closure, 94%; skin, cyst, and osteophyte excision with skin grafting, 94%; skin and cyst excision with skin grafting, 97%; cyst and osteophyte excision with primary closure, 98%; skin, cyst, and osteophyte excision with local flap closure, 98%; and osteophyte excision, 98%. The total cure rate for these techniques is 95%.[14]

A surgical technique based on the excision of the digital mucous cyst and reconstruction using self-grafting from the overlying skin lesion has been described recently. This technique is a new option for the reconstruction of digital mucous cyst defects that decreases the surgical time and avoids graft removal of healthy skin and consequently a new scar (Figures 14.7 and 14.8).[17]

Surgical options are more related with nail dystrophy when compared to other techniques, so the patient should be advised of this before the procedure.[3,14]

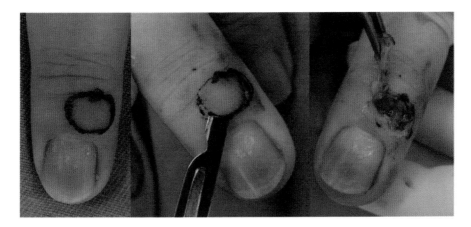

FIGURE 14.7 Delimitation of the cyst, followed by the removal of the underlying skin, and the removal of the cyst to its most proximal part (connection to the joint).

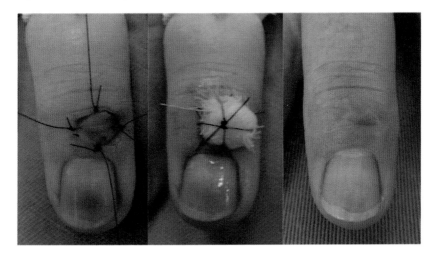

FIGURE 14.8 The same skin that was removed is placed back as a graft into the wound. A Brown's dressing is performed, and the result after 8 months.

The level of evidence of nonsurgical and the surgical techniques described in the literature ranges from B to C (Tables 14.1 and 14.2).[13,18–55]

In conclusion, surgery is considered as a first-line therapy with a 95% cure rate. According to surgeon or patient preferences, or in cases of contraindications to surgery, a second-line therapy can be chosen, which is sclerotherapy or cryotherapy. The third option is corticosteroid injection, expression of the cyst content, and infrared coagulation.[14,18]

TABLE 14.1

Conservative Treatments and Levels of Evidence

Conservative or Nonsurgical Options	Level of Evidence
Sclerotherapy	B[42–45], C[41]
Cryotherapy	B[46–48], C[49]
Corticosteroid injection	B[33,50]
Expression of the cyst	B[26,53], C[51]
CO_2 laser	C[20,54]
Infrared coagulation	C[19,21]

TABLE 14.2

Surgical Treatments and Levels of Evidence

Surgical Techniques	Level of Evidence
Simple cyst excision	B[13,18,26], C[25,27]
Destruction of cyst pedicle	B[22,28]
Osteophyte excision	B[31,32]
Cyst and osteophyte excision with primary closure	B[29,33,34], C[30]
Skin and cyst excision with local flap closure	B[18], C[24]
Skin and cyst excision with skin grafting	C[25]
Skin, cyst, and osteophyte excision with primary closure	B[55]
Skin, cyst, and osteophyte excision with skin grafting	B[34,35]
Skin, cyst, and osteophyte excision with local flap closure	B[36,38,40], C[23,37,39]

REFERENCES

1. Hernandez-Lugo AM, Dominguez-Cherit J, Vega-Memije ME. Digital mucoid cyst: The ganglion type. *Int J Dermatol.* 1999;38:533–535.
2. Haneke E. Tumors with adipocyte, myxoid, muscular, osseous, and cartilaginous features. In: Haneke E (ed), *Histopathology of the Nail—Onychopathology.* Boca Raton, FL: Taylor & Francis Group; 2017, pp. 233–234.
3. de Berker D, Baran R. Clinical features of subungual myxoid cysts. *Br J Dermatol.* 1999;141:111–112.
4. Seok HY, Eun MY, Yang HW, Lee HJ. Medial plantar proper digital neuropathy caused by a ganglion cyst. *Am J Phys Med Rehabil.* 2013;92:1119.
5. Sonnex TS. Digital myxoid cysts: A review. *Cutis.* 1986;37:89–94.
6. Ferreli C, Caravano M, Fumo G, Rongioletti F. Digital myxoid cysts: 12 years' experience from two Italian dermatology units. *G Ital Dermatol Venereol.* 2018 July 18 [Epub].
7. Lin YC, Wu YH, Scher RK. Nail changes and association of osteoarthritis in digital myxoid cyst. *Dermatol Surg.* 2008 March;34(3):364–369.
8. De Berker DA, Lawrence CM. Treatment of myxoid cysts. *Dermatol Surg.* 2001 March;27(3):296–299.
9. Salerni G, Alonso C. Images in clinical medicine. Digital mucous cyst. *N Engl J Med.* 2012 April 5;366(14):1335.
10. Chae JB, Ohn J, Mun JH. Dermoscopic features of digital mucous cysts: A study of 23 cases. *J Dermatol.* 2017;44:1309–1312.
11. Pagliarello C, Paradisi A, Dianzani C, Paradisi M, Persichetti P. Flash-powered transillumination: Old concept, new technology. *Arch Dermatol.* 2012 May;148(5):Cover 3.
12. Wortsman X, Jemec GB. Ultrasound imaging of nails. *Dermatol Clin.* 2006 July;24(3):323–328.
13. Lawrence C. Skin excision and osteophyte removal is not required in the surgical treatment of digital myxoid cysts. *Arch Dermatol.* 2005;141:1560–1564.
14. Jabbour S, Kechichian E, Haber R, Tomb R, Nasr M. Management of digital mucous cysts: A systematic review and treatment algorithm. *Int J Dermatol.* 2017 July;56(7):701–708.
15. de Berker D, Lawrence C. Surgical treatment of myxoid cysts guided by methylene blue joint injection. *Br J Dermatol.* 1998;139 (Suppl 51):72.
16. Eaton RG, Dobranski AI, Littler JW. Marginal osteophyte excision in treatment of mucous cysts. *J Bone Joint Surg.* 1973;55A:570–574.
17. Di Chiacchio NG, Fonseca Noriega L, Ocampo-Garza J, Di Chiacchio N. Digital mucous cyst: Surgical closure technique based on self-grafting using skin overlying the lesion. *Int J Dermatol.* 2017 April;56(4):464–466.
18. Crawford RJ, Gupta A, Risitano G et al. Mucous cyst of the distal interphalangeal joint: Treatment by simple excision or excision and rotation flap. *J Hand Surg Edinb Scotl.* 1990;15:113–114.
19. Lonsdale-Eccles AA, Langtry JA. Treatment of digital myxoid cysts with infrared coagulation: A retrospective case series. *Br J Dermatol.* 2005;153:972–975.
20. Huerter CJ, Wheeland RG, Bailin PL et al. Treatment of digital myxoid cysts with carbon dioxide laser vaporization. *J Dermatol Surg Oncol.* 1987;13:723–727.

21. Kemmett D, Colver GB. Myxoid cysts treated by infra-red coagulation. *Clin Exp Dermatol.* 1994;19:118–120.
22. de Berker D, Lawrence C. Ganglion of the distal interphalangeal joint (myxoid cyst): Therapy by identification and repair of the leak of joint fluid. *Arch Dermatol.* 2001;137:607–610.
23. Young KA, Campbell AC. The bilobed flap in treatment of mucous cysts of the distal interphalangeal joint. *J Hand Surg Edinb Scotl.* 1999;24:238–240.
24. Imran D, Koukkou C, Bainbridge LC. The rhomboid flap: A simple technique to cover the skin defect produced by excision of a mucous cyst of a digit. *J Bone Joint Surg Br.* 2003;85:860–862.
25. Constant E, Royer JR, Pollard RJ et al. Mucous cysts of the fingers. *Plast Reconstr Surg.* 1969;43:241–246.
26. Abe Y, Watson HK, Renaud S. Flexor tendon sheath ganglion: Analysis of 128 cases. *Hand Surg Int J.* 2004;9:1–4.
27. Arenas-Prat J. Digital mucous cyst excision using a proximally based skin flap. *J Plast Surg Hand Surg.* 2015;49:189–190.
28. Kanaya K, Wada T, Iba K et al. Total dorsal capsulectomy for the treatment of mucous cysts. *J Hand Surg.* 2014;39:1063–1067.
29. Brown RE, Zook EG, Russell RC et al. Fingernail deformities secondary to ganglions of the distal interphalangeal joint (mucous cysts). *Plast Reconstr Surg.* 1991;87:718–725.
30. Hoshino Y, Saito N, Kuroda H. Surgical treatment of mucous cysts on fingers without skin excision. *Hand Surg Int J.* 2010;15:145–148.
31. Gingrass MK, Brown RE, Zook EG. Treatment of fingernail deformities secondary to ganglions of the distal interphalangeal joint. *J Hand Surg.* 1995;20:502–505.
32. Lee H-J, Kim P-T, Jeon I-H et al. Osteophyte excision without cyst excision for a mucous cyst of the finger. *J Hand Surg Eur.* 2014;39:258–261.
33. Rizzo M, Beckenbaugh RD. Treatment of mucous cysts of the fingers: Review of 134 cases with minimum 2-year follow-up evaluation. *J Hand Surg.* 2003;28:519–524.
34. Baazil H, Dalemans A, De Smet L et al. Comparison of surgical treatments for mucous cysts of the distal interphalangeal joint. *Acta Orthop Belg.* 2015;81:213–217.
35. Jamnadas-Khoda B, Agarwal R, Harper R et al. Use of Wolfe graft for the treatment of mucous cysts. *J Hand Surg Eur.* 2009;34:519–521.
36. Hojo J, Omokawa S, Shigematsu K et al. Patient-based outcomes following surgical debridement and flap coverage of digital mucous cysts. *J Plast Surg Hand Surg.* 2016;50:111–114.
37. Jager T, Vogels J, Dautel G. The Zitelli design for bilobed flap applied on skin defects after digital mucous cyst excision. A review of 9 cases. *Tech Hand Up Extrem Surg.* 2012;16:124–126.
38. Johnson SM, Treon K, Thomas S et al. A reliable surgical treatment for digital mucous cysts. *J Hand Surg Eur.* 2014;39:856–860.
39. MacCollum MS. Mucous cysts of the fingers. *Br J Plast Surg.* 1975;28:118–120.
40. Blanc S, Candelier G, Bonnan J, Faure P. [Use of a bilobed flap for the treatment of mucous cysts]. *Chir Main.* 2004;23:137–141.
41. Cordoba S, Romero A, Hernandez-Nunez A et al. Treatment of digital mucous cysts with percutaneous sclerotherapy using polidocanol. *Dermatol Surg.* 2008;34:1387–1388;discussion 1388.
42. Esson GA, Holme SA. Treatment of 63 subjects with digital mucous cysts with percutaneous sclerotherapy using polidocanol. *Dermatol Surg.* 2016;42:59–62.
43. Park SE, Park EJ, Kim SS et al. Treatment of digital mucous cysts with intralesional sodium tetradecyl sulfate injection. *Dermatol Surg.* 2014;40:1249–1254.
44. Sung JY, Roh MR. Efficacy and safety of sclerotherapy for digital mucous cysts. *J Dermatol Treat.* 2014;25:415–418.
45. Tanaka Y, Takakura Y, Kumai T et al. Sclerotherapy for intractable ganglion cyst of the hallux. *Foot Ankle Int.* 2009;30:128–132.
46. Bohler-Sommeregger K, Kutschera-Hienert G. Cryosurgical management of myxoid cysts. *J Dermatol Surg Oncol.* 1988;14:1405–1408.
47. Dawber RP, Sonnex T, Leonard J et al. Myxoid cysts of the finger: Treatment by liquid nitrogen spray cryosurgery. *Clin Exp Dermatol.* 1983;8:153–157.
48. Kuflik EG. Specific indications for cryosurgery of the nail unit. Myxoid cysts and periungual verrucae. *J Dermatol Surg Oncol.* 1992;18:702–706.

49. Minami S, Nakagawa N, Ito T et al. A simple and effective technique for the cryotherapy of digital mucous cysts. *Dermatol Surg.* 2007;33:1280–1282.
50. Dodge LD, Brown RL, Niebauer JJ et al. The treatment of mucous cysts: Long-term follow-up in sixty-two cases. *J Hand Surg.* 1984;9:901–904.
51. Epstein E. A simple technique for managing digital mucous cysts. *Arch Dermatol.* 1979;115:1315–1316.
52. Esteban JM, Oertel YC, Mendoza M et al. Fine needle aspiration in the treatment of ganglion cysts. *South Med J.* 1986;79:691–693.
53. Rollins KE, Ollivere BJ, Johnston P. Predicting successful outcomes of wrist and finger ganglia. *Hand Surg Int J.* 2013;18:41–44.
54. Karrer S, Hohenleutner U, Szeimies RM et al. Treatment of digital mucous cysts with a carbon dioxide laser. *Acta Derm Venereol.* 1999;79:224–225.
55. Calder JDF, Buch B, Hennessy MS et al. Treatment of mucous cysts of the toes. *Foot Ankle Int.* 2003;24:490–493.

15

Onycholysis

Shari R. Lipner and Carlton Ralph Daniel, III

15.1 Introduction

Onycholysis is defined as the distal separation of the nail plate from its underlying hyponychium/nail bed. There are a myriad of causes including inflammatory disorders, such as psoriasis and lichen planus; systemic disease; systemic drugs and chemotherapies; and neoplasms, including warts and squamous cell carcinoma. Simple onycholysis is defined as onycholysis that is not due to the aforementioned etiologies, but instead due to contactants or more commonly trauma.

Simple onycholysis is commonly seen in clinical practice, but the true incidence is unknown. Fingernail and toenail onycholysis affect both sexes, but fingernail involvement is much more common in women than men. If the separation is mild, it is typically asymptomatic. However, when moderate-to-severe detachment occurs, patients may experience pain and difficulty performing activities of daily living. Simple onycholysis is most commonly caused by physical trauma. Etiologies of fingernail onycholysis include manicuring, onychophagia, and onychotillomania, while toenail onycholysis is usually due to pressure of the closed shoes on the toes secondary to asymmetric gait.

15.2 How to Confirm Diagnosis

A full medical history and dermatologic examination is performed in evaluating onycholysis. This requires removal of nail cosmetics and artificial nails followed by an examination of the skin, hair, mucosa, and all 20 nails. Separation of the nail plate from the nail bed typically begins at the distal lateral border of the nail plate and then progresses to involve the entire distal border. Clinically, the separated nail plate appears white or slightly yellow due to light transmitted through the transparent plate (Figure 15.1a,b). Onycholysis creates a moist and warm environment, which may be colonized by *Candida* species (Figure 15.2). Secondary infection with *Pseudomonas aeruginosa* is also relatively common, and the nail plate appears green-brown due to the pigments pyoverdine and pyocyanin (Figure 15.3). Grading of onycholysis can be useful for documentation.

Simple onycholysis has a broad differential diagnosis. Recognition of specific patterns are helpful in ruling in/out other nail disorders. For example, involvement of one nail may indicate an infection, or a benign or malignant neoplasm (Figure 15.4). If only one hand is affected, the patient should be questioned about trauma, handedness, and contactants. If one hand and both feet are involved, a fungal infection is suspected. Involvement of the feet only is typically common for trauma or fungal infection. Table 15.1 summarizes etiologies of simple onycholysis, and Table 15.2 summarizes other causes of onycholysis.

Simple onycholysis is a diagnosis of exclusion. A careful history, the absence of characteristic clinical findings, and observation of the patient in the examination room will rule in/out onychophagia and onychotillomania (Figure 15.2). Phototoxic or allergic dermatitis can often be confirmed or negated by taking a careful contactant and drug history. Nail clippings with histopathology and staining (PAS [periodic acid–Schiff], GMS [Grocott's methenamine silver], gram stains) are helpful in ruling out nail psoriasis, onychomycosis, and *P. aeruginosa* infections. Scrapings from under the nail plate can also be analyzed with microscopy and KOH, fungal culture, or polymerase chain reaction to confirm or negate

(a)

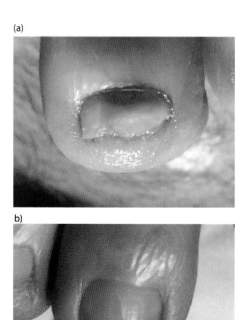

FIGURE 15.1 Simple onycholysis. (a) A 66-year-old man with significant separation of the nail plate from the nail bed of his left second toenail due to repeated trauma from walking during golfing. His chronic onycholysis led to a disappearing nail bed. (b) Right second toenail from same patient showing a relatively normal nail for comparison.

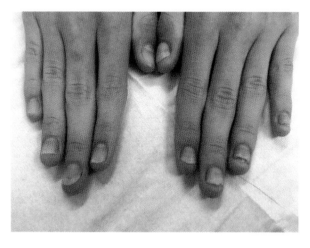

FIGURE 15.2 Onycholysis secondary to onychotillomania. A 15-year-old boy with a known history of nail picking who presented with a several-month history of separation of nail plate from the nail bed. PAS and GMS staining of nail clippings showed colonizing spores.

presence of a nail fungal infection. Although *Candida* species may be cultured, they are almost always colonizers rather than pathogenic. A wound culture can be used to confirm the presence of *P. aeruginosa* when the nail plate appears green-brown (Figure 15.3). Subungual exostosis can easily be eliminated from the differential diagnosis by obtaining an x-ray. If there is any suspicion of a malignant nail tumor, a nail biopsy must be performed.

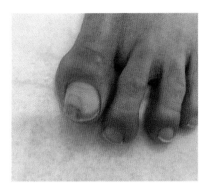

FIGURE 15.3 Onycholysis secondary to trauma and infection with *Pseudomonas aeruginosa*. A 49-year-old woman with a history of wearing tight shoes; left great toenail with separation of nail plate from nail bed and green-brown discoloration of nail plate.

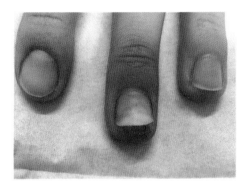

FIGURE 15.4 Onycholysis secondary to verruca vulgaris. A 33-year-old man; left third fingernail with separation of the nail plate from nail bed due to verrucous nodule. A biopsy confirmed the presence of verruca vulgaris.

TABLE 15.1

Etiologies of Simple Onycholysis

Condition	Nail Findings in Addition to Onycholysis
Onychophagia	Extremely short and uneven nail plates, ragged cuticles
Onychotillomania	Uneven nail plates, erosion of nail folds, parallel transverse grooves in nail plates
Allergic contact dermatitis	"Roller coaster" onycholysis, eczematous changes on nail folds, exposure to gasoline, paint removers, thioglycolate, nail cosmetics

TABLE 15.2

Other Causes of Onycholysis

Condition	Nail Findings in Addition to Onycholysis
Nail psoriasis	Pitting, splinter hemorrhages, salmon patches, oil spots
Onychomycosis	Nail plate yellowing/thickening, subungual hyperkeratosis
Phototoxic dermatitis	Onycholytic area follows shape of cuticle, history of UV exposure and tetracycline derivative, psoralen, aminolevulinic acid, griseofulvin, oral contraceptives, capecitabine, 5-fluorouracil, paclitaxel, olanzapine
Subungual exostosis	Firm nodule under the nail plate
Subungual verruca	Verrucous papule under the nail plate, pinpoint bleeding
Squamous cell carcinoma	Varied presentation, including ulceration, hyperkeratosis, leukonychia, melanonychia
Nail unit melanoma	Longitudinal melanonychia, up to one-third are amelanotic

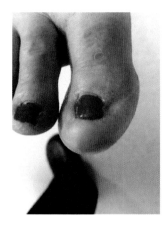

FIGURE 15.5   Disappearing nail bed. A 70-year-old woman with short and narrow nail bed from years of wearing high-heeled shoes, a consequence of prolonged onycholysis.

TABLE 15.3

Treatments and Levels of Evidence

Treatment	Level of Evidence
Ciclopirox lotion daily or oral fluconazole 150 mg weekly for several months	B[2]
Calcipotriene/betamethasone	B[12]
2%–4% thymol in chloroform	E[13]
Custom-made insoles	B[14]

15.3 Evidence-Based Treatment

Management of simple onycholysis requires careful and thorough explanation of the treatment plan by the dermatologist, and strict patient compliance and adherence. Written instructions are helpful. Frequent hand washing and frequent use of hand sanitizers may worsen the onycholysis. Onycholysis should be diagnosed and treated as early as possible to avoid secondary infections and permanent sequelae.[1–5] When the nail bed is uncovered for prolonged periods, it may develop a granular layer (epithelialize) and form dermatoglyphics. When this occurs, especially in toenails, it becomes less likely that the nail plate will reattach, and this has been named the disappearing nail bed (Figures 15.1a and 15.5).[6–8]

Patients are instructed to keep nails as short as possible; avoid physical trauma, irritants, and moisture; and to cut the nails straight across without rounding at the edges.[1,9] Patients should avoid artificial nails and nail cosmetics until nails have been normal for at least 1 month. Lightweight cotton gloves are worn under heavy-duty vinyl gloves for wet work and heavy-duty cotton gloves are used for dry work. In most immunocompetent individuals, *Candida* is not likely a primary pathogen but is cultured from many patients with simple onycholysis.[10] This topic is controversial[10] and some believe that ciclopirox lotion[2,11] daily or oral fluconazole 150 mg weekly for several months may be helpful.[11] Calcipotriene/betamethasone has also been tried topically with varying success.[12] A topical antiseptic solution (2%–4% thymol in chloroform twice daily) applied to the nail bed may be helpful in preventing infections.[13] For toenail onycholysis due to asymmetric gait, custom-made insoles serve to even out plantar surfaces and correct the gait.[14] See further Table 15.3.

REFERENCES

1. Daniel CR, 3rd, Daniel MP, Daniel CM, Sullivan S, Ellis G. Chronic paronychia and onycholysis: A thirteen-year experience. *Cutis.* 1996;58(6):397–401.
2. Daniel CR, 3rd, Daniel MP, Daniel J, Sullivan S, Bell FE. Managing simple chronic paronychia and onycholysis with ciclopirox 0.77% and an irritant-avoidance regimen. *Cutis.* 2004;73(1):81–85.

3. Zaias N, Escovar SX, Zaiac MN. Finger and toenail onycholysis. *J Eur Acad DermatolVenereol.* 2015;29(5):848–853.
4. Velez NF, Jellinek NJ. Simple onycholysis: A diagnosis of exclusion. *J Am Acad Dermatol.* 2014;70(4):793–794.
5. Daniel CR, 3rd, Iorizzo M, Piraccini BM, Tosti A. Grading simple chronic paronychia and onycholysis. *Int J Dermatol.* 2006;45(12):1447–1448.
6. Daniel CR, 3rd, Tosti A, Iorizzo M, Piraccini BM. The disappearing nail bed: A possible outcome of onycholysis. *Cutis.* 2005;76(5):325–327.
7. Daniel R, Meir B, Avner S. An update on the disappearing nail bed. *Skin Appendage Disord.* 2017;3(1):15–17.
8. Dominguez-Cherit J, Daniel CR. Simple onycholysis: An attempt at surgical intervention. *Dermatol Surg.* 2010;36(11):1791–1793.
9. Daniel CR, 3rd. Onycholysis: An overview. *Semin Dermatol.* 1991;10(1):34–40.
10. Daniel CR, 3rd, Gupta AK, Daniel MP, Sullivan S. Candida infection of the nail: Role of Candida as a primary or secondary pathogen. *Int J Dermatol.* 1998;37(12):904–907.
11. Daniel CR, 3rd, Iorizzo M, Piraccini BM, Tosti A. Simple onycholysis. *Cutis.* 2011;87(5):226–228.
12. Park JM, Mun JH, Jwa SW et al. Efficacy and safety of calcipotriol/betamethasone dipropionate ointment for the treatment of simple onycholysis: An open-label study. *J Am Acad Dermatol.* 2013;69(3):492–493.
13. Iorizzo M. Tips to treat the 5 most common nail disorders: Brittle nails, onycholysis, paronychia, psoriasis, onychomycosis. *Dermatol Clin.* 2015;33(2):175–183.
14. Zaias N, Rebell G, Casal G, Appel J. The asymmetric gait toenail unit sign. *Skinmed.* 2012;10(4):213–217.

16

Onychomatricoma

Glaysson Tassara Tavares

16.1 Introduction

Onychomatricoma (OM) is part of a group of nail tumors originating at the matrix, together with onychopapilloma, acantholytic dyskeratotic acanthoma, onychocytic matricoma, and onychocytic carcinoma. In addition, the matrix may be affected by melanoma and in some cases squamous cell carcinoma and Bowen disease, although the two latter more often originate at the nail bed.[1] OM is a tumor predominantly affecting women, fingers, adults, and mean age of 57 years; it rarely affects children. Usually, the diagnosis is late, either because it takes long for patients to seek medical attention or because it is still somehow unknown by the medical community.[2]

OM manifests as xanthonychia, increased nail thickness, splinter hemorrhage, increased transversal or longitudinal curvature of the nail plate (Figure 16.1), and presence of cavitations (honeycomb-like or woodworm-caused perforations) on the nail plate free edge. Other less commonly seen signs include edema and erythema at the proximal fold, pain upon compression, and longitudinal melanonychia.[2]

16.2 How to Confirm the Diagnosis

Dermatoscopy is an important aid in diagnosing OM. It may be performed on the nail plate, as well as the free edge. On the nail plate, longitudinal, parallel lines can be visualized, which may be white (in most cases), but might also be yellowish or grayish. Splinter hemorrhage may be better visualized, particularly at the proximal portion of the nail plate. The presence of parallel white lines as well as well-demarcated tumor lateral margins, characterized by the parallelism of these lines, may be considered as characteristic of onychomatricoma (Figure 16.2). At the free edge, dermatoscopy makes the visualization of honeycomb-like cavitations or woodworm-caused perforations easier (Figure 16.3), in addition to evidencing the nail's thickening and overcurvature. The presence of multiple perforations at the free edge is considered as pathognomonic by some authors.[3,4]

Regarding imaging methods, upon ultrasound, the oblique image can show solid hypoechogenic areas at the nail matrix and hyperechogenic linear sites, representing the digitiform projections at the nail plate.

Nuclear magnetic resonance can show the Y-shaped tumoral digitiform projections with high-intensity signal, and in the axial image it can show perforations in the plate and projections.[5]

Nail clipping should be performed through the nail plate free edge, by containing 4 mm of plate. Upon H&E staining histology, cavitations can be visualized at the transversal plane (which correspond to the honeycomb appearance apparent upon clinical examination or dermatoscopy), some of which are filled with serous fluid and delineated by nail matrix epithelium. To evidence the matrix epithelium, pan-cytokeratin staining may be used. Periodic acid–Schiff (PAS) staining may be useful to rule out onychomycosis, which may be associated with the tumor.[6]

The diagnosis can basically be confirmed following nail plate avulsion, when it is possible to visualize the filiform, digitiform projections from the matrix toward the nail plate, resembling the "medusa-head appearance projections or intestinal villi," and the resulting cavitations caused by them in the plate (Figure 16.4).

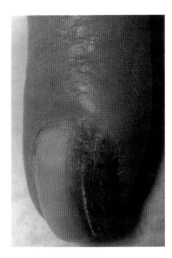

FIGURE 16.1   Xanthonychia, overcurvature, nail thickening, splinter hemorrhage.

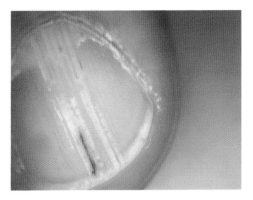

FIGURE 16.2   Well-demarcated parallel white lines at the tumor's lateral margins.

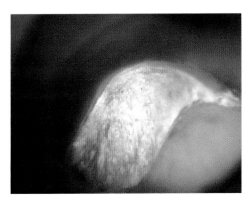

FIGURE 16.3   Cavitations at the nail plate free edge.

Histology shows a fibroblastic tumor, with dense, highly cellular stroma, and delicate or thin collagen fibers. The filiform projections are coated by the matrix epithelium, which extends deeply into the tumor, causing fissures. The longitudinal sections reveal parallel channels containing nail matrix epithelium and edematous, little structured connective tissue. The cross-sections show the cavitations, as mentioned in clippings.[1]

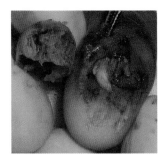

FIGURE 16.4   Filiform digitiform projections and its cavitations at the nail plate.

TABLE 16.1

Treatments and Levels of Evidence

Surgical Treatments	Level of Evidence
Regular surgical excision	E[8]
Tangential excision of the tumor	D[1]
Mohs surgery	E[10]

16.3 Evidence-Based Treatment

The treatment is surgical. The goal is tumor excision, which, however, if performed as an en bloc excision, may cause nail dystrophy[8] (level of evidence E). Therefore, tangential excision of the tumor may provide full remission and less damage to the nail[1] (level of evidence D). For this approach, following antisepsis, digital block, and the use of a tourniquet, relaxation incisions at the proximal fold junction with the lateral folds, nail plate avulsion, visualization of the tumor, and its filiform projections are performed, followed by tangential excision (superficial shaving similar to what is done for longitudinal melanonychia biopsy). Next, the proximal fold must be repositioned and sutured. A hydrocolloid dressing or a screen or the nail plate itself (out of the onychomatricoma area) must be kept between the proximal fold and the matrix, in order to avoid a scar forming at the matrix, resulting in dystrophy.[7,9]

Mohs micrographics for OM is reported with the objective of saving the matrix tissue; however, in the case published, although no relapse has occurred, there was nail plate dystrophy at the surgery site. Therefore, there is no advantage over the tangential excision technique[10] (level of evidence E). See further Table 16.1.

REFERENCES

1. Haneke E. Important malignant and new nail tumors. *J Dtsch Dermatol Ges.* 2017;5(4):367–386.
2. Di Chiacchio N, Tavares GT, Tosti A et al. Onychomatricoma: Epidemiological and clinical findings in a large series of 30 cases. *Br J Dermatol.* 2015;173(5):1305–1307.
3. Lesort C, Debarbieux S, Duru G et al. Dermoscopic features of onychomatricoma: A study of 34 cases. *Dermatology.* 2015;231(2):177–183.
4. Schneider SL, Tosti A. Tips to diagnose uncommon nail disorders. *Dermatol Clin.* 2015;33(2):197–205.
5. Cinotti E, Veronesi G, Labeille B et al. Imaging technique for the diagnosis of onychomatricoma. *J Eur Acad Dermatol Venereol.* 2018;32(11):1874–1878.
6. Stephen S, Tosti A, Rubin AI. Diagnostic applications of nail clippings. *Dermatol Clin.* 2015;33(2):289–301.
7. Becerro de Bengoa R, Gates JR, Losa Iglesias ME et al. Rare toenail onychomatricoma: Surgical resolution of five cases. *Dermatol Surg.* 2011 May;37(5):709–711.
8. Fierro-Arias L, Corrales-Rosas B, Mercadillo-Pérez P et al. Giant onychomatricoma in third toe: Exceptional condition with surgical resolution. *J Eur Acad Dermatol Venereol.* 2016;30(3):525–527.
9. Richert B, André J. Onychomatricoma. *Ann Dermatol Venereol.* 2011;138(1):71–74.
10. Graves MS, Anderson JK, LeBlanc KG Jr et al. Utilization of Mohs micrographic surgery in a patient with onychomatricoma. *Dermatol Surg.* 2015 June;41(6):753–755.

17

Onychomycosis

Roberto Arenas-Guzmán, Sabrina Escandón-Pérez, and Eder R. Juárez-Durán

17.1 Introduction

Onychomycosis are nail infections caused mainly by dermatophytes and yeasts such as *Trichophyton rubrum*, *T. interdigitale*, and *Candida* spp. Also non-dermatophytes mold (NDMs) are increasing as etiological agents. Distal or lateral subungual onychomycosis and total dystrophic onychomycosis are the most frequent clinical presentations. Frequency is higher in adults and increases with age, and also associated with diseases like diabetes mellitus, peripheral vascular insufficiency, and immunosuppression.[1]

Diagnosis is supported by mycological study, mainly direct examination with KOH–Chlorazol-Black® and dermoscopic or histopathological findings, and recently by molecular biology tests (polymerase chain reaction [PCR])[2–4] (Figures 17.1 and 17.2).

17.2 How to Confirm the Diagnosis

Evidence level: Evidence-based strength of recommendation B[10], D/A[9], D[11]

A retrospective cohort study including 541 patients' toenail clippings sent for confirmatory periodic acid-Schiff (PAS) demonstrated that clinical diagnostic accuracy between dermatologists and podiatrists mainly is comparable to accuracy with KOH testing, which shows a sensitivity of 80% and specificity of 72%, although it supports confirmatory testing prior to treatment.

Another review of different therapies for onychomycosis (oral therapy, chemical avulsion, topical therapy, device-based treatments) shows the advantages and disadvantages of each method and supports the proper mycological diagnosis before the initiation of therapy. In all cases, personalized treatment should be considered since a recurrence rate of 10%–50% has been observed due to reinfection or lack of mycological cure.

17.3 Evidence-Based Treatment

First-line treatment is mainly based on two oral drugs: terbinafine or itraconazole with a daily dose or pulse therapy. Potential side effects are infrequent (Table 17.1).[5] Topical treatment can be an option in children, during pregnancy, breastfeeding, or when one or few nails are affected. Combined therapy with oral and topical drugs is more effective and can reduce length of treatment.[6,7] Alternative therapies can include surgery, laser, and photodynamic therapy.[8,9]

17.3.1 Topical Treatment

17.3.1.1 Efinaconazole

Evidence level: Evidence-based strength of recommendation A[13], B[12]

A compilation of various clinical trials shows the efficacy of efinaconazole 10% topical solution for the treatment of mild-to-moderate distal lateral subungual onychomycosis (DLSO) on different

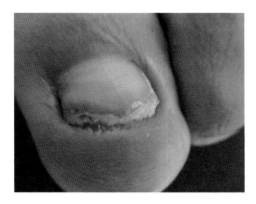

FIGURE 17.1   Dermatophytic onychomycosis before treatment with itraconazole.

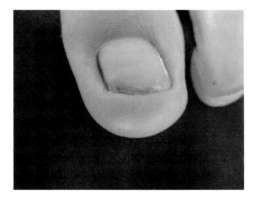

FIGURE 17.2   Dermatophytic onychomycosis after treatment with itraconazole.

TABLE 17.1

Most Commonly Used Oral Drugs for Onychomycosis

Drug	Indication	Adult Dose	Pediatric Dose	Mycological and Complete Cure
Terbinafine	Fingernail/toenail onychomycosis by dermatophytes	250 mg/day per 6 weeks for fingernails and 12 weeks for toenails	<20 kg: 62.5 mg/day 20–40 kg: 125 mg/day >40 kg: 250 mg/day per 6 weeks for fingernails and 12 weeks for toenails	Mycological Fingernails: 79%, Toenails: 70% Complete Fingernails: 59%, Toenails: 38%
Itraconazole	Fingernails/toenails	200 mg twice daily/ week per month for 2 months for fingernails and 200 mg/day for 12 weeks for toenails	5 mg/kg/day for one week per month, 2 months fingernails and 3 months toenails	Mycological Fingernails: 61%, Toenails: 54% Complete Fingernails: 47%, Toenails: 14%
Fluconazole	Not FDA approved. Off-label for treatment of fingernail and toenail onychomycosis	150 mg/week for 6–9 months for fingernails and 12–18 months for toenails	150 mg/week for 6–9 months for fingernails and 12–18 months for toenails	—

patient populations, including diabetic patients in where 13% showed complete clinical cure and 56.5% mycological cure, whereas only 17.8% in nondiabetic patients.[12]

The analysis of two identical multicenter, double-blind, vehicle-controlled, 48-week studies including 1655 patients, evaluated efficacy and safety of efinaconazole topical solution 10%. Quality of life was assessed using a validated OnyCOE-t™ questionnaire. Patients with clinical improvement between weeks 24 and 52 showed higher satisfaction scores (79.9%–89.2%) compared to patients who did not improve, with a satisfaction score of 65.3%–58%.[13]

17.3.1.2 Amorolfine versus Ciclopirox

Evidence level: Evidence-based strength of recommendation D[14], C[15,16]

Various series of patients were analyzed and, in conclusion, efficacy of amorolfine and ciclopirox as monotherapy couldn't be properly evaluated because of the different criteria for recruiting patients. Analyzing two randomized studies comparing the usage of the aforementioned drugs showed certain limitations such as the high proportion of screening failures, which added up to 60%. Plus, not only does an improper diagnosis limit the study of the drugs' efficacy, but also the lack of adherence to the regimen by the patients compromised their outcomes. Combined therapy with oral antifungal and topical lacquers is advised for a better outcome.[14–16]

17.3.1.3 Tavaborole 5% Topical Solution

Evidence level: Evidence-based strength of recommendation B[17]

Two clinical trials uncovered the efficacy and safety of tavaborole topical solution in the treatment of onychomycosis after 52 weeks of treatment. It was found that 31.1%–35.9% had a negative mycological test, 6.5%–9.1% a complete cure, and 26.1%–27.5% a clear nail presentation.[17]

17.3.2 Invasive and Device-Based Therapy

17.3.2.1 Laser

Evidence level: Evidence-based strength of recommendation B, C[8,18]

A clinical trial performed on 67 patients with onychomycosis, using as single therapy Q-Switched laser Nd:YAG 1064 nm, with a pulse duration of 9 ns. Thirty-seven participants presented with distal subungual onychomycosis (DSO) and 30 with total dystrophic onychomycosis (TDO). No improvement was observed after 3 months in 51% of DSO patients and 44% at 6 months, while in TDO patients it was 40% and 39%, respectively. In conclusion, the study demonstrates only clinical improvement on 55% and showed no mycological cure in any patient.[18]

In a comparison between different clinical trials that applied laser therapy for the treatment of onychomycosis, results were unclear because of the lack of a control group among most studies.[8]

17.3.2.2 Nail Poration

Evidence level: Evidence-based strength of recommendation C[19]

Flores et al. investigated the impact of formulation including in vitro release profile on the ex vivo nail delivery performance of antifungal formulations. Porating the nails enhanced tioconazole delivery in single-dose experiments only, and the depth of penetration of Nile Red into the nails clippings ranged between 90 and 160 mm. This research suggests that ensuring prolonged release of a drug is fundamental to developing efficacious topical nail formulations.[19]

17.3.2.3 Photodynamic Therapy

Evidence level: Evidence-based strength of recommendation D[20]

Various series of patients were analyzed and, in conclusion, photodynamic therapy appears to be a promising alternative to conventional antifungal therapy, although its main problem is the inadequate penetration of the drug (photosensitizer) through the nail plate. Randomized multicenter clinical trials are necessary.[20]

17.3.2.4 Plasma Device

Evidence level: Evidence-based strength of recommendation C[21]

A pilot study on 13 participants with toenail onychomycosis treated with a plasma pen device evaluated clinical efficacy, mycological cure, and safety. The overall clinical cure was 53.8%, mycological cure was 15.4%, and tolerability was 100%. Limitations of this study are small sample size and lack of a control group.[21]

17.3.3 Oral Treatment

17.3.3.1 Terbinafine

Evidence level: Evidence-based strength of recommendation D[22], C[23]

Oral treatment with terbinafine was shown to be more cost effective than performing confirmatory testing, while confirmatory testing before treatment with topical efinaconazole was shown reduce costs ($53 versus $2307). Confirmatory testing with KOH before treatment should be considered for the patient's economy ($123 versus $1548).[22]

A review comparing different studies explained the differences between oral therapy treatments, topical antifungal agents, surgical removal of the nail, laser and photodynamic therapy, and their efficacy in the resolution of this infection. In conclusion, oral treatment with terbinafine pulse therapy (4 pulses 250 mg) showed complete cure in 54%, while topical treatment with efinaconazole, tavaborole, and ciclopirox showed 18%, 9.1%, and 8.5%, respectively.[23]

17.3.3.2 Itraconazole

Evidence level: Evidence-based strength of recommendation D[24], A[4], C[9]

In one study response to treatment and prognosis of drugs approved by the U.S. Food and Drug Administration (FDA) were reviewed. It was demonstrated that pulse itraconazole as monotherapy

TABLE 17.2

Therapy Options for Onychomycosis and Their Evidence-Based Levels

Treatment	Level of Evidence
Topical Treatment	
Amorolfine	D[14], C[15,16]
Ciclopirox	D[14], C[15,16]
Tavaborole solution 5%	B[17]
Efinaconazole 10%	B[12], A[13]
Terbinafine	D[22,23]
Tioconazole	C[14]
Invasive and Device-Based Therapy	
Laser therapy	C[8], B[18]
Photodynamic therapy	D[20]
Surgical removal of the nail	D[7], A[7]
Nail poration	C[19]
Plasma pin device	C[21]
Oral Treatment	
Terbinafine	D[22,23]
Itraconazole	D[24], A[4], C[9]
Fluconazole	D[24], C[25]

showed similarity in odds ratios of mycological and clinical cure compared to topical treatment. It also showed fewer side effects and a higher patient satisfaction compared to terbinafine.[24]

Itraconazole pulse therapy is recommended in cases of onychomycosis caused by non-dermatophyte molds and *Candida* spp. showing a mycological and clinical cure rate of 84% within a population of 19 patients with mixed-infection onychomycosis.[4,9]

17.3.3.3 Fluconazole

Evidence level: Evidence-based strength of recommendation D[24], C[25]

A review portraying the advantages of choosing fluconazole over other oral therapies found its absorption is not dependent on gastric pH and may be an adequate alternative for patients unable to tolerate itraconazole or terbinafine. It showed higher patient compliance because of its once-weekly dosing regimen. However, it has been demonstrated to be less effective than itraconazole or terbinafine in achieving mycological cure with a percentage of 47%–62% in toenail infections with a low recurrence rate of 4%.[24,25] See previous—Table 17.2.

REFERENCES

1. Arenas R, Torres-Guerrero E. Onychomycosis. In: Tosti A (ed.), *Nail Disorders.* Ann Arbor, MI: Elsevier; 2018, pp. 31–35.
2. Jesus-Silva MA, Roldán-Marin R, Asz-Sigall D, Arenas R. Dermoscopy. In: Tosti A, Vlahovic TC, Arenas R (eds), *Onychomycosis: An Illustrated Guide to Diagnosis and Treatment.* Springer; 2017, pp. 131–140.
3. Piraccini BM, Balestri R, Starance M, Rech G. Nail digital dermoscopy (onychoscopy) in the diagnosis of onychomycosis. *J Eur Acad Dermatol Venereol.* 2013;27:509–513.
4. Lipner SR, Scher RK. Part II: Onychomycosis: Treatment and prevention of recurrence. *J Am Acad Dermatol.* 2019;80(4):853–867.
5. Gupta AK, Korotzer A. Topical treatment of onychomycosis and clinically meaningful outcomes. *J Drugs Dermatol.* 2016;15(10):1260–1266.
6. Tosti A, Elewki BE. Onychomycosis: Practical approaches to minimize relapse and recurrence. *Skin Appendage Disord.* 2016;2(1–2):83–87.
7. Moreno-Coutiño G, Arenas R. New topical and systemic antifungals. In: Tosti A, Vlahovic TC, Arenas R (eds), *Onychomycosis: An Illustrated Guide to Diagnosis and Treatment.* Springer; 2017, pp. 205–213.
8. Lidell LT, Rosen T. Laser therapy for onychomycosis: Fact or fiction? *J. Fungi (Basel).* 2015;1(1):44–54.
9. Gupta AK, Paquet M, Simpson F. Therapies for the treatment of onychomycosis. *Clin Dermatol.* 2013;31(5):544–554.
10. Li DG, Cohen JM, Mikailov A, Williams R, Laga A, Mostaghimi A. Clinical diagnostic accuracy of onychomycosis: A multispecialty comparison study. *Dermatol Res Practice.* 2018:2630176.
11. Westerberg DP, Voyack MJ. Onychomycosis: Current trends in diagnosis and treatment. *Am Fam Physician.* 2013;88(11):762–770.
12. Lipner S, Scher R. Efinaconazole in the treatment of onychomycosis. *Infect Drug Resist.* 2015;8:163–172.
13. Tosti A, Elewski B. Treatment of onychomycosis with efinaconazole 10% topical solution and quality of life. *J Clin Aesthet Dermatol.* 2014 Nov;7(11):25–30.
14. Tabara K, Szewczyk A, Bienias W, Wojciechowska A, Pastuszka M, Oszukowska M, Kaszuba A. Amorolfine vs. ciclopirox—Lacquers for the treatment of onychomycosis. *Postepy Dermatol Alergol.* 2015;32(1):40–45.
15. Paul C, Coustou D, Lahfa M et al. A multicenter, randomized, open-label, controlled study comparing the efficacy, safety and cost-effectiveness of a sequential therapy with RV4104A ointment, ciclopiroxolamine cream and ciclopirox film-forming solution with amorolfine nail lacquer alone in dermatophytic onychomycosis. *Dermatology.* 2013;227(2):157–64.
16. Schaller M, Sigurgeirsson B, Sarkany M. Patient-reported outcomes from two randomised studies comparing once-weekly application of amorolfine 5% nail lacquer to other methods of topical treatment in distal and lateral subungual onychomycosis. *Mycoses.* 2017;60(12):800–807.

17. Elewski BE, AlyR, Baldwin SL, González Soto RF. Efficacy and safety of tavaborole topical solution, 5%, a novel boron-based antifungal agent, for the treatment of toenail onychomycosis: Results from 2 randomized phase III studies. *J Am Acad Dermatol.* 2015;73(1):62–69.

18. Rodríguez NJ, Fernández RF, Ávila A, Arenas R. Tratamiento láser en onicomicosis. *Dermatología cosmética, médica y quirúrgica.* 2014;12(1):7–12.

19. Flores FC, Chiu WS, Beck RCR, Da Silva CB, Delgado-Charro MB. Enhancement of tioconazole ungual delivery: Combining nanocapsule formulation and nail poration approaches. *Int J Pharm.* 2018;535(1–2):237–244.

20. Kalinowska K, Hryncewicz-Gwóźdź A. Photodynamic therapy in the treatment of onychomycosis—A review. *Dermatol Rev/Przegl Dermatol.* 2017;4:290–299.

21. Lipner SR, Friedman G, Scher RK. Pilot study to evaluate a plasma device for the treatment of onychomycosis. *Clin Exp Dermatol.* 2017;42(3):295–298.

22. Mikailov A, Cohen J, Joyce C, Mostaghimi A. Cost-effectiveness of confirmatory testing before treatment of onychomycosis. *JAMA Dermatology.* 2017;152(3):276–281.

23. Pariser DM, Jellinek N, Phoebe R. Efficacy and safety of onychomycosis treatments: An evidence-based overview. *Dermatology News.* 2015:1–19.

24. Gupta A, Foley A, Mays R, Shear N, Piguet V. Monotherapy for toenail onychomycosis: A systematic review and network meta-analysis. *Br J Dermatol.* 2019 [Epub].

25. Roberts DT, Taylor WD, Boyle J. Guidelines for treatment of onychomycosis. *Br J Dermatol.* 2003 Mar;148(3):402–10.

18

Onychotillomania

Sarah Azarchi and Evan A. Rieder

18.1 Introduction

Onychotillomania, also known as nail-picking disorder, is the recurrent, compulsive manipulation of the nail apparatus via picking, pulling, rubbing, and tearing. This self-induced disorder manifests as the repetitive use of fingers, fingernails, and occasionally instruments, resulting in dystrophy of the fingernail or toenail.

While traditionally separated from other behavioral disorders of the nail unit, onychotillomania can be conceptualized as an umbrella term, with many shared and some contrasting features with other self-induced nail disorders such as habit tic deformity, onychophagia, and median nail dystrophy (Figure 18.1). Habit tic deformity is a variant of onychotillomania that results from compulsive rubbing of the thumbnail and proximal nail fold by the adjacent index finger, causing horizontal ridges and depressions (Figures 18.2 through 18.4). Other self-induced nail disorders include onychophagia (biting or chewing of the distal nail plate and nail folds) and median nail dystrophy (repeated manipulation of cuticle and nail fold resulting in a midline, longitudinal canal formation or split) (Figure 18.2). Self-inflicted nail disorders have traditionally been categorized as a subset of traumatic nail abnormalities, but occur independently of external insults.[1] A novel classification scheme of onychotillomania was proposed in 2015 to encompass all self-induced nail disorders.[2] Although relatively misunderstood, these disorders are thought to be associated with underlying psychological dysfunction or psychiatric disease, and may be better classified as body-focused repetitive behaviors (BFRBs).[3–7]

Although the true incidence of self-induced nail disorders is unknown, it is likely uncommon as well as underreported.[2] The majority of literature dedicated to onychotillomania and other self-induced nail disorders is limited to case reports. The only study to attempt to characterize the prevalence of onychotillomania was a 2014 questionnaire-based study of 339 Polish medical students, which identified a 0.9% prevalence (3 cases) of onychotillomania based on behavioral and physical stigmata.[2,8] Additionally, a 2000 study that assessed prevalence of dermatillomania (skin-picking disorder) in 105 American psychology students found that onychotillomania was frequently comorbid ($n = 46$, 59.0%) with dermatillomania.[9]

Distinguishing clinical findings of onychotillomania include atypical architecture of the nail apparatus with an asymmetric distribution of nail findings (Figures 18.5 and 18.6). The nail plate may be distorted resulting in brachyonychia (exceedingly short nails, Figure 18.7) or anonychia (absence of nails), as well as melanonychia and macrolunula (enlarged distal lunula, Figures 18.2 through 18.4) thought to result from repetitive pushing back of the cuticle. Nail bed findings may include pinpoint hemorrhages. The proximal nail fold may be characterized by hyperpigmentation. Additionally, secondary changes to the periungual tissues as a result of repetitive trauma are common (Figure 18.8). While these findings are fairly nonspecific, the nails are usually asymmetrically affected in onychotillomania, compared to characteristic symmetric involvement seen in onychophagia.

Diagnoses that should be considered in the context of suspected onychotillomania include onychophagia, paronychia, onychomycosis, and trachyonychia (twenty-nail dystrophy). Nail findings seen in psoriasis, lichen planus, and epidermolysis bullosa acquisita should also be considered in the differential.[2] Accurate assessment of the etiology of a nail condition is essential given distinctive treatment modalities for self-induced nail disorders.

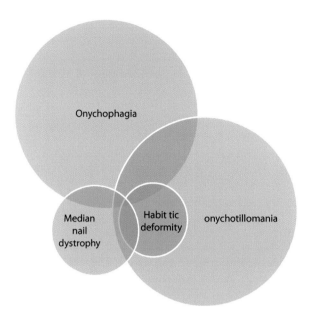

FIGURE 18.1   Self-induced nail disorders have overlapping features.

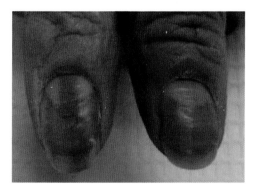

FIGURE 18.2   Horizontal ridging (Beau's lines) seen in habit tic deformity, a subtype of onychotillomania, as a result of repetitive rubbing. Note the presence of concomitant melanonychia.

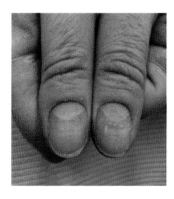

FIGURE 18.3   Horizontal ridging and macrolunula in habit tic deformity.

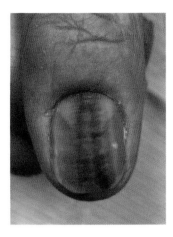

FIGURE 18.4 Horizontal ridging, melanonychia, and macrolunula.

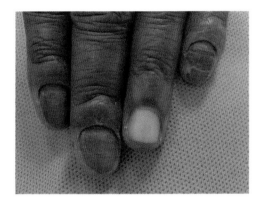

FIGURE 18.5 Characteristic findings of onychotillomania seen here include asymmetric nail involvement and melanonychia.

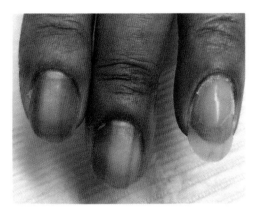

FIGURE 18.6 Asymmetric nail involvement and longitudinal melanonychia in onychotillomania.

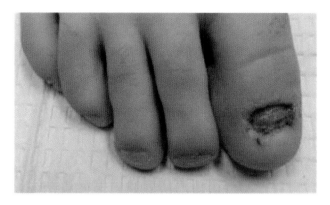

FIGURE 18.7   Brachyonychia and periungual crusting limited to one digit, consistent with onychotillomania.

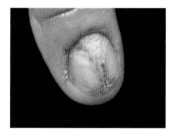

FIGURE 18.8   Another common clinical feature of onychotillomania is an enlarged distal lunula (macrolunula). Note the concomitant cuticular erosions.

18.2 How to Confirm the Diagnosis

Characteristic yet nonspecific clinical findings of onychotillomania include anonychia, brachyonychia, and abnormal appearance of the nail plate (including macrolunula and melanonychia) of the fingernails or toenails. Evidence of traumatic changes to the periungual tissues as a result of repetitive nail picking may include erosions, erythema, excoriations, crusting, and paronychia.[2,10] Common histopathological findings include acanthosis, epithelial hyperplasia, hypergranulosis, and hyperkeratosis (Figure 18.9). However, these findings lack specificity for onychotillomania and require additional clinical correlation.[2] Finally, dermoscopic features may help the physician when diagnosis is uncertain. Dermoscopic features are invariably disorganized and may include the absence of nail plate and the presence of scales, crusts, wavy lines in uneven planes, speckled dots, pinpoint hemorrhages of the nail bed, and nail bed pigmentation[10] (Figures 18.10 and 18.11).

Patients may not necessarily present to a dermatologist for their nail changes, but stigmata of onychotillomania may be recognized during a thorough physical examination that encompasses the fingernails and toenails. Second only to physical examination, the most useful diagnostic tool is a patient interview that assesses their thoughts and behaviors. Focused questioning should include inquiry about the presence of unrelenting or obsessive thoughts about picking, overwhelming compulsions to pick, and the repetitive or cyclical nature of these thoughts and compulsions. Though a mild degree of nail picking or biting is common in the general population, a true case of onychotillomania would include meaningful effects on patient social or occupational functioning, and potentially, quality of life. Evidence can be seen in behaviors that continue despite adverse effects such as pain, bleeding, and undesirable changes in physical appearance. The manner (fingers, teeth, instruments, frictional force) and frequency of manipulation can help identify the specific variety of self-induced nail disorder. Additionally, given that BFRBs such as skin picking disorder and trichotillomania may coexist with onychotillomania, a thorough examination of the skin and scalp is highly advised.[2,6,9,11]

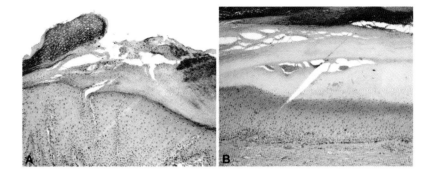

FIGURE 18.9 Histopathologic images of the (A) nail plate and (B) nail bed. (A) Crusting, parakertosis, compact orthokeratosis, and extravasated erythrocytes. (B) Epithelial hyperplasia. (Hematoxylin–eosin stain; original magnification: ×20.) (Images used with permission, courtesy of Dr. Cosimo Misciali.)

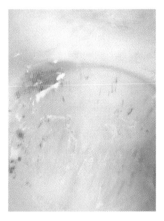

FIGURE 18.10 Dermoscopic view of pinpoint hemorrhages of the nail bed as a result of repetitive trauma.

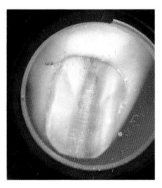

FIGURE 18.11 Pinpoint hemorrhages of the nail bed on a background of longitudinal melanonychia and horizontal ridging (dermoscopic view).

18.3 Evidence-Based Treatment

18.3.1 Topical

- Application of bitter-tasting lacquer to discourage nail biting—*Evidence level E*
  - This treatment modality has been studied for use in onychophagia, but not onychotillomania, and relies on frequent application of the lacquer by the patient.[1,12]

- Application of a nonpermanent physical barrier (such as adhesive dressing) to the nail to discourage manipulation of the nail—*Evidence level E*
  - Utility of this treatment modality is largely anecdotal; superiority to placebo has yet to be proven.[1,3,13,14]
- Application of an occlusive barrier (such as glue) to the nail to obstruct manipulation of the nail—*Evidence level E*
  - Utility of this treatment modality is limited to nominal case reports to date.[2,13,15–17]

18.3.2 Systemic

Various psychoactive medications (antidepressants and antipsychotics) from the following classes have been posited for use in treating onychotillomania: N-acetylcysteine (NAC), selective serotonin reuptake inhibitors (SSRIs), tricyclic antidepressants (TCAs), dopamine agonists, and lithium.

- N-acetyl cysteine—*Evidence level E*
  - Available studies and case reports to date have assessed NAC only for the treatment of onychophagia. Those data have not demonstrated statistically significant success of NAC for the treatment of self-induced nail disorders.[18–21]
- Selective serotonin reuptake inhibitors (SSRIs), tricyclic antidepressants (TCAs), and antipsychotics—*Evidence level E*
  - Studies of SSRIs (fluoxetine, citalopram), TCAs (clomipramine, amitriptyline), and antipsychotics (pimozide, thioridazine) have only been conducted for onychophagia and have not demonstrated statistically significant clinical efficacy. Literature of the use of SSRIs and TCAs for the treatment of onychotillomania is limited to case reports without sufficient evidence for dosage or indication.[3,4,11,14,22]

18.3.3 Behavioral

- Behavioral modification and habit reversal training (HRT)—*Evidence level E*
  - This treatment option is a type of psychotherapy in which patients learn to predict and modify or replace behaviors. HRT has had documented success in the treatment of other BFRBs.[7,23] Although evidence specific to onychotillomania remains anecdotal, referral to a mental health provider for psychotherapeutic intervention may be considered.[2] See further Table 18.1.

TABLE 18.1

Treatments and Levels of Evidence

Treatment	Level of Evidence
Topical	
Application of bitter-tasting lacquer	E[1,12]
Application of a nonpermanent physical barrier	E[1,3,13,14]
Application of an occlusive barrier	E[2,13,15,17]
Systemic	
N-acetyl cysteine	E[18,21]
Selective serotonin reuptake inhibitors (SSRIs), tricyclic antidepressants (TCAs), and antipsychotics	E[3,4,11,14,22]
Behavioral	
Behavioral modification and habit reversal training	E[2,7,23]

REFERENCES

1. Tosti APB. Traumatic nail disorders. In: Bolognia JL, Schaffer J (eds), *Dermatology. Vol. 2.* New York: Elsevier Saunders; 2012, pp. 1142–1143.
2. Rieder EA, Tosti A. Onychotillomania: An underrecognized disorder. *J Am Acad Dermatol.* 2016;75(6):1245–1250.
3. Inglese M, Haley HR, Elewski BE. Onychotillomania: 2 case reports. *Cutis.* 2004;73(3):171–174.
4. Reese J, Hudacek K, Rubin A. Onychotillomania: Clinicopathologic correlations. *J Cutan Pathol.* 2013;40(4):419–23.
5. Wilhelm S, Keuthen NJ, Deckersbach T et al. Self-injurious skin picking: Clinical characteristics and comorbidity. *J Clin Psychiatry.* 1999;60(7):454–459.
6. Houghton DC, Alexander JR, Bauer CC, Woods DW. Body-focused repetitive behaviors: More prevalent than once thought? *Psychiatry Res.* 2018;270:389–393.
7. Snorrason I, Woods DW. Nail picking disorder (onychotillomania): A case report. *J Anxiety Disord.* 2014;28(2):211–214.
8. Pacan P, Grzesiak M, Reich A, Kantorska-Janiec M, Szepietowski J. Onychophagia and onychotillomania: Prevalence, clinical picture, and comorbidities. *Acta Derm Venereol.* 2014;94(1):67–71.
9. Keuthen NJ, Deckersbach T, Wilhelm S et al. Repetitive skin-picking in a student population and comparison with a sample of self-injurious skin-pickers. *Psychosomatics.* 2000;41(3):210–215.
10. Maddy AJ, Tosti A. Dermoscopic features of onychotillomania: A study of 36 cases. *J Am Acad Dermatol.* 2018;79(4):702–705.
11. Halteh P, Scher RK, Lipner SR. Onychotillomania: Diagnosis and management. *Am J Clin Dermatol.* 2017;18(6):763–770.
12. Allen KW. Chronic nailbiting: A controlled comparison of competing response and mild aversion treatments. *Behav Res Ther.* 1996;34(3):269–272.
13. Najafi S, Aronowitz P, Thompson GR, 3rd. The habit tic: Onychotillomania. *J Gen Intern Med.* 2015;30(2):264.
14. Singal A, Daulatabad D. Nail tic disorders: Manifestations, pathogenesis and management. *Indian J Dermatol Venereol Leprol.* 2017;83(1):19–26.
15. Ring DS. Inexpensive solution for habit-tic deformity. *Arch Dermatol.* 2010;146(11):1222–1223.
16. Colver GB. Onychotillomania. *Br J Dermatol.* 1987;117(3):397–399.
17. Sidiropoulou P, Sgouros D, Theodoropoulos K, Katoulis A, Rigopoulos D. Onychotillomania: A chameleon-like disorder: Case report and review of literature. *Skin Appendage Disord.* 2019;5(2):104–107.
18. Ghanizadeh A, Derakhshan N, Berk M. N-acetylcysteine versus placebo for treating nail biting, a double blind randomized placebo controlled clinical trial. *Antiinflamm Antiallergy Agents Med Chem.* 2013;12(3):223–228.
19. Odlaug BL, Grant JE. N-acetyl cysteine in the treatment of grooming disorders. *J Clin Psychopharmacol.* 2007;27(2):227–229.
20. Berk M, Jeavons S, Dean OM, Dodd S, Moss K, Gama CS, et al. Nail-biting stuff? The effect of N-acetyl cysteine on nail-biting. *CNS Spectr.* 2009;14(7):357–360.
21. Halteh P, Scher R, Lipner S. A nail-biting conundrum for physicians. *J Dermatol Treat.* 2017;28(2):166–172.
22. Vittorio CC, Phillips KA. Treatment of habit-tic deformity with fluoxetine. *Arch Dermatol.* 1997;133(10):1203–1204.
23. Shenefelt PD. Biofeedback, cognitive-behavioral methods, and hypnosis in dermatology: Is it all in your mind? *Dermatol Ther.* 2003;16(2):114–122.

19

Psoriasis

Stamatis Gregoriou, Eftychia Platsidaki, and Dimitris Rigopoulos

19.1 Introduction

Nail psoriasis is the clinical manifestation of cutaneous psoriasis in the nail. It has significant impact on the patient, both functionally and psychologically. Nail psoriatic signs are present in 7%–56% of patients with cutaneous psoriasis. However, the lifetime incidence may be as high as 80%–90%. The prevalence of nail psoriasis without skin involvement or arthritis ranges from 1% to 6%. Nail lesions may appear several years later than cutaneous lesions, which may explain the fact that nail psoriasis is observed less frequently in children.

Inflammation associated with nail psoriasis may involve other structures, including distal interphalangeal joints, digital extensor tendons, and the enthesis, which is thought to be a continuation of the supporting fascia of the nail (enthesopathy). Psoriatic arthritis can also be considered as part of the natural progression of the same disease.

Clinical features in patients with nail psoriasis are divided into nail matrix and nail bed signs. Fingernails are more frequently affected than toenails. Effects on the nail matrix include pitting, onychomadesis, leukonychia, Beau's lines, red spots in the lunula, and crumbling. Effects on the nail bed include onycholysis, splinter hemorrhages, subungual hyperkeratosis, and oil-drop (salmon) patches. The prevalence of the specific nail features varies in different studies. Pitting and onycholysis are very common and characteristic in psoriatic fingernails. Subungual hyperkeratosis and onycholysis are common in the toenails, while pitting and leukonychia are relatively rare in the toenails (Figures 19.1 and 19.2).

Psoriatic nail disease can resemble several other nail disorders. Although the oil-drop sign and the red lunula spots are more specific for nail psoriasis, the presence of the rest of the psoriatic nail signs can make the diagnosis more difficult to establish. Nail pitting has been described in alopecia areata, eczema, trauma, and less often in parakeratosis pustulosa, pemphigus vulgaris, sarcoidosis, dermatomyositis, drug-induced erythroderma, secondary syphilis, Reiter disease, chronic renal disease, and chronic paronychia. Subungual hyperkeratosis may be seen in eczema, lichen planus, pityriasis rubra pilaris, and even cutaneous T-cell lymphomas. Onycholysis is commonly idiopathic, observed in women dealing with household tasks, but also observed in hand eczema, lichen planus, tumors, hyperthyroidism, bullous disease, and connective tissue disorders. Splinter hemorrhages are most commonly seen in trauma. Proximal splinter hemorrhages may be indicative of systemic disorders, such as infective endocarditis, renal or pulmonary disease, diabetes mellitus, vasculitis, and antiphospholipid syndrome. On the other hand, distal splinter hemorrhages can be found in onychomycosis and eczema.

19.2 How to Confirm the Diagnosis

In most cases, diagnosis of nail psoriasis is easy and based on clinical findings. However, many clinical features of nail psoriasis are not disease-specific, and several diagnostic tools have been found to be especially helpful to confirm the diagnosis. Histopathology of nail psoriasis includes findings similar to cutaneous psoriasis but also some unique features. When performing such a biopsy, it is important to remember that matrix lesions cause changes on the nail plate, while those of the nail bed are seen

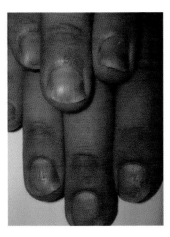

FIGURE 19.1 Fingernail psoriasis. Multiple pits, splinter hemorrhages, and onycholysis are evident in several nails.

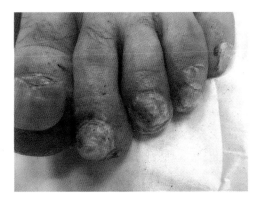

FIGURE 19.2 Toenail psoriasis. Hyperkeratosis and onycholysis affect all nails. A Beau line resulting in onychomadesis is evident on the first toenail.

under the nail plate. Biopsy should be considered when diagnosis is not possible by other means, since obtaining a biopsy specimen from the nail matrix might be complicated with adverse events. Pits are areas of spongiosis and parakeratosis. Red lunula spots present as mild acanthosis, spongiosis, neutrophilic exocytosis, and parakeratosis in the matrix. Munro's microabscesses formed by widespread parakeratosis containing neutrophils are often observed. The spongiform pustule that is characteristic of pustular psoriasis might also be present in nail psoriasis.

Dermoscopy can clarify clinical signs of nail psoriasis. It allows confirmation of the psoriatic pits when using a polarized dermoscope. In cases of onycholysis as the only sign present, dermoscopy can be useful in diagnosis, showing a white homogeneous area. Multiple thin longitudinal white striae might also be visible. It also allows seeing the erythematous border as a red or orange discoloration surrounding the onycholytic areas. Using videodermoscopy, the evolution of dermoscopy, the capillaries of the hyponychium of nails affected by psoriasis are visible, dilated, tortuous, elongated, and irregularly distributed. Nail fold capillaroscopy shows the dilated tortuous capillaries of the proximal nail fold. Ultrasonography may reveal hypervascularity in the nail bed, increased distance from the ventral plate to the bony margin of the distal phalanx, increased nail plate thickness, and enthesopathy. Optical coherence tomography is able to demonstrate even higher resolution changes, with prominent thickening in the ventral plate at the nail bed, which presents as inhomogeneous, "eroded," and irregularly fused. Finally, nail clippings are diagnostic for the most important differential diagnosis, onychomycosis, which has many clinical and histopathological features in common with nail psoriasis.

19.3 Evidence-Based Treatment

Treating nail psoriasis is a challenge. The clinician should take into account that agents effective in the treatment of nail bed signs often have poor efficacy in nail matrix signs. Involvement of skin or joints, quality of life, comorbidities, age and gender, and productivity or ability to work might also influence treatment choices. Behavioral interventions such as the use of cotton gloves when performing household tasks, frequent use of nail moisturizers, cutting onycholytic nail parts, and avoidance of trauma are also a key part of the treatment.

Topical therapies might have poor results, due to their limited penetration to the lesional tissue. However, they are indicated in mild nail psoriasis, not associated with psoriatic arthritis, if only few nails are affected, if the nail bed is affected, when systemic treatment is contraindicated, and in combination with systemic treatment.

19.3.1 Topical Treatment

Topical treatment includes topical steroids, vitamin D analogues, tazarotene, tacrolimus, photodynamic, laser, and intense pulsed light (IPL).

19.3.1.1 Topical Steroids (Evidence-Based Strength of Recommendation A)

Potent or superpotent steroids are used for a period of 4–6 months at the nail bed or at the nail folds. In case of prolonged use, skin atrophy, telangiectasia on the surrounding skin, tachyphylaxis, and atrophy of the underlying phalanx may occur as side effects. Intralesionally administered steroids is a popular therapeutic choice despite being a rather painful procedure. Triamcinolone acetonide is used monthly or bimonthly for 5–6 months at the proximal nail fold, at concentrations ranging from 2.5 to 5 mg/mL and quantity per site injected between 0.05 and 0.1 mL at up to four injection areas. In one study a more potent triamcinolone acetonide solution (10 mg/mL) in a dosage of 0.1 mL was used for bimonthly injections with excellent results regarding subungual hyperkeratosis (100% reduction), pitting (57.7%), and onycholysis (40.5%).[1]

When the nail bed is affected, injections must be performed at the lateral nail folds in the nail bed.[2] Side effects include skin atrophy, depigmentation, cyst formation, tendon rupture, and subungual hemorrhage.[3] Iontoforesis with triamcinolone acetonide once per month might be a good alternative to reduce adverse events.[4] Several studies consider 8% clobetasol nail lacquer used twice a week for 16 weeks as an effective and safe treatment for both nail matrix and nail bed signs of psoriasis.[5–7]

19.3.1.2 Vitamin D Analogues (Calcipotriol and Tacalcitol) (Evidence-Based Strength of Recommendation: Calcipotriol, A; Tacalcitol, B)

Calcipotriol (synthetic vitamin D analogue) is used twice a day for 4–6 months, at the nail plate, the hyponychium, the nail bed, and nail folds, with improvement mainly reported for hyperkeratosis.

A randomized double-blind study reported a 49% reduction of subungual hyperkeratosis after 5 months of calcipotriol topical application.[8] Another study using calcipotriol showed that the symptoms that responded better were hyperkeratosis, onycholysis, and discoloration. In addition, fingernails responded better than toenails.[9] Combined treatment (calcipotriol on weekdays and clobetasol on weekends) on the nail plate, nail folds, and hyponychium has been used with excellent results after 6 and 12 months of patient evaluation.[10] Calcipotriol was used in a study on 15 patients with pustular psoriasis and nail involvement. It was effective in 60% of them after 3–6 months of treatment.[11] A randomized, double-blind trial, calcitriol (3 mcg/g) ointment was compared with betamethasone dipropionate (64 mg/g) ointment in 10 patients with nail psoriasis. Absolute reduction of the thickness (38% and 35%, respectively) of the nail was noted with no statistical significant difference between the two groups.[12]

Tacalcitol (synthetic analogue of vitamin D3) has been used in 15 patients with psoriatic onychodystrophy once a day for 6 months demonstrating a significant improvement in all nail parameters.[13]

19.3.1.3 Tazarotene (Evidence-Based Strength of Recommendation A)

Tazarotene 0.1% gel, a synthetic retinoid, downregulates hyperproliferation of keratinocytes, differentiation, and inflammation.

In a controlled, randomized, parallel-group study, patients received either the active tazarotene gel or the vehicle applied on two target fingernails at bedtime (one with and the other without occlusion) for 21 weeks. A significantly greater reduction of onycholysis was observed in patients treated with tazarotene.[14] Another study used tazarotene 0.1% gel, which was applied at bedtime for 48 weeks. A good to very good response was noted in 76% of the patients. Fingernails responded better than toenails and tolerability was excellent.[15] Tazarotene 0.1% gel was also used in 23 patients, while 23 others used clobetasol cream 0.05% under occlusion for 12 weeks. The Nail Psoriasis Severity Index (NAPSI) score was improved in both groups, but at the end of the 12-week follow-up period, patients in the tazarotene group appeared with minor relapse rate, as far as hyperkeratosis is concerned.[16] Tazarotene gel may cause mild skin irritation with burning sensation and desquamation of the area.

19.3.1.4 Tacrolimus (Evidence-Based Strength of Recommendation A)

Tacrolimus 0.1% ointment has been proven effective for both nail matrix and bed signs in a study enrolling 21 patients who applied the medication on the nail folds at bedtime, for 12 weeks, in a left-right randomly used application of the drug. No topical or systemic side effects were reported.[17]

19.3.1.5 Laser and Intense Pulsed Light (IPL) Treatment (Evidence-Based Strength of Recommendation B)

A study with 20 patients showed that pulsed dye laser (PDL) may be considered as an effective and well-tolerated therapeutic option of both nail bed and nail matrix psoriasis after 6 months of first treatment.[18] In another study, PDL 595 nm once monthly for 3 months proved also to be effective and safe for both nail matrix and nail bed signs (the latter responded better).[19]

A single blinded left-to-right study compared excimer laser versus PDL in patients with nail psoriasis. Authors reported excellent response of the PDL in treating these patients, whereas results of the excimer laser were poor.[20]

Intense pulsed light treatment can be considered a promising effective and safe treatment modality. In a study, 20 patients were treated with IPL every 2 weeks for 6 months, demonstrating nail bed improvement by 71.2% and nail matrix by 32.2%.[21]

19.3.1.6 Photodynamic Treatment (Evidence-Based Strength of Recommendation B)

In a study with 14 patients, photodynamic treatment (PDT) with the application on the nail plate of methylaminolaevulinic acid (MAL) under occlusion for 3 hours, followed by PDL 595 nm irradiation (7 mm, 6 ms, 9 J/cm^2, three pulses on each nail) once a month for 6 months was compared with PDL 595 nm as monotherapy on the other hand of the same patient, with the same parameters. Both treatments were equally effective, suggesting that MAL does not increase the beneficial effect of PDL.[22]

19.3.1.7 Combination Treatment (Evidence-Based Strength of Recommendation A)

The NAPSI score was significantly improved in a study where patients were treated with a combination of calcipotriol and betamethasone ointment. It was used at bedtime for 7 days a week and for a period of 12 weeks at the nail folds, the nail plate, and the hyponychium.[23] Clobetasol 8% nail lacquer (at bedtime on weekends) has been used in combination with tacalcitol ointment (on weekdays under occlusion) on 15 patients with both matrix and bed nail psoriasis. NAPSI scores improved by 78% while tolerability was excellent.[24] A single-blind, intrapatient left-to-right study including 19 patients evaluated the efficacy of PDL plus topical tazarotene 0.1% gel once a month for 6 months versus tazarotene 0.1% gel alone in nail psoriasis. The combination was proven a significantly superior treatment option.[25]

19.3.2 Systemic Treatment

Systemic treatment, including acitretin, cyclosporin A, methotrexate, and biologic medication, is indicated in nail psoriasis involving many or all nails when it is associated with moderate or severe skin symptoms and in cases of pustular psoriasis of the nail. It can be used either as monotherapy or combined with topical treatment in order to achieve a reduced dose and duration of systemic treatment or to maintain disease remission.

19.3.2.1 Acitretin (Evidence-Based Strength of Recommendation B)

Acitretin is used in lower dose than that used in skin psoriasis (0.2–0.3 mg/kg/day) in order to reduce the risk of side effects like nail fragility, reduction of nail thickness, pseudopyogenic-type granuloma, and anonychia-like lesions. In a study, a low dose of acitretin was used in 36 patients for a 6-month period and the NAPSI score was reduced on average by 41%.[26]

In another study, acitretin 0.5 mg/kg/day was used to treat a small number of patients with pustular psoriasis of the nails demonstrating good response. However, the relapse rate was high.[27]

19.3.2.2 Cyclosporin A (Evidence-Based Strength of Recommendation A)

Cyclosporin A (CyA) acts by inhibition of T-cell activity and decrease of inflammatory mediators. It is considered an effective treatment modality for nail psoriasis. A multicenter study with 90 psoriasis patients with nail disease treated with CyA showed a significant decrease of the nail involvement.[28] In a recent retrospective study, seven patients with nail psoriasis were treated with CyA 3 mg/kg/day. NAPSI scores were reduced by 37.9%, 71.8%, and 89.1% after 12, 24, and 48 weeks of treatment, respectively.[29] Long-term improvement of both matrix and bed affection was noted in a series of 70 patients treated with 3 mg/kg of CyA for 8 weeks.[30] Another study included 54 patients divided into two groups: one receiving CyA (3.5 and 4.5 mg/kg/day) as monotherapy and the other combining CyA with calcipotriol cream applied twice daily. After 12 weeks of treatment, 79% improvement of subungual hyperkeratosis, onycholysis, and pitting was observed in the combination group of patients, whereas the monotherapy group showed 47.6% reduction of the same symptoms.[31] In 16 patients with psoriatic nail changes, CyA was used in a dosage of 3 mg/kg/day, and after improvement reduction to 1.5 mg/kg/day was administrated. Over 90% of the patients improved and were satisfied.[32] On the other hand, a blind randomized study including 17 patients with nail psoriasis received CyA (5 m/kg/day) for 24 weeks, with a moderate result (reduction of NAPSI, mainly nail bed signs, up to 45.2% for fingernails and 37.2% for toenails).[33] Serious adverse reactions such as renal dysfunction, hypertension, fatigue, headache, paresthesia, hypertrichosis, gingival hyperplasia, and gastrointestinal disorders have been reported in patients treated with CyA.

19.3.2.3 Methotrexate (Evidence-Based Strength of Recommendation A)

There are only a few studies using methotrexate (MTX) to treat nail psoriasis. In a one-blind, randomized study, 17 patients with nail psoriasis were treated with MTX 15 mg/day for 24 weeks. A reduction of NAPSI up to 49.3% for fingernails and 43.1% for toenails was noted.[33] A retrospective study using MTX 5 mg/week as initial dosage and thereafter 7.5–25 mg/week for 48 weeks, demonstrated a 30.8% reduction of the NAPSI score at week 24 and to 34.9% at week 48.[29] Another study using MTX for nail psoriasis reported a 36.8% reduction of NAPSI after 24 weeks.[34] Potential side effects of this treatment include hepatotoxicity, ulcerative stomatitis, lymphopenia, nausea, and low white blood cell count. Intralesional injections in the proximal nail fold with 0.1 mL of a 5 mg/2 mL solution of methotraxate might also be effective.[35]

19.3.2.4 Biologics and Small Molecules

Biologic agents that have been employed in the treatment of cutaneous psoriasis and arthritis have also been used to treat nail psoriasis. These agents include anti-TNF-α, anti-IL-12,-23 drugs, phosphodiesterase

4 inhibitors, and anti-IL-17A drugs. Retrospective studies comparing the efficacy of multiple anti-TNF-α agents suggest that etanercept, infliximab, and adalimumab result in a significant improvement in the NAPSI score in patients with nail psoriasis.[36,37]

19.3.2.4.1 Etanercept (Evidence-Based Strength of Recommendation A)

Etanercept (fusion protein) is considered an effective and safe treatment for nail psoriasis. Five hundred sixty-four psoriasis patients received subcutaneously 25 mg etanercept twice/week for 54 weeks or 50 mg twice/week for 12 weeks. The NAPSI score was improved by 51% at week 24, while complete resolution was seen in 30% of patients at week 54.[38] In an open randomized study, 69 patients with psoriasis and nail involvement were treated with etanercept 50 mg twice/week for 12 weeks followed by 50 mg once/week for 12 more weeks or 50 mg once/week for 24 weeks. On week 24, NAPSI 75 was reached by 57.0% of patients in the first group and 68.6% of patients in the second group.[39]

19.3.2.4.2 Adalimumab (Evidence-Based Strength of Recommendation A)

A prospective, open-label, uncontrolled study including 244 patients with psoriatic arthritis and nail involvement showed that adalimumab (human monoclonal antibody) provided significant improvement in nail psoriasis. By week 12, a 57% decrease in the mean NAPSI score was demonstrated, while by week 20 (optional extension period of treatment for 103 patients), the decrease was almost 91%.[40] Another cohort study included 7 patients with psoriasis and nail disease and 14 patients with psoriatic arthritis and nail affection. Patients were treated with adalimumab 45 mg twice a month subcutaneously. At week 24, a decrease of the NAPSI score by 85% on the fingernail psoriasis and 71.5% on the toenail psoriasis was observed in patients of the first group, while 86% for fingernails and 64% for the toenails in the patients of the second group. Statistically significant improvement on patients' quality of life was also seen.[41] A randomized, placebo-controlled, double-blind trial study with 36 patients demonstrated an improvement in NAPSI score as high as 54% at week 28.[42]

A subanalysis of the effect of adalimumab on scalp and nail psoriasis in the population of the BELIEVE study showed improvement of nail psoriasis by 39.5% at week 16 and a reduction of 74.31% in the impact on patients' quality of life.[43] All the aforementioned studies confirmed a good response of the drug in cases of nail psoriasis. A recent randomized, placebo-controlled trial with 217 randomized patients (108 received placebo and 109 received adalimumab) showed statistically significant improvement in signs and symptoms of moderate-to-severe nail psoriasis versus with placebo. In almost half of the patients being treated with adalimumab (46.6%), NAPSI 75 was seen on week 26. No new safety risks were identified.[44]

19.3.2.4.3 Infliximab (Evidence-Based Strength of Recommendation A)

Infliximab is a chimeric monoclonal antibody. In a 50-week, phase III, randomized, double-blind trial in 373 patients with moderate-to-severe psoriasis, infliximab demonstrated improvement in NAPSI from baseline to week 24 was 56.3%.[45] Twenty-five patients with nail psoriasis were treated with infliximab (5 mg/kg), and NAPSI 75 at week 22 was achieved by all patients.[46] In an unblinded, nonrandomized, open-label study, 18 patients with nail involvement (13 patients with psoriatic arthritis and 5 with severe plaque psoriasis) were treated with infliximab infusions. All patients demonstrated almost complete clearance (94% improvement) and an improvement in quality of life with a significant reduction of the score of the international quality of life questionnaire was reported in all patients.[47] In a randomized, double-blind, placebo-controlled multicenter study, improvement in NAPSI score at week 10 was 1.4 ± 2.2 in the infliximab group compared with 0.3 ± 1.0 in the placebo group.[48]

An open-labeled study including 48 patients with nail psoriasis involvement showed a rapid response. There was an almost 81% improvement in the NAPSI score at week 22 of infliximab treatment.[49]

19.3.2.4.4 Certolizumab (Evidence-Based Strength of Recommendation A)

A double-blind, randomized, placebo-controlled study (RAPID PsA) in patients with psoriatic arthritis treated with certolizumab pegol (CZP) showed statistical significant improvement of mNAPSI at week 24. The reduction in mNAPSI was −1.6 with CZP 200 mg Q2W and −2.0 with CZP 400 mg Q4W versus −1.1 with placebo.[50]

19.3.2.4.5 Golimumab (Evidence-Based Strength of Recommendation A)

A randomized, double-blind, placebo-controlled trial with golimumab in patients with psoriatic arthritis reported an improvement of target median NAPSI by 25% and 33% at weeks 12 and 24 for patients receiving 50 mg of golimumab, and 43% and 54% at weeks 12 and 24 for patients receiving 100 mg of golimumab. Both improvements were statistically significant compared to the placebo groups.[51]

19.3.2.4.6 Ustekinumab (Evidence-Based Strength of Recommendation A)

A large double-blind, randomized, placebo-controlled, multicenter trial including 545 psoriasis patients with nail involvement were treated with ustekinumab (recombinant, completely human, monoclonal antibody). A significant improvement of the NAPSI score was observed from baseline to week 12 by 26.7% in the 45 mg group and by 24.9% in the 90 mg group of patients, highlighting the early drug's efficacy. This improvement was further increased at week 24 (46.5% and 48.7%, respectively).[52] This quick response on nail psoriasis with ustekinumab was impressively recorded in a case report. The authors reported a significant improvement at week 4 and a complete cure at week 8 of treatment. Another study including 27 patients with nail disease, reported a 90% reduction of NAPSI score and an improvement of patients' quality of life by 80% after 40 weeks of treatment with ustekinumab.[53]

In a double-blind, placebo-controlled study, 158 patients with moderate-to-severe plaque-type psoriasis were randomized to receive ustekinumab 45 or 90 mg at weeks 0, 4, and every 12 weeks, or placebo with crossover to ustekinumab at week 12.[54] The authors stated that in week 64, the patients with nail involvement had a mean percentage of improvement in NAPSI 56.6% ± 43.2% and 67.8% ± 37.5% for the 45 and 90 mg of ustekinumab, respectively.

A study by Vittiello et al. included 13 patients with moderate-to-severe psoriasis and psoriatic arthritis with nail involvement who had previously tried multiple therapeutic modalities with poor results.[55] Five patients received ustekinumab 90 mg as monotherapy because they exceeded the 90 kgr range. According to the results of this study, the average NAPSI score and modified NAPSI for the 13 patients was reduced from 22.3 and 6.3 at week 0, and to 14.8 and 5.2 at week 12, respectively, demonstrating a reduction of the NAPSI score and mNAPSI score of 31.8% and 13.3%. A 37.6% reduction of the NAPSI score was noted in the 5 patients with ustekinumab administration monotherapy. The 6 patients with the combination of ustekinumab and MTX had a 27% reduction of NAPSI score, while in the 2 patients with the combination of ustekinumab and cyclosporin complete resolution of nail disease was noted. An open-label, uncontrolled study evaluated the effectiveness of ustekinumab in 27 patients with nail psoriasis (administered with the standard regimen). The 49% reduction of the NAPSI score was noted at week 16, which was increased to 88% at week 28, confirming the quick positive effect of the drug on nail disease.[56]

19.3.2.4.7 Secukinumab (Evidence-Based Strength of Recommendation A)

A subanalysis of a randomized, double-blind, placebo-controlled, regimen-finding phase 2 trial demonstrated a beneficial effect of secukinumab (fully human monoclonal antibody) on psoriasis of the hands, feet, and nails. Subjects were randomized (1:2:2:1) to one of three subcutaneous secukinumab 150 mg induction regimens (single [week 0]; monthly [weeks 0, 4, 8]; early [weeks 0, 1, 2, 4]) or placebo.[57] At week 12, a significantly higher percentage of subjects with hand or foot psoriasis achieved an Investigator's Global Assessment (IGA) response with the early regimen versus placebo (54.3% vs. 19.2%, $P = 0.005$). The composite fingernail score improved with the early and monthly regimens, but worsened with placebo. A recent randomized placebo control trial showed a NAPSI improvement of 45.3% and 37.9% for patients receiving 300 and 150 mg of secukinumab, respectively, after 16 weeks of treatment.[58] Improvement of NAPSI has been reported to be even more rapid in a case series of 15 patients with a 50% reduction at 6 weeks and an 80% reduction at 12 weeks.[59] A recent case report suggests that secukinumab might also have good efficacy in children with nail psoriasis.[60]

19.3.2.4.8 Ixekizumab (Evidence-Based Strength of Recommendation A)

Ixekizumab treatment (a fully humanized monoclonal anti-IL-17A drug) and its effect on psoriatic nail disease were evaluated in a post hoc analysis of a phase 2 study comprising a 20-week randomized, placebo-controlled period and 48 weeks of an open-label extension period.[61] There were 142 patients with moderate-to-severe plaque psoriasis who were randomized to receive placebo, 10, 25, 75, or 150 mg of ixekizumab injected subcutaneously at weeks 0, 2, 4, 8, 12, and 16. In week 48, all patients received 120 mg ixekizumab every 4 weeks. Patients with nail psoriasis in the 75 and 150 mg groups had significant improvements from baseline NAPSI. By week 48, 51.0% of patients with nail psoriasis experienced complete resolution of lesions, suggesting ixekizumab as a possible option for the treatment of patients with skin and nail psoriasis. A poster on the results of the IXORA-S trial suggested superior efficacy of ixekizumab over ustekinumab in nail psoriasis.[62]

19.3.2.4.9 *Apremilast (Evidence-Based Strength of Recommendation A)*

Apremilast was prescribed orally in a dosage of 30 mg twice daily, in patients with psoriasis and nail involvement. At week 16, a reduction of the NAPSI score was seen (22.5% for patients in ESTEEM 1 and 29% for patients in ESTEEM 2 study), with improvement in both matrix and bed disease. At week 32 the mean reduction of NAPSI was 43.6% and 60%, respectively, while at week 52, 60.2% and 59.7%.[63] Therefore, apremilast can be considered an effective oral treatment for psoriatic patients with nail disease.

19.3.2.4.10 *Tofacitinib (Evidence Based Strength of Recommendation A)*

Tofacitinib is an oral Janus kinase inhibitor. A randomized, controlled phase 3 study evaluated the efficacy and safety of tofacitinib in patients with moderate-to-severe plaque psoriasis and nail psoriasis. At week 16, significantly more patients receiving tofacitinib 5 mg and tofacitinib 10 mg versus placebo twice daily achieved NAPSI 50 (32.8%, 44.2% vs. 12.0%), NAPSI 75 (16.9%, 28.1% vs. 6.8%), and NAPSI 100 (10.3%, 18.2% vs. 5.1%), respectively.[64] In subgroup analyses from a randomized, placebo-controlled phase 3 trial, reductions from baseline in NAPSI score were observed at week 16 with both tofacitinib 5 and 10 mg twice daily versus placebo. NAPSI scores continued to decrease through week 52 with both tofacitinib dose groups. By week 52, 22.2% and 47.6% of the patients who received tofacitinib 5 and 10 mg, respectively, achieved NAPSI 75.[65] The most common adverse events related to laboratory parameter abnormalities were noted. Both studies showed that oral tofacitinib demonstrates efficacy on nail psoriasis, sustained over 52 weeks, with a manageable safety profile.

A recent consensus striving to provide recommendations for the treatment of nail psoriasis suggested that few nail diseases should be considered as nail psoriasis affecting three or fewer nails as a general rule for deciding on topical or systemic therapy. Intralesional steroids should be employed as the treatment of choice in nail matrix disease, and topical steroids alone or in combination with vitamin D analogues for nail bed disease affecting up to three nails. If more nails are affected or systemic therapy is indicated for other reasons acitretin, methotrexate, cyclosporine, small molecules, and biologics can be prescribed.[66] See further Tables 19.1 and 19.2.

TABLE 19.1

Topical Treatments and Levels of Evidence

Topical Treatment	Level of Evidence
Topical steroids	A[1]
Intralesional steroids	A[1]
Iontoforesis with triamcinolone acetonide	A[4]
8% Clobetasol nail lacquer	A[5–7]
Vitamin D analogues—Calcipotriol	B[8,9,11,12]
Calcipotriol with clobetasol	B[10]
Tacalcitol (synthetic analogue of vitamin D3)	B[13]
Tazarotene	A[14,15]
Tacrolimus	A[17]
Laser and IPL	B[19–21]
Photodynamic therapy	B[19–21]
Combination Treatment	
Calcipotriol and betamethasone ointment	A[23]
Clobetasol 8% nail lacquer with tacalcitol ointment	A[24]
PDL plus topical tazarotene 0.1% gel	A[25]

TABLE 19.2

Systemic Treatments and Levels of Evidence

Systemic Treatment	Level of Evidence
Acitretin	B[26,27]
Cyclosporin A	A[28–33]
Methotrexate	A[3–35,29]
Biologics	
Etanercept	A[38,39]
Adalimumab	A[40–44]
Infliximab	A[45–49]
Certolizumab	A[50]
Golimumab	A[51]
Ustekinumab	A[52–56]
Secukinumab	A[57–60]
Ixekizumab	A[61,62]
Apremilast	A[63]
Tofacitinib	A[64–66]

REFERENCES

1. Saleem K, Azim W. Treatment of nail psoriasis with a modified regimen of steroid injections. *J Coll Physicians Surg Pak*. 2008;18:78–81.
2. De Berker D, Lawrence CM. A simplified protocol of steroid injection for psoriatic nail dystrophy. *Br J Dermatol*. 1998;138:90–95.
3. De Berker D. Management of nail psoriasis. *Clin Exp Dermatol*. 2000;25:357–362.
4. Saki N, Hosseinpoor S, Heiran A et al. Comparing the efficacy of triamcinolone acetonide iontophoresis versus topical calcipotriol/betamethasone dipropionate in treating nail psoriasis: A bilateral controlled clinical trial. *Dermatol Res Pract*. 2018 November 21;2018:2637691
5. Baran R, Tosti A. Treatment of nail psoriasis with a new corticoid-containing nail lacquer formulation. *J Dermatol Treatm*. 1999;10:201–204.
6. Sanchez Regana M, Martin Ezwuerra G, Millet U et al. Treatment of nail psoriasis with 8% clobetasol nail lacquer: Positive experience in 10 patients. *J Eur Acad Dermatol Venereol*. 2005;19:573–577.
7. Nakamura R, Duque-Estrada B, Pizzaro Leverone A et al. Comparison of nail lacquer clobetasol efficacy at 0, 05%, 1% and 8% in nail psoriasis treatment: Prospective, controlled and randomized pilot study. *An Bras Dermatol*. 2012;87(2):203–211.
8. Gladman DD, Schentag CT, Tom BD et al. Development and initial validation of a screening questionnaire for psoriatic arthritis: The Toronto Psoriatic Arthritis Screen (ToPAS). *Ann Rheum Dis*. 2009;68:497–501.
9. Husni ME, Meyer KH, Cohen DS, Mody E, Qureshi AA. The PASE questionnaire: Pilot-testing a psoriatic arthritis screening and evaluation tool. *J Am Acad Dermatol*. 2007;57:581–587.
10. Alenius GM, Stenberg B, Stenlund H, Lundblad M, Dahlqvist SR. Inflammatory joint manifestations are prevalent in psoriasis: Prevalence study of joint and axial involvement in psoriatic patients, and evaluation of a psoriatic and arthritic questionnaire. *J Rheumatol*. 2002;29:2577–2582.
11. Tinazzi I, Adami S, Zanolin EM et al. The early psoriatic arthritis screening questionnaire: A simple and fast method for the identification of arthritis in patients with psoriasis. *Rheumatology (Oxford)*. 2012;51:2058–2063.
12. Ash Z, Aydin SZ, Tan AL, McGonagle D. Arthritis. In: Rigopoulos D, Tosti A (eds), *Nail Psoriasis from A to Z*. Switzerland: Springer International Publishing; 2014, pp. 34–41.
13. Ash Z, Gaujoux-Viala C, Gossec L et al. A systematic literature review of drug therapies for the treatment of psoriatic arthritis: Current evidence and meta-analysis informing the EULAR recommendations for the management of psoriatic arthritis. *Ann Rheum Dis*. 2012;71:319–326.
14. Scher RK, Stiller M, Zhu YI. Tazarotene 0.1% gel in the treatment of fingernail psoriasis: A double-blind, randomized, vehicle-controlled study. *Cutis*. 2001;68:355–358.
15. Bianchi L, Soda R, Diluvio L et al. Tazarotene 0.1% gel for psoriasis of the fingernails and toenails: An open, prospective study. *Br J Dermatol*. 2003;149:207–209.

16. Rigopoulos D, Gregoriou S, Katsambas A. Treatment of psoriatic nails with tazarotene 0.1% gel vs clobetasol propionate 0.05% cream: A double-blind study. *Acta Derm Venereol*. 2007;87:167–168.
17. De Simone C, Maiorino A, Tassone F et al. Tacrolimus 0.1% ointment in nail psoriasis: A randomized, controlled, open-label study. *J Eur Acad Dermatol Venereol*. 2013;27:1003–1006.
18. Trieewittayapoon C, Sigvahamont P, Chanprapaph K et al. The effect of different pulse durations in the treatment of nail psoriasis with 595-nm pulsed dye laser: A randomized, doubleblind, intrapatient left-to-right study. *J Am Acd Dermatol*. 2012;66:807–812.
19. Oram Y, Karincaoğlu Y, Koyuncu E et al. Pulsed dye laser in the treatment of nail psoriasis. *Dermatol Surg*. 2010;36:377–381.
20. Al-Mutairi N, Noor T, Al-Haddad. Single blinded left-to-right comparison study of excimer laser versus PDL for the treatment of nail psoriasis. *Dermatol Ther*. 2014;4:197–205.
21. Tawifik AA. Novel treatment of nail psoriasis using the IPL: A 1-year follow-up study. *Dermatol Surg*. 2014;1:1–6.
22. Fernández-Guarino M, Harto A, Sánchez-Ronco M et al. Pulsed dye laser vs photodynamic therapy in the treatment of refractory nail psoriasis: A comparative pilot study. *J Eur Acad Dermatol Venereol*. 2009;23:891–895.
23. Rigopoulos D, Gregoriou S, Daniel CR et al. Treatment of nail psoriasis with a two compound formulation of calcipotriol plus betamethasone dipropionate ointment. *Dermatology*. 2009;218:338–341.
24. Sanchez Regana M, Marquez Balbas G, Millet Umbert P. Nail psoriasis: A combined treatment with8% clobetasol nail laquer and tacalcitol ointment. *J Eur Acad Dermatol Venereol*. 2008;22:963–969.
25. Huang YC, Chou CL, Chiang YY. Efficacy of pulsed dye laser plus topical tazarotene versus topical tazarotene alone in psoriatic nail disease: A single-blind, intrapatient left-to-right controlled study. *Lasers Surg Med*. 2013;45:102–107.
26. Tosti A, Ricotti C, Romanelli P et al. Evaluation of the efficacy of acitretin therapy for nail psoriasis. *Arch Dermatol*. 2009;145:269–271.
27. Piraccini BM, Tosti A, Iorizzo M et al. Pustular psoriasis of the nails: Treatment and long-term follow-up of 46 patients. *Br J Dermatol*. 2001;144:1000–1005.
28. Mahrle G, Schultze HG, Farber L et al. Low- dose short-term cyclosporine versus etretinate in psoriasis: Improvement of skin, nails and joint involvement. *J Am Acad Dermatol*. 1995;32:78–88.
29. Sanchez-Regana M, Sola-Ortigosa J, Gibert-Alsina J et al. Nail psoriasis: A retrospective study on the effectiveness of systemic treatment (classical and biological therapy). *J Eur Acad Dermatol Venereol*. 2011;25:57–586.
30. Ojeda R, Sanchez-Regana M, Massana J et al. Clinical experience with the use of cyclosporine A in psoriasis. Results of a retrospective study. *J Dermatol Treat*. 2005;16:338–341.
31. Feliciani C, Zampetti A, Forleo P et al. Nail psoriasis: Combined therapy with systemic cyclosporine and topical calcipotriol. *J Cutan Med Surg*. 2004;8:122–125.
32. Syuto T, Abe M, Ishibuchi H et al. Successful treatment of psoriatic nails with low-dose cyclosporine administration. *Eur J Dermatol*. 2007;17:248–249.
33. Gumusel M, Ozdemir M, Mevlitoglou I et al. Evaluation of the efficacy of methotrexate and cyclosporine therapies on psoriatic nails: A one-blind, randomized study. *J Eur Acad Dermatol Venereol*. 2011;25:1080–1084.
34. Reich N, Nestle FO, Papp K et al. Infliximab induction and maintenance therapy for moderate-to-severe psoriasis: A phase III multicentre double-blind trial. *Lancet*. 2005;366:1367–1374.
35. Mokni S, Ameur K, Ghariani N et al. A case of nail psoriasis successfully treated with intralesional methotrexate. *Dermatol Ther (Heidelb)*. 2018;8:647–651.
36. Kyriakou A, Patsatsi A, Sotiriadis D. Anti-TNF agents and nail psoriasis: A single-center, retrospective, comparative study. *J Dermatol Treat*. 2013;24:162–168.
37. Bardazzi F, Antonucci V, Odorici G et al. A 36-week retrospective open trial comparing the efficacy of biological therapies in nail psoriasis. *J Dtsch Dermatol Ges*. 2013;11:1065–1070.
38. Luger TA, Barker J, Lambert J et al. Sustained improvement in joint pain and nail symptoms with Etanercept therapy in patients with moderate-to-severe psoriasis. *J Eur Acad Dermatol Venereol*. 2009;23:896–904.
39. Ortonne JP, Paul C, Berardesca E et al. A 24-week randomized clinical trial investigating the efficacy and safety of two doses of etanercept in nail psoriasis. *Br J Dermatol*. 2013;168:1080–1087.

40. Van den Bosch F, Manger B, Goupille P et al. Effectiveness of adalimumab in treating patients with active psoriatic arthritis and predictors of good clinical responses for arthritis, skin and nail lesions. *Ann Rheum Dis.* 2010;69:394–399.

41. Rigopoulos D, Gregoriou S, Lazaridou E et al. Treatment of nail psoriasis with adalimumab. An open label, uncontrolled study. *J Eur Acad Dermatol Venereol.* 2010;24:530–534.

42. Leonardi C, Langley RG, Papp K et al. Adalimumab for the treatment of moderate to severe chronic plaque psoriasis of the hands and feet: Efficacy and safety results from REACH a randomized, placebo-controlled, double-blind trial. *Arch Dermatol.* 2011;147:429–436.

43. Thaci D, Unnebrink K, Sundaram M et al. Adalimumab for the treatment of moderate to severe psoriasis: Subanalysis of effects on scalp and nails in the BELIEVE study. *JEADV.* 2015;29:353–360.

44. Elewski BE, Okun MM, Papp K et al. Adalimumab for nail psoriasis: Efficacy and safety from the first 26 weeks of a phase 3, randomized, placebo-controlled trial. *J Am Acad Dermatol.* 2018;78:90–99.e1.

45. Rich P, Griffiths C, Reich K et al. Baseline nail disease in patients with moderate to severe psoriasis and response to treatment with Infliximab during 1 year. *J Am Acad Dermatol.* 2008;58:224–231.

46. Bianchi L, Bergamin A, de Felice C et al. Remission and time of resolution of nail psoriasis during infliximab therapy. *J Am Acad Dermatol.* 2005;52:736–737.

47. Rigopoulos D, Gregoriou S, Stratigos A et al. Evaluation of the efficacy and safety of infliximab on psoriatic nails: An unblinded, non-randomized, open-label study. *Br J Dermatol.* 2008;159:453–456.

48. Torii H, Nakagawa H. Infliximab monotherapy in Japanese patients with moderate-to-severe plaque psoriasis and psoriatic arthritis. A randomized, double-blind, placebo-controlled multicenter trial. *J Dermatol Sci.* 2010;59:40–49.

49. Fabroni C, Gori A, Troiano M et al. Infliximab efficacy in nail psoriasis. A retrospective study in 48 patients. *J Eur Acad Dermatol Venereol.* 2011;25:549–563.

50. Mease PJ, Fleischmann R, Deodhar AA et al. Effect of certolizumab pegol on signs and symptoms in patients with psoriatic arthritis: 24-week results of a phase 3 double-blind randomised placebo-controlled study (RAPID-PsA). *Ann Rheum Dis.* 2014;73:48–55.

51. Kavanaugh A, McInnes I, Mease P et al. Golimumab, a new human tumor necrosis factor alpha antibody, administered every 4 weeks as a subcutaneous injection in psoriatic arthritis: 24-week efficacy and safety results of a randomized, placebo-controlled study. *Arthritis Rheum.* 2009;60(4):976–986.

52. Rich P, Bourcier M, Sofen H et al. Ustekinumab improves nail disease in patients with moderate-to-severe psoriasis: Results from PHOENIX 1. *Br J Dermatol.* 2014;170:398–407.

53. Rigopoulos D, Gregoriou S, Makris M, Ioannides D. Efficacy of ustekinumab in nail psoriasis and improvement in nail associated QoL in a population treated with ustekinumab for cutaneous psoriasis. An open prospective unblinded study. *Dermatology.* 2011;223:325–329.

54. Igarashi A, Kato T, Kato M et al. Efficacy and safety of ustekinumab in Japanese patients with moderate-to-severe plaque-type psoriasis: Long-term results from a phase 2/3 clinical trial. *J Dermatol.* 2012;39:242–252.

55. Vitiello M, Tosti A, Abuchar A et al. Ustekinumab for the treatment of nail psoriasis in heavily treated psoriatic patients. *Int J Dermatol.* 2013;52:358–362.

56. Patsatsi A, Kyriakou A, Sotiriadis D. Ustekinumab in nail psoriasis: An open-label, uncontrolled, nonrandomized study. *J Dermatolog Treat.* 2013;24:96–100.

57. Paul C, Reich K, Gottlieb AB. Secukinumab improves hand, foot and nail lesions in moderate-to-severe plaque psoriasis: Subanalysis of a randomized, double-blind, placebo-controlled, regimen-finding phase 2 trial. *J EADV.* 2014;28:1670–1675.

58. Reich K, Sullivan J, Arenberger P et al. Effect of secukinumab on the clinical activity and disease burden of nail psoriasis: 32-week results from the randomized placebo-controlled TRANSFIGURE trial. *Br J Dermatol.* 2018 October 26. doi: 10.1111/bjd.17351. [Epub].

59. Pistone G, Gurreri R, Tilotta G et al. Secukinumab efficacy in the treatment of nail psoriasis: A case series. *J Dermatolog Treat.* 2018;29:21–24.

60. Wells LE, Evans T, Hilton R et al. Use of secukinumab in a pediatric patient leads to significant improvement in nail psoriasis and psoriatic arthritis. *Pediatr Dermatol.* 2019 February 27. doi: 10.1111/pde. [Epub].

61. Langley GR, Rich P, Menter A et al. Improvement of scalp and nail lesions with ixekizumab in a phase 2 trial in patients with chronic plaque psoriasis. *JEADV.* 2015;29:1763–1770.

62. Ghislain P-D, Conrad C, Dutronc Y et al. Comparison of ixekizumab and ustekinumab efficacy in the treatment of nail lesions of patients with moderate-to-severe plaque psoriasis: 24-week data from a phase 3 trial. *Abstract 1827;2017 ACR/ARHP Annual Meeting*, November 3–8, 2017, San Diego, CA.

63. Rich P, Gooderham M, Bachelez H et al. Apremilast, an oral phosphodiesterase 4 inhibitor, in patients with difficult-to-treat nail and scalp psoriasis: Results of 2 phase III randomized, controlled trials (ESTEEM 1 and ESTEEM 2). *JAAD*. 2016;74:134–142.

64. Merola JF, Elewski B, Tatulych S et al. Efficacy of tofacitinib for the treatment of nail psoriasis: Two 52-week, randomized, controlled phase 3 studies in patients with moderate-to-severe plaque psoriasis. *J Am Acad Dermatol*. 2017;77:79–87.e1.

65. Abe M, Nishigori C, Torii H et al. Tofacitinib for the treatment of moderate to severe chronic plaque psoriasis in Japanese patients: Subgroup analyses from a randomized, placebo-controlled phase 3 trial. *J Dermatol*. 2017;44:1228–1237.

66. Rigopoulos D, Baran R, Chibeb S et al. Recommendations for the definition, evaluation, and treatment of nail psoriasis in adult patients with no or mild skin psoriasis: A dermatologist and nail expert group consensus. *J Am Acad Dermatol*. 2019 February 4. doi: 10.1016/j.jaad.2019.01.072. [Epub].

20

Retronychia

Thomas Knackstedt and Nathaniel J. Jellinek

20.1 Introduction

Retronychia is a rare nail disorder that presents with proximal ingrowing of the nail plate with the resulting triad of proximal nail fold inflammation, thickening of the nail with multiple nail plate layers, and nail growth arrest.[1] Retronychia remains a rare and likely underrecognized diagnosis. In the literature of 2018, a search for "retronychia" reveals only 29 publications since its first description by de Berker and Renall in 1999.[2] This chapter will review the pathophysiology, epidemiology, diagnostics, treatment, and prevention of retronychia.

Previous studies have identified retronychia to frequently occur in young individuals with mean or median ages 28–39.[1,3,4] Patients as young as 8 and as mature as 84 have been reported.[1] The majority of cases (84%–88%) occur in females.[1,4] In most studies, the great toe(s) are affected (96%, study of $n = 25$). Up to 30% of cases may be bilateral[3] and involvement of multiple nails has been reported.[5] Retronychia is not always readily diagnosed and median durations from 5 to 24 months prior to diagnosis are reported.[1,3] The distribution on the halluces is probably due to trauma commonly affecting these digits.[6] Repetitive microtrauma from physical activity or ill-fitting shoes can precipitate retronychia.[3] In one study, 44% of patients had a responsible hobby, 28% wore tight shoes, and 24% recalled overt trauma to the affected digit.[1] This may be exacerbated by underlying "claw toe" or "hammertoe" with reflex compensatory hyperextension of the hallux in up to half of the patients[3] and lateral malalignment of the toenails in 20% of patients.[1] Systemic illness including arthritis, thrombophlebitis, and postpartum state have been associated with retronychia.[5] Indeed, any cause of prolonged matrix hypoxia including severe illness such as Guillain-Barré syndrome may be contributory.[7]

Normally, the nail grows outward from its production in the matrix with an oblique distal and upward course from the matrix over the nail bed. Trauma may interrupt this process, which usually results in Beau's line formation or onychomadesis (complete shedding of the nail) as the nail matrix tissue recovers from insult. Indeed, Beau's lines, onychomadesis, and retronychia all have their origin in a temporary cessation of cell growth in the affected nail matrix.[8] In normal circumstances, such as in a Beau's line, onychomadesis, or crush injury, the original nail would remain aligned in the horizontal axis so that the new, forming nail is able to push the separated original nail out distally. The proximal nail fold plays a part in maintaining this alignment by preventing the old nail from rising up in response to pressure from behind. In retronychia, something disrupts the alignment growth resulting in partial separation of the old plate from the matrix and nail bed, with vertical growth of the new nail plate into the ventral surface of the proximal nail fold. The nail is not completely shed because the nail plate remains attached at the lateral matrix horns.[5] At the same time, onycholysis of the distal nail plate occurs. Once no longer attached to the nail bed, the nail plate is pushed proximally by normal biomechanic pressures and, through a rocking motion, cause irritation and injury of the proximal nail fold. It remains unclear if retropulsion of the nail unit is the result of low interstitial pressure or the product of an active mechanism, such as a fibroblastic reaction.[7] Ultimately, the oldest, most superficial nail plate, with a sharp edge, is pushed into the ventral aspect of the proximal nail fold or eponychium. With this disruption in longitudinal growth, a new nail consequently passes beneath the remnants of old nail plate. A vicious cycle with repetitive disruption of nail matrix growth occurs with subsequent stacking of multiple sheets of nail plate.[6] Chronic

TABLE 20.1

Patient and Examination Findings Suggestive of Retronychia

Patient Characteristics

Single affected nail—rarely bilateral

History of trauma including repetitive microtrauma—inappropriate footwear, athletic activity, biomechanical gait
  abnormalities

Female

Young age

Toenails, favoring great toe

Exam Findings

Proximal nail fold inflammation (paronychia)

Thickened nail with multiple layers

Transverse nail ridging

Onycholysis

Yellow-white discoloration

Granulation tissue

Pain

Nail plate growth arrest

---

inflammation with pain, paronychia, and granulation tissue may ensue. These findings correspond with
the sonographic hypoechogenicity seen in the central portion of the nail matrix in retronychia suggesting
liquefaction, fluid content, the presence of inflammation, and tissue digestion.[7] See further Table 20.1.

20.2 How to Confirm the Diagnosis

The presentation of retronychia relates to the triad of proximal nail fold inflammation, thickening of the
nail with multiple nail plate layers, and nail growth arrest (Figure 20.1). Oftentimes patients report not
needing to cut the nails for months.[3]

Yellow discoloration of the nail, xanthonychia, is seen in almost all patients (Figure 20.2).[1] This
discoloration is probably secondary to a thickened proximal nail plate, onycholysis, and air introduced
underneath the free nail plate as well as the accumulation of serous or serosanguineous inflammatory

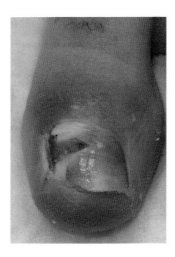

FIGURE 20.1   Retronychia of the left great toenail. In the area of nail fragmentation, multiple layers of stacked nail plate
are apparent proximally.

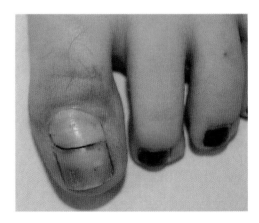

FIGURE 20.2   Retronychia of the left great toenail presenting with prominent xanthonychia. (Courtesy of Bianca Maria Piraccini, MD.)

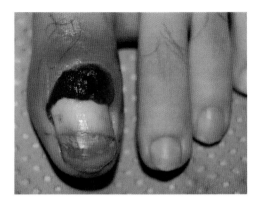

FIGURE 20.3   Retronychia of the left great toenail. In addition to xanthonychia and onycholysis, a crescentic band of friable granulation tissue is apparent at the proximal nail fold. (Courtesy of Bianca Maria Piraccini, MD.)

exudate.[5] When avulsed, a Y-shaped proximal margin of split multiple nail plates is apparent.[6] Nail ridging (76% frequency) and pain (40% frequency) can also occur.[1] One-third of patients will present with exuberant granulation tissue,[4] oftentimes as a crescentic plaque of granulation tissue between the proximal and lateral nail folds (Figure 20.3).[5] This friable tissue can be visualized by gently elevating the proximal nail fold.[6]

In recent years, high-frequency ultrasound imaging has been utilized for the diagnosis of retronychia. Criteria for retronychia include the presence of more than two overlapping nail plates, decreased distance between the origin of the nail plates and the base of the distal phalanx (level of the distal interphalangeal joint compared with the contralateral digit), decreased echogenicity, and increased blood flow in the dermis of the posterior nail fold and proximal nail bed.[7,9] Ultrasound may also provide chronology to establish the date of the initial insult by comparing the nail plate length of new and old fragments with the normal growth rate established for the referenced digit.[7,9]

The differential diagnosis for retronychia is broad as it includes most other causes of chronic paronychia such as bacterial infection, candidiasis, inflammatory arthritis including psoriatic and rheumatoid arthritis, subungual tumors, and myxoid cysts.[5]

Early in the disease course, the patient may present simply with a paronychia, with marked swelling and inflammation of the proximal nail fold (Figure 20.4). Palpably, the proximal nail fold feels hard (representing the multiple nail plate layers) and demonstrates tenderness. At this earliest stage, the nail plate has not penetrated the proximal nail fold's ventral surface but is applying pressure. As the inflammation and foreign-body reaction progresses, the nail unit demonstrates more typical features

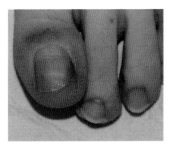

FIGURE 20.4 Retronychia of the left great toenail. Prominent xanthonychia is accompanied by paronychia presenting with erythema of the proximal and lateral nail folds. (Courtesy of Bianca Maria Piraccini, MD.)

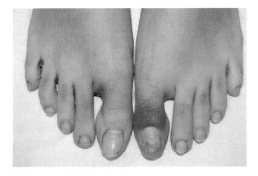

FIGURE 20.5 Absence of the left great toe nail plate shortly after proximal avulsion with resolving erythema of the proximal and lateral nail folds. (Courtesy of Bianca Maria Piraccini, MD.)

of ingrown nail (however, localized primarily to the proximal nail fold): granulation tissue; secondary infection; and increased pain, tenderness, and drainage.

20.3 Evidence-Based Treatment

Conservative treatment may be appropriate for mild retronychia.[1] This may include clipping back the onycholytic nail plate, treatment of concurrent nail infections, and moisturizer to the nail folds. Laird et al. reported partial improvement in 55% of patients. Further measures with topical steroids, orthesis, or taping have been described.[3,10–12] Exuberant granulation tissue may be managed with curettage and laser ablation but is oftentimes unsuccessful until the irritant (retronychia nail plate) has been addressed.[4]

Unless chronic paronychia with secondary acute infection ensues, antibiotics are unnecessary for the treatment of retronychia and should be avoided, especially in the absence of positive culture data. Up to 70% of cases may have been inadequately treated with oral antibiotics or oral antifungals.[3] Indeed, even inappropriate hospitalization for intravenous antibiotics for misdiagnosed osteomyelitis has occurred when retronychia was not appropriately diagnosed.[12]

Proximal nail plate avulsion remains the therapeutic procedure of choice (Figure 20.5). Proximal avulsion works best when the proximal margin of the uppermost nail plate is visible at the proximal nail fold.[4] When proximal ingrowing is painful, avulsion results in rapid pain relief.[5] Microscopic examination of the avulsed nail plate or histologic evaluation of the proximal nail fold is occasionally necessary to rule out an underlying neoplasm or concomitant fungal infection (including non-dermatophyte mold organisms). Ultrasound has also been used to rule out an inciting tumor.[9] While considered the treatment of choice, up to 16% of cases may recur after proximal avulsion.[10] Micronychia or pincer nail deformity may occur due to postoperative retraction[10] and 33% of patients may have permanent nail dystrophy according to Poveda-Montoyo et al.[12] Fortunately, the majority of patients have an uneventful recovery with nail plate regrowth (Figure 20.6).

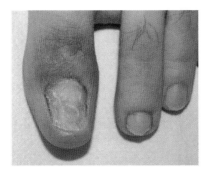

FIGURE 20.6 Regrowth of a nondystrophic nail plate after proximal nail plate avulsion without surrounding features of inflammation or paronychia. (Courtesy of Bianca Maria Piraccini, MD.)

TABLE 20.2

Treatments and Levels of Evidence

Treatment	Level of Evidence
Conservative Treatment	D[1]
Clipping back the onycholytic nail plate	D[1]
Topical steroids	D[3]
Orthesis	D[10]
Taping	E[12]
Curettage and laser ablation	E[4]
Antibiotics	E[12]
Surgical Treatment	
Proximal nail plate avulsion	E[4]

Anchor taping is integral to avoid formation of a distal nail fold and painful distal ingrowing during the recovery period after plate avulsion.[3] Indeed, loss of counterpressure from an absent nail plate may result in distal embedding or nail bed hyperkeratosis. This requires treatment with emollients, massage, taping, keratolytics, and rarely surgery to allow for appropriate adhesion of the newly growing nail plate.[5]

Opportunities for prevention are limited, as retronychia is oftentimes caused by repeat microtrauma, which is not easily avoidable in the passionate runner, hiker, athlete, or in anyone otherwise with predisposing biomechanics and high-risk activities. The importance of appropriate footwear should be stressed to patients and with relevant education, patients may be able to identify retronychia recurrence at the earliest onset. See further Table 20.2.

REFERENCES

1. Laird ME, Lo Sicco KI, Rich P. Conservative treatment of retronychia: A retrospective study of 25 patients. *Dermatol Surg.* 2018:1–13.
2. de Berker DAR, Renall JRS. Retronychia-proximal ingrowing nail. *J Eur Acad Dermat Venereol.* 1999;12:S126.
3. Ventura F, Correia O, Duarte AF, Barros AM, Haneke E. Retronychia—Clinical and pathophysiological aspects. *J Eur Acad Dermat Venereol.* 2016;30(1):16–19.
4. de Berker DA, Richert B, Duhard E, Piraccini BM, Andre J, Baran R. Retronychia: Proximal ingrowing of the nail plate. *J Eur Acad Dermat Venereol.* 2008;58(6):978–983.
5. Mello C, Souza M, Noriega LF, Chiacchio ND. Retronychia. *Anais brasileiros de dermatologia.* 2018;93(5):707–711.

6. Baumgartner M, Haneke E. Retronychia: diagnosis and treatment. *Dermatol Surg.* 2010;36(10):1610–1614.

7. Wortsman X, Wortsman J, Guerrero R, Soto R, Baran R. Anatomical changes in retronychia and onychomadesis detected using ultrasound. *Dermatol Surg.* 2010;36(10):1615–1620.

8. Braswell MA, Daniel CR 3rd, Brodell RT. Beau lines, onychomadesis, and retronychia: A unifying hypothesis. *J Am Acad Dermatol.* 2015;73(5):849–855.

9. Wortsman X, Calderon P, Baran R. Finger retronychias detected early by 3D ultrasound examination. *J Eur Acad Dermat Venereol.* 2012;26(2):254–256.

10. Gerard E, Prevezas C, Doutre MS, Beylot-Barry M, Cogrel O. Risk factors, clinical variants and therapeutic outcome of retronychia: A retrospective study of 18 patients. *Eur J Dermatol.* 2016;26(4):377–381.

11. Piraccini BM, Richert B, de Berker DA et al. Retronychia in children, adolescents, and young adults: A case series. *J Am Acad Dermatol.* 2014;70(2):388–390.

12. Poveda-Montoyo I, Vergara-de Caso E, Romero-Perez D, Betlloch-Mas I. Retronychia a little-known cause of paronychia: A report of two cases in adolescent patients. *Pediatr Dermatol.* 2018;35(3):e144–e146.

21

Squamous Cell Carcinoma

Adriana Guadalupe Peña-Romero and Judith Dominguez-Cherit

21.1 Introduction

Squamous cell carcinoma of the nail unit (SCCnu) is the most common malignant tumor of the nail unit. It has a male predominance (sex ratio 2:1). Location is predominant in fingers, mainly the thumb and index. This could be due the more frequent exposure of the hands to trauma and oncogenic agents. It occurs most commonly in the fifth decade of life. They are usually single lesions, but polydactylous involvement has also been reported. Risk factors for SCCnu include trauma; immunosuppression; chronic paronychia; oral exposure to arsenic or pesticides; ionizing radiation exposure; dyskeratosis congenita; and infection with HPV subtypes 2, 11, 18, 26, 31, 34, 35, 52, 56, 58, 73, and especially type 16 (in 60%–80% of cases). Previous studies have shown that some *Candida* species produce carcinogenic nitrosamine compounds, thus chronic candida infection has also been proposed as a risk factor for SCCnu.

SCCnu has nonspecific clinical features and is often misdiagnosed leading to an average delay of 4 years for definitive treatment. The spectrum of the clinical features includes onycholysis, leukonychia, subungual and periungual hyperkeratosis, trachyonychia, subungual tumor, longitudinal melanonychia, and erythronychia (Figure 21.1). The warty type is one of the most common clinical types and is associated with longitudinal melanonychia in 11.8% of cases (Figure 21.1c,d). Bony invasion is observed in approximately 20% of cases SCCnu. Lymph nodal involvement is rare, occurring in 2% of patients. Metastases due to SCCnu are extremely rare; there are less than 10 cases reported in the worldwide literature.

Differential diagnosis includes viral warts, onychomycosis, benign tumors (pyogenic granuloma, subungual exostosis, fibrokeratoma, onychopapilloma, and onychomatricoma), subungual keratoacanthoma, paronychia, melanoma, and posttraumatic dystrophy.

21.2 How to Confirm the Diagnosis

Accurate diagnosis is made by surgical biopsy. The histological features are irregularly thickened and disorganized epithelium with impaired maturation; atypical keratinocytes with large, irregularly shaped nuclei; and scattered mitotic figures. The depth of invasion (distance from the basal layer to the deepest carcinoma cell) should be measured, and histological changes related to HPV should be reported. Depth of invasion and histopathologic signs of human papilloma virus infection are related with an unfavorable prognosis.

Radiography and computed tomography (CT) show SCCnu as a crescent-shaped soft tissue mass with invasive osteolytic defect of the affected phalanx without periosteal reaction. Radiography of the finger is recommended in all cases. Ultrasonography (US) shows a heterogeneous hypoechoic focal mass with irregular contours and posterior acoustic enhancement; erosions of the bone may be seen with tumor infiltration of adjacent tissue. In examination with color Doppler, the tumor shows low-resistance pulsatile flow both at the center and periphery. Magnetic resonance imaging (MRI) is superior to other radiologic imaging methods for soft tissue masses and should be performed in doubtful cases. The tumor shows homogeneous hypointensity on T1-weighted images, intermediate signal intensity on T2-weighted images, and heterogeneous enhancement after contrast material administration. Increased intramedullary signal intensity can be seen due to marrow edema, which may be secondary to reactive change, direct

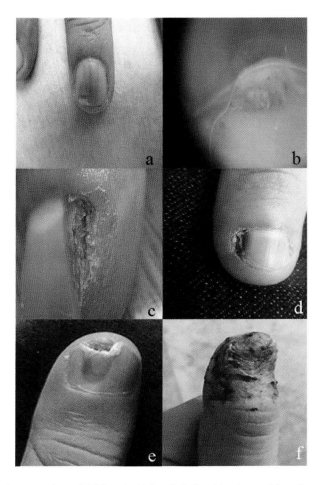

FIGURE 21.1 Clinical presentations of SCCnu: (a, b) Onycholysis with subungual hyperkeratosis, (c, d) periungual hyperkeratosis with longitudinal melanonychia. (e) SCCnu in the thumb, (f) 10 days post–en bloc nail excision with full-thickness skin graft.

tumor invasion, or combined infection and other factors. The distinction between tumor infiltration and other causes of marrow edema in the underlying bone can be difficult with radiologic imaging. Therefore, when marrow edema is present without definite bone erosion or destruction, it is important to consider the possibility of minimal invasion. In our experience and in case of doubt of bone invasion, a bone biopsy during the whole nail apparatus excision is done.

Onychoscopy can be useful for the diagnosis showing onycholysis, polymorphous vessels, hemorrhages, or white structures. In subungual SCC, intraoperative dermoscopic findings of structureless white areas, polymorphous vascular patterns, and yellow dots and scales strongly suggest subungual invasive SCC. Ex vivo fluorescence confocal microscopy (FCM) has shown a good correlation of malignant epithelial tumors with the observation of marked cytological and architectural atypia. Furthermore, this technique can be used intraoperatively to assess the surgical margins.

21.3 Evidence-Based Treatment

The treatment method depends on the extension of the tumor in or underneath the nail bed.[1] All treatment modalities with their evidence levels are listed in Table 21.1. First-line treatment of SCCnu is surgical resection.[2] Surgical treatments include limited surgical excision, Mohs micrographic surgery (MMS), en bloc excision of the nail unit with 4–6 mm margins, and digital amputation.[1–3,5–12] Limited surgical

TABLE 21.1

Treatments and Levels of Evidence

Tumor		Treatment	Recurrence Rates (%)	Evidence Level
Surgical Treatments				
Without evidence of bone invasion	Lateral cases involving <50% of the nail apparatus	Mohs micrographic surgery (MMS)	0%–22%	C[1,5,10,11]
		Limited surgical excision	56%	C[1]
	Medial invasive nail apparatus SCC or in lateral cases involving >50% of the nail apparatus	En bloc excision of the nail unit with 4–6 mm margins	4%	C[1,12]
With evidence of bone invasion or with involved inferior margin at pathological examination of the MMS or en bloc excision specimen		Digit amputation	5%	C[1]
Nonsurgical Treatments				
Imiquimod cream, fluorouracil 5% cream, curettage and cryosurgery and photodynamic therapy, radiation				E[4,6–9,14]

excision seems to have higher recurrence rates. Dalle et al. reported a recurrence rate of 56% in nine patients treated with limited surgical excision.[1,3] Reported recurrence rates of MMS range from 0% to 25%.[3,5,10,11] En bloc nail excision with full-thickness skin graft is an efficient method for SCCnu without bone involvement, with a recurrence rate of 4%. This technique consists of an en bloc wide excision of the nail unit including the lateral and proximal nail folds and the hyponychium. A proximal transverse incision is made from 3 to 5 mm beyond the interphalangeal joint at the base of the distal phalanx. This incision is prolonged laterally and distally to the hyponychium down to the bone with a margin from 4 to 5 mm beyond these structures. Then distal to proximal dissection of the nail bed is performed, directly down to the periosteum. Matricial horns are then destructed with electrocautery. A full-thickness skin graft is harvested from the internal aspect of the nondominant arm and inset over the wound with nonabsorbable nylon sutures (Figure 21.1e,f).[12,13] In case of doubt of bone invasion, we recommend a bone biopsy beforehand to place the graft in the wound. On the basis of our experience, to fenestrate and place a tie-over on the graft helps to improve the adherence of the graft on the wound.

Digit amputation is recommended if bone invasion is evidenced by x-ray, MRI, or bone biopsy, or in tumors involving inferior margin at pathological examination in MMS or en bloc excision specimen.[1] Sentinel lymph node biopsy is not recommended since axillary lymph node involvement and metastases are rare.[13]

Other nonsurgical treatments that have been proposed are imiquimod cream, curettage with or without fluorouracil 5% cream, curettage and cryosurgery, bleopuncture, and photodynamic therapy.[6–9,14] Radiation can be used in unresectable lesions after pathological confirmation.[4,13] Most recurrences occur during the first 3 years. Therefore, follow-up twice a year during the first year, then once a year for the following 2 years is recommended.[12]

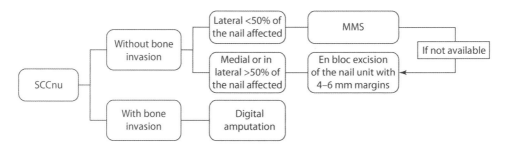

FIGURE 21.2 Treatment algorithm for SCCnu.

In conclusion, for tumors without bone invasion: if the lesion is lateral and involves less than 50% of the nail apparatus, MMS is the first-line therapy; if MMS is not available, in medial lesions or in lateral cases involving more than 50% of the nail apparatus en bloc excision of the nail unit with 4–6 mm margins should be done. Limited surgical excision is not recommended due its high recurrence rate. Tumors with bone invasion should be treated with digital amputation (Figure 21.2, Table 21.1).

REFERENCES

1. Dalle S, Depape L, Phan A, Balme B, Ronger-Savle S, Thomas L. Squamous cell carcinoma of the nail apparatus: Clinicopathological study of 35 cases. *Br J Dermatol*. 2007 May;156:871–874.
2. Lecerf P, Richert B, Theunis A, André J. A retrospective study of squamous cell carcinoma of the nail unit diagnosed in a Belgian general hospital over a 15-year period. *J Am Acad Dermatol*. 2013;69:253–261.
3. Lee TM, Jo G, Kim M et al. Squamous cell carcinoma of the nail unit: A retrospective review of 19 cases in Asia and comparative review of Western literature. *Int J Dermatol*. 2018 November 27 [Epub].
4. Yu NY, Sanghvi P. Nonmelanoma subungual malignancies: A case-based review of radiation therapy. *Pract Radiat Oncol*. 2016;6:126–128.
5. Dika E, Piraccini BM, Balestri R et al. Mohs surgery for squamous cell carcinoma of the nail: Report of 15 cases. Our experience and a long-term follow-up. *Br J Dermatol*. 2012 December;167(6):1310–1314.
6. Laffitte E, Saurat J-H. Recurrent Bowen's disease of the nail: Treatment by topical imiquimod (Aldara). *Ann Dermatol Venereol*. 2003;130:211–213.
7. Sturm HM. Bowen's disease and 5-fluorouracil. *J Am Acad Dermatol*. 1979;1:513–522.
8. Tan B, Sinclair R, Foley P. Photodynamic therapy for subungual Bowen's disease. *Australas J Dermatol*. 2004;45:172–174.
9. Usmani N, Stables GI, Telfer NR, Stringer MR. Subungual Bowen's disease treated by topical aminolevulinic acidphotodynamic therapy. *J Am Acad Dermatol*. 2005;53:S273–S276.
10. Young LC, Tuxen AJ, Goodman G. Mohs' micrographic surgery as treatment for squamous dysplasia of the nail unit. *Australas J Dermatol*. 2012;53:123–127.
11. Dika E, Fanti PA, Patrizi A, Misciali C, Vaccari S, Piraccini BM. Mohs surgery for squamous cell carcinoma of the nail unit: 10 years of experience. *Dermatol Surg*. 2015;41:1015–1019.
12. Topin-Ruiz S, Surinach C, Dalle S, Duru G, Balme B, Thomas L. Surgical treatment of subungual squamous cell carcinoma by wide excision of the nail unit and skin graft reconstruction: An evaluation of treatment efficiency and outcomes. *JAMA Dermatol*. 2017;153:442–448.
13. Inkaya E, Sayit E, Sayit AT, Zan E, Bakirtas M. Subungual squamous cell carcinoma of the third finger with radiologic and histopathologic findings: A report of case. *J Hand Microsurg*. 2015;7:194–198.
14. Nordin P, Stenquist BC. Aggressive curettage-cryosurgery for human papillomavirus-16 associated subungual squamous cell carcinoma in situ. *J Cutan Aesthet Surg*. 2013;6:155–157.

22

Subungual Exostosis

Leandro Fonseca Noriega

22.1 Introduction

Subungual exostosis (SE) is a relatively uncommon benign osteocartilaginous tumor.[1–4] Trauma, chronic irritation, and chronic infection may be implicated in some cases, but the pathogenesis remains unknown.[2,5] It usually occurs in adolescents and young adults, with the female:male ratio being approximately equal. Toes are most commonly affected, especially the hallux.[1–3,6]

The suggestive clinical presentation is a slow growth, painful, pink or flesh-colored, hard nodule on the dorsal tip of the terminal phalanx, with an epidermal collarette and hyperkeratotic smooth surface. It often elevates the nail plate, and the overlying nail can become brittle, with or without onycholysis (Figure 22.1a).[4,5,7–9] A porcelain white hue with telangiectasia may be observed (Figure 22.1b).[10]

Conditions to be considered in the differential diagnosis are subungual wart, onychoclavus, ingrown toenail, osteochondroma, osteosarcoma, chondrosarcoma, epidermoid cyst, pyogenic granuloma, acquired digital fibrokeratoma, glomus tumor, squamous cell carcinoma, keratoacanthoma, and amelanotic melanoma.[1,4,5]

22.2 How to Confirm the Diagnosis

Imaging tests are very helpful to the diagnostic investigation, in which radiography is paramount. X-ray suggests the diagnosis by demonstrating an exophytic bony growth (composed of trabecular bone) on the distal phalanx, protruding from its dorsal or dorsomedial region (Figure 22.2).[2,5,8,9,11] The same findings, in more detail, can be observed in computed tomography. Ultrasonography shows a heterogeneously hyperechoic lesion with well-defined margins and a hypoechoic fibrocartilaginous cap.[12] Magnetic resonance imaging can be used for preoperative assessment because is the best radiologic modality for depicting the effect of SE on surrounding tissues. An hypointense fibrocartilaginous cap (all imaging sequences) allows to differentiate the SE from the osteochondroma (hyaline cartilage cap, high signal intensity on T2-weighted images).[11,12]

Histological examination confirms the diagnosis, differentiating from other osseous tumors. SE is characterized by a trabecular bone covered by a fibrocartilaginous cap.[1,4,5]

22.3 Evidence-Based Treatments

Complete surgical resection is the treatment of choice. However, there are several surgical techniques described.[1,2,4,6,13] Lesion topography and the preservation or destruction of the nail bed may influence the choice of surgery procedure. Usually the longitudinal fish-mouth-type incision was described for cases when the lesion does not destroy the nail bed (Figure 22.3a), whereas if the SE destroys the nail bed, then a direct dorsal approach is preferable (Figure 22.3b).[6,13]

General anesthesia may be considered for children, whereas digital block is commonly used in adolescents and adults.[14] After surgery, a bupivacaine injection may be used to prolong the duration of anesthesia.[15]

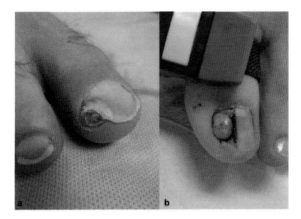

FIGURE 22.1   (a) Nodule on the dorsal tip of the terminal phalanx, with an epidermal collarette and hyperkeratotic smooth surface. SE elevates the nail plate and causes onycholysis. (b) A porcelain white hue with telangiectasia is observed after partial nail plate avulsion. (Courtesy Dr. Nilton Di Chiacchio.)

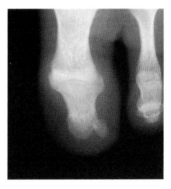

FIGURE 22.2   X-ray—Exophytic bony growth on the distal phalanx.

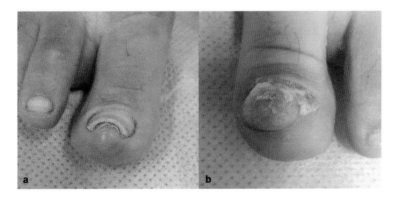

FIGURE 22.3   (a) SE does not destroy the nail bed and hyponychium. (b) Destruction of the nail bed.

The key points of treatment are:

1. Excision of the entire lesion including the fibrocartilaginous cap: Fundamental to reduce the recurrence rate (varies between 10% and 20%).[4,6,13]
2. Preservation of the nail matrix: Crucial to avoid nail deformity/onychodystrophy, which is the most prevalent complication (16%).[6,11]

Surgical techniques include the following:

- Nail plate preservation or removal followed by a longitudinal fish-mouth-type incision. Lift the nail bed and remove the tumor. Healing by first intention (Figure 22.4).[11,13]
- Partial nail plate removal followed by L-shaped incision (longitudinal on the nail bed and transverse on the tip). SE is excised with the pedicle from the distal phalanx. The nail bed is carefully repaired using a 6-0 absorbable suture, and the excised nail is fixed onto its bed.[14]
- Partial or total nail plate removal followed by complete tumor excision—directly from the dorsal surface—by rasparator, bone rongeur, nail nippers, and curettage; or bone rongeur and curettage.[4,13,15] Postoperative wound closure strategies described for this surgical approach:
  - Healing by second intention (Figure 22.5)[4,13,15]
  - Artificial skin (collagen matrix substitute dermis)—if the defect is larger than 5 mm[13]
  - Vacuum-assisted closure dressing for 12 days[2]
  - An in situ thin split-thickness graft that is harvested from the midportion of the adjacent nail bed (thickest part); suture with 6-0 vicryl[16]
  - Healing by first intention (Figure 22.6)[7]
- Remove the nail plate and make an incision through the nail bed. The nail elevator is used to dissect the nail bed off the bony lesion. An osteotome is used to remove the exostosis. A fine rongeur is used to aid in removal of any residual lesion and to smooth the bony surface. The nail bed should then be approximated and repaired with a suture. The nail plate is replaced (physiological dressing).[17] See further Table 22.1.

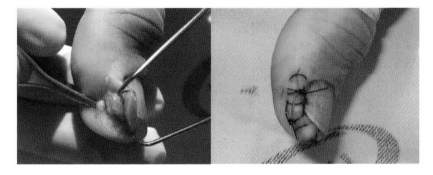

FIGURE 22.4 Longitudinal fish-mouth-type incision and primary wound closure. (Courtesy Dr. Nilton Di Chiacchio.)

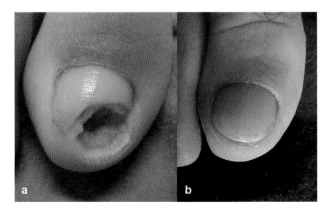

FIGURE 22.5 (a) Complete tumor excision (direct dorsal approach) and healing by second intention. (b) One year after the surgical procedure. (Courtesy Dr. Nilton Di Chiacchio.)

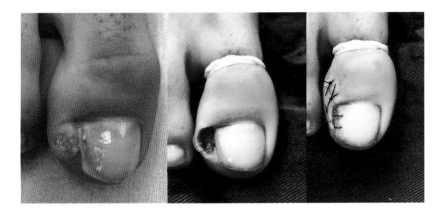

FIGURE 22.6 Complete tumor excision (direct dorsal approach) and healing by first intention. (Courtesy Dr. Letícia Valandro.)

TABLE 22.1

Treatments with Levels of Evidence

Surgical Treatment	Level of Evidence
Longitudinal fish-mouth-type incision	D[11–13]
L-shaped incision	D[14]
Partial or total nail plate removal followed by complete tumor excision	D[4–13–15]
• Healing by second intention	D[4–13–15]
• Artificial skin (collagen matrix substitute dermis)	E[13]
• Vacuum-assisted closure dressing	E[2]
• An in situ thin split-thickness graft	E[16]
• Healing by first intention	E[7]
Remove the nail plate and make an incision through the nail bed	E[17]

REFERENCES

1. Russell JD, Nance K, Nunley JR, Maher IA. Subungual exostosis. *Cutis.* 2016;98(2):128–129.
2. DaCambra MP, Gupta SK, Ferri-de-Barros F. A novel management strategy for subungual exostosis. *BMJ Case Rep.* 2013;2013. pii: bcr2013200396.
3. Piccolo V, Argenziano G, Alessandrini AM, Russo T, Starace M, Piraccini BM. Dermoscopy of subungual exostosis: A retrospective study of 10 patients. *Dermatology.* 2017;233(1):80–85.
4. Wollina U, Baran R, Schönlebe J. Dystrophy of the great toenail by subungual exostosis and hyperostosis: Three case reports with different clinical presentations. *Skin Appendage Disord.* 2016;1(4):213–216.
5. Demirdag HG, Tugrul Ayanoglu B, Akay BN. Dermoscopic features of subungual exostosis. *Australas J Dermatol.* 2018;60(2):e1380–e141.
6. DaCambra MP, Gupta SK, Ferri-de-Barros F. Subungual exostosis of the toes: A systematic review. *Clin Orthop Relat Res.* 2014;472(4):1251–1259.
7. Haneke E. Nail surgery. *Clin Dermatol.* 2013;31(5):516–525.
8. Calligaris L, Berti I. Subungual exostosis. *J Pediatr.* 2014;165(2):412.
9. Miguel-Gómez L, Fonda-Pascual P, Vañó-Galván S, Jaen-Olasolo P. [Subungual exostosis]. *An Pediatr (Barc).* 2015;82(6):443–444.
10. Richert B, André J. Nail disorders in children: Diagnosis and management. *Am J Clin Dermatol.* 2011;12(2):101–112.
11. Higuchi K, Oiso N, Yoshida M, Kawada A. Preoperative assessment using magnetic resonance imaging for subungual exostosis beneath the proximal region of the nail plate. *Case Rep Dermatol.* 2011;3(2):155–157.

12. Baek HJ, Lee SJ, Cho KH et al. Subungual tumors: Clinicopathologic correlation with US and MR imaging findings. *Radiographics.* 2010;30(6):1621–1636.
13. Suga H, Mukouda M. Subungual exostosis: A review of 16 cases focusing on postoperative deformity of the nail. *Ann Plast Surg.* 2005;55(3):272–275.
14. Malkoc M, Korkmaz O, Keskinbora M, Seker A, Oltulu I, Bulbul AM, Say F, Cakir A. Surgical treatment of nail bed subungual exostosis. *Singapore Med J.* 2016;57(11):630–633.
15. Göktay F, Atış G, Güneş P, Macit B, Çelik NS, Gürdal Kösem E. Subungual exostosis and subungual osteochondromas: A description of 25 cases. *Int J Dermatol.* 2018;57(7):872–881.
16. Choi CM, Cho HR, Lew BL, Sim WY. Subungual exostosis treated with an in situ thin split-thickness toenail bed graft. *Dermatol Ther.* 2011;24(4):452–454.
17. Starnes A, Crosby K, Rowe DJ, Bordeaux JS. Subungual exostosis: A simple surgical technique. *Dermatol Surg.* 2012;38(2):258–260.

23

Trachyonychia

Jacob Griggs, Brandon Burroway, and Antonella Tosti

23.1 Introduction

Trachyonychia, also called twenty-nail dystrophy and sandpaper nails, is a disorder characterized by thin, rough, brittle nails with excessive longitudinal ridging.[1] The name twenty-nail dystrophy is misleading, as not all nails need to be affected in trachyonychia, and other nail disorders that can affect all 20 nails are sometimes misidentified as twenty-nail dystrophy (Figure 23.1). The pediatric population is most frequently affected, with a peak age of onset between 3 and 12 years old.[2] Trachyonychia can occur in association with alopecia areata, where it is usually seen in children with severe disease, or it can be idiopathic.[2,3]

In trachyonychia, any number of nails can be affected, and severity can be variable between different nails. There are two main varieties of clinical features: opaque and shiny.[4] The opaque variety is considered more severe and is characterized by brittle nails that are thin and rough with longitudinal ridging, often described as having a "sandpaper-like" appearance (Figure 23.2). Onychoschizia, or nail splitting, is frequently present. The shiny variety is considered a milder presentation.[1] The nails keep their luster and demonstrate many small geometric pits arranged longitudinally. The shiny variety nails are not as thin and fragile as the opaque variety. Both varieties frequently exhibit superficial scaling of the nail plate as well as hyperkeratosis of the cuticles and koilonychia (Figure 23.3).

The cause of trachyonychia is thought to be inflammation of the nail matrix.[5] Mild and intermittent inflammation may result in localized damage, allowing the nails to maintain their luster as seen in the shiny variety, whereas severe and persistent inflammation causes diffuse nail damage resulting in the opaque variety. Trachyonychia has been reported to be hereditary in some cases, which suggests a genetic component to the disease.[2] Table 23.1 shows a differential diagnosis of trachyonychia.[1]

23.2 How to Confirm the Diagnosis

Trachyonychia can be diagnosed clinically; there is no need for a nail biopsy.[1] The disease is nonscarring even when due to lichen planus; thus, there is no reason to subject the patient to a nail matrix punch or longitudinal nail biopsy, both of which can cause scarring.

23.3 Evidence-Based Treatment

23.3.1 Treatment Overview

Trachyonychia is a nonscarring disease process that usually causes only cosmetic symptoms and has been reported to resolve regardless of treatment type in a high proportion of cases when given sufficient time (often several months to years).[8,9] Thus, the best treatment is often reassurance and expectant management. If patients or their parents are significantly bothered by the symptoms and request treatment, a number of options can be attempted.

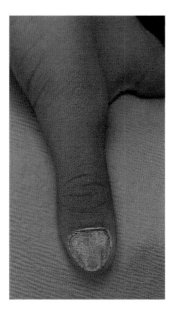

FIGURE 23.1   Opaque trachyonychia affecting the first digit.

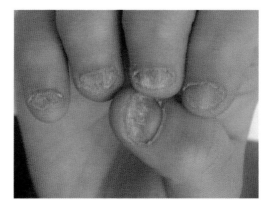

FIGURE 23.2   Trachyonychia with associated hyperkeratosis of the cuticles and koilonychia.

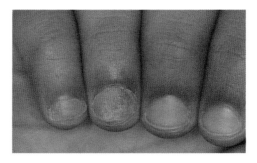

FIGURE 23.3   Trachyonychia only affecting the fourth and fifth digits.

TABLE 23.1

Differential Diagnosis of Trachyonychia

Diagnosis	Distinguishing Features
Brittle nails	Longitudinal ridging and superficial splitting, but without rough texture or excessive ridging seen in trachyonychia.
Lichen planus	Longitudinal fissures and pterygium.[6]
Nail psoriasis	Large, deep, irregularly distributed pits. Distinct from superficial, small, regular pits seen in shiny trachyonychia. Nails also exhibit onycholysis, nail bed discoloration, spots, subungual keratosis, and splinter hemorrhages.[7]
Senile nails	Only mild longitudinal ridging and does not involve the entire nail plate.

To this point, no randomized control trials have been attempted to identify the best treatment for trachyonychia, and no gold standard, evidence-based treatment approach exists. A summary of reported treatment options can be seen in Table 23.2.

23.3.2 Topical

The most conservative approaches to treatment include mild emollients and nail polish, which can help hide signs of the disease.[10] Outside of these measures, topical treatments represent a good first line of medications especially in cases of idiopathic trachyonychia.

A number of case reports and case series have reported some success in using petroleum jelly;[9] corticosteroids;[9,11] tazarotene gel;[12] 5% 5-fluorouracil cream;[13] psoralen plus ultraviolet A (PUVA);[14]

TABLE 23.2

Treatments and Levels of Evidence

Treatment	Study Type (Quality Level)
Topical	
Topical calcipotriol and betamethasone dipropionate	B[16]
Topical corticosteroids (fluocinonide, triamcinolone, clobetasol)	D[9,11]
Topical tazarotene 0.1% gel	E[12]
Topical 5% 5-fluorouracil cream	E[13]
Psoralen plus ultraviolet A (PUVA)	E[14]
Nail plate dressings of ultrathin adhesive bandages with lactic acid, silicon dioxide, aluminum acetylacetonate, copolymer of vinyl acetate with acrylic acid, and azelaic acid	E[15]
Topical petroleum jelly	E[9]
Systemic	
Alitretinoin	B[29]
Cyclosporine	C[26–28]
Tofacitinib citrate	E[20,21]
Biotin	E[25]
Oral prednisolone	E[17]
Mini-pulse betamethasone	E[18]
Chloroquine phosphate	E[19]
Acitretin	E[22–24]
Injections	
Intralesional injections of triamcinolone acetonide	C[30,31,33]
Intralesional injection of triamcinolone and hydrocortisone with oral griseofulvin	E[32]

and nail plate dressings of ultra-thin adhesive bandages with lactic acid, silicon dioxide, aluminum acetylacetonate, copolymer of vinyl acetate with acrylic acid, and azelaic acid.[15] In addition, one case report described increased success of topical steroid treatment by occluding clobetasol propionate ointment with paper tape, which is suggested to help ensure absorption by the nail matrix, the site of the inflammation in trachyonychia.[11]

A larger-scale, prospective, open-label trial with 39 patients and a total of 432 affected nails reported success with the use of a combination of calcipotriol and betamethasone ointment applied to the proximal nail fold.[16] After 6 months, 94.4% of nails showed some improvement with 4.2% showing complete recovery.[16] The side effects of these medications were mild including one patient with mild erythema and one patient with pruritus, both of which were self-limited. Dosages of medications were not reported in the study, and there was no control group.[16]

23.3.3 Systemic

Systemic treatments are best utilized when trachyonychia is associated with another disorder such as lichen planus or psoriasis. Recurrences are common when the treatment is discontinued.

Oral steroids including 4 weeks of prednisolone taper[17] and 2 months of mini-pulse betamethasone[18] have had reported success in one patient each. In the authors' personal experience, pulse intramuscular triamcinolone acetonide (0.5 mg/kg every 30 days) can be useful in cases of severe trachyonychia in adults.

Chloroquine phosphate 250 mg used twice daily in one patient also showed success after 10 weeks of therapy, but recurrence occurred after treatment was discontinued.[19]

Tofacitinib citrate at a dose of 10–15 mg daily allowed for improvement after 5–6 months in three patients with trachyonychia with concomitant alopecia areata universalis, two of whom also experienced improved hair growth.[20] An additional case reports a patient with trachyonychia and alopecia areata universalis who received 10 mg tofacitinib daily with improvement in nails and hair growth within 10 months.[21] Tofacitinib use has not been reported in trachyonychia without concomitant alopecia areata.

Acitretin has shown success after 2–6 months of using between 0.3 and 0.5 mg/kg/day to treat trachyonychia associated with lichen planus and psoriasis in three case reports.[22–24]

Biotin 2.5 mg daily for 6 months resulted in nail improvement in two pediatric patients.[25] Patients exhibited a reduction in longitudinal ridging, thinning, and distal notching, with no observed adverse events.

Cyclosporine showed improvement in five patients with comorbid psoriasis after 2–3 months of treatment with 3 mg/kg/day.[26] In another retrospective study, cyclosporine (2–3.5 mg/kg/day) was used in 15 patients that all showed at least slight improvement after one month of treatment.[27] Thirteen of these 15 patients (87%) had significant improvement and 2 (13%) showed complete recovery after completing 6 months of treatment.[27] After 6 months, dosage was decreased to 1.5 mg/kg/day until complete recovery or treatment cessation.[27] Pruritus and pain secondary to trachyonychia significantly improved, and no side effects such as hypertension, gastrointestinal irritation, or elevated creatinine were reported.[27]

In addition, cyclosporine was studied in combination with a pantothenic acid complex-based dietary supplement (Pantogar®).[28] In this retrospective study, 38 patients taking both the supplement and 3–5 mg/kg/day of cyclosporine were compared to control patients taking only the supplement. After a mean treatment length of 16.75 months, about 13% of patients taking both the supplement and cyclosporine showed greater than 75% improvement.[28]

Alitretinoin showed success in an open-label, prospective study of 21 patients and 210 nails affected by idiopathic trachyonychia.[29] All patients were refractory to at least one previous treatment and the length of their disease process exceeded that of spontaneous resolution. After 1 month and 3 months, about 74% and 98% of nails, respectively, showed some improvement. Eight of the 12 patients that remained in the study for 6 months demonstrated at least 90% recovery. No nails were disease free after 1 month, but upon further treatment, about 69% were disease free after 6 months. Headache was the most common side effect reported in the study, occurring in 6 of 21 patients and forcing 2 of 21 to withdraw from the study. Other side effects included flushing (2/21), dry eyes (1/21), and high cost, which caused 5 patients to withdraw from the study. Recurrence was common, occurring in 5 of 9 patients studied at a mean of 6 months after treatment cessation.[29]

23.3.4 Injections

Intralesional injections should generally be avoided, especially in pediatric patients, due to the pain associated with the procedure that leads to low compliance as well as insufficient evidence to show its superiority over other treatments. In addition, the high relapse rates indicate that it is likely only a temporary solution.[30] Topical anesthetics are used in some methods[31] and withheld in others.[30] The largest-scale study using the method described using a 26-gauge needle and injecting the steroid into the proximal nail fold.[30]

Nail unit steroid injections of triamcinolone acetonide have been described in a number of studies.[30,31,33] Dosing schedule of triamcinolone varied between studies and included 2.5–10 mg/mL single injection,[31] 5 mg/mL monthly,[30] and 10 mg/mL twice a week.[33] In a study of 19 patients with trachyonychia who completed 6 months of treatment with monthly intralesional injections of 5 mg/mL (0.1–0.2 mL) of triamcinolone acetonide, 11 of the patients showed at least 75% improvement.[30] Relapse occurred in about 62% of patients within 6 months, but relapse was also responsive to treatment. Side effects of treatment included pain (36%), proximal nail fold atrophy (24%), subungual hematoma (20%), and vasovagal syncope (4%).[30] In a case report, a patient suffered mild atrophy and telangiectasias of the proximal nail fold as well as a subungual hematoma as side effects to nail unit steroid injections.[33]

REFERENCES

1. Jacobsen AA, Tosti A. Trachyonychia and twenty-nail dystrophy: A comprehensive review and discussion of diagnostic accuracy. *Ski Appendage Disord*. 2016;2(1–2):7–13.
2. Haber JS, Chairatchaneeboon M, Rubin AI. Trachyonychia: Review and update on clinical aspects, histology, and therapy. *Ski Appendage Disord*. 2017;2(3–4):109–115.
3. Tosti A, Fanti PA, Morelli R, Bardazzi F. Trachyonychia associated with alopecia areata: A clinical and pathologic study. *J Am Acad Dermatol*. 1991;25(2 Pt 1):266–270.
4. Baran R, Dupré A, Christol B, Bonafé JL, Sayag J, Ferrère J. [Vertical striated sand-papered twenty-nail dystrophy (author's transl)]. *Ann Dermatol Venereol*. 1978;105(4):387–392.
5. Tosti A, Bardazzi F, Piraccini BM, Fanti PA. Idiopathic trachyonychia (twenty-nail dystrophy): A pathological study of 23 patients. *Br J Dermatol*. 1994;131(6):866–872.
6. Tosti A, Ghetti E, Piraccini BM, Fanti PA. Lichen planus of the nails and fingertips. *Eur J Dermatol*. 1998;8(6):447–448.
7. Reich K. Approach to managing patients with nail psoriasis. *J Eur Acad Dermatology Venereol*. 2009;23:15–21.
8. Sakata S, Howard A, Tosti A, Sinclair R. Follow up of 12 patients with trachyonychia. *Australas J Dermatol*. 2006;47(3):166–168.
9. Kumar MG, Ciliberto H, Bayliss SJ. Long-term follow-up of pediatric trachyonychia. *Pediatr Dermatol*. 2015;32(2):198–200.
10. Tosti A, Piraccini BM, Iorizzo M. Trachyonychia and related disorders: Evaluation and treatment plans. *Dermatol Ther*. 2002;15(2):121–125.
11. Sakiyama T, Chaya A, Shimizu T, Ebihara T, Saito M. Spongiotic trachyonychia treated with topical corticosteroids using the paper tape occlusion method. *Ski Appendage Disord*. 2016;2(1–2):49–51.
12. Soda R, Diluvio L, Bianchi L, Chimenti S. Treatment of trachyonychia with tazarotene. *Clin Exp Dermatol*. 2005;30(3):301–302.
13. Schissel DJ, Elston DM. Topical 5-fluorouracil treatment for psoriatic trachyonychia. *Cutis*. 1998;62(1):27–28.
14. Halkier-Sørensen L, Cramers M, Kragballe K. Twenty-nail dystrophy treated with topical PUVA. *Acta Derm Venereol*. 1990;70(6):510–511.
15. Arias-Santiago S, Fernández-Pugnaire MA, Husein El-Ahmed H, Girón-Prieto MS, Naranjo Sintes R. A 9 year-old child with trachyonychia: A good response with nail plate dressings. *An Pediatr (Barc)*. 2009;71(5):476–477.
16. Park J-M, Cho H-H, Kim W-J et al. Efficacy and safety of calcipotriol/betamethasone dipropionate ointment for the treatment of trachyonychia: An open-label study. *Ann Dermatol*. 2015;27(4):371–375.
17. Evans A V, Roest MA, Fletcher CL, Lister R, Hay RJ. Isolated lichen planus of the toe nails treated with oral prednisolone. *Clin Exp Dermatol*. 2001;26(5):412–414.

18. Mittal R, Khaitan BK, Sirka CS. Trachyonychia treated with oral mini pulse therapy. *Indian J Dermatol Venereol Leprol.* 2001;67(4):202–203.
19. Mostafa WZ. Lichen planus of the nail: Treatment with antimalarials. *J Am Acad Dermatol.* 1989;20(2 Pt 1):289–290.
20. Dhayalan A, King BA. Tofacitinib citrate for the treatment of nail dystrophy associated with alopecia universalis. *JAMA Dermatology.* 2016;152(4):492–493.
21. Ferreira SB, Scheinberg M, Steiner D, Steiner T, Bedin GL, Ferreira RB. Remarkable improvement of nail changes in alopecia areata universalis with 10 months of treatment with tofacitinib: A case report. *Case Rep Dermatol.* 2016;8(3):262–266.
22. Kolbach-Rengifo M, Navajas-Galimany L, Araneda-Castiglioni D, Reyes-Vivanco C. Efficacy of acitretin and topical clobetasol in trachyonychia involving all twenty nails. *Indian J Dermatol Venereol Leprol.* 2016;82(6):732–734.
23. Tosti A, Bellavista S, Iorizzo M, Vincenzi C. Occupational trachyonychia due to psoriasis: Report of a case successfully treated with oral acitretin. *Contact Dermatitis.* 2006;54(2):123–124.
24. Brazzelli V, Martinoli S, Prestinari F, Borroni G. An impressive therapeutic result of nail psoriasis to acitretin. *J Eur Acad Dermatology Venereol.* 2004;18(2):229–230.
25. Möhrenschlager M, Schmidt T, Ring J, Abeck D. Recalcitrant trachyonychia of childhood—Response to daily oral biotin supplementation: Report of two cases. *J Dermatolog Treat.* 2000;11(2):113–115.
26. Piérard GE, Piérard-Franchimont C. Dynamics of psoriatic trachyonychia during low-dose cyclosporin a treatment: A pilot study on onychochronobiology using optical profilometry. *Dermatology.* 1996;192(2):116–119.
27. Lee YB, Cheon MS, Eun YS, Cho BK, Park YG, Park HJ. Cyclosporin administration improves clinical manifestations and quality of life in patients with 20-nail dystrophy: Case series and survey study. *J Dermatol.* 2012;39(12):1064–1065.
28. Oh SJ, Kim JE, Ko JY, Ro YS. Therapeutic efficacy of combination therapy using oral cyclosporine with a dietary supplement (Pantogar®) in twenty-nail dystrophy. *Ann Dermatol.* 2017;29(5):608–613.
29. Shin K, Kim T-W, Park S-M et al. Alitretinoin can be a good treatment option for idiopathic recalcitrant trachyonychia in adults: An open-label study. *J Eur Acad Dermatology Venereol.* 2018;32(10):1810–1814.
30. Grover C, Bansal S, Nanda S, Reddy BSN. Efficacy of triamcinolone acetonide in various acquired nail dystrophies. *J Dermatol.* 2005;32(12):963–968.
31. Khoo BP, Giam YC. A pilot study on the role of intralesional triamcinolone acetonide in the treatment of pitted nails in children. *Singapore Med J.* 2000;41(2):66–68.
32. Sehgal VN, Sharma S, Khandpur S. Twenty-nail dystrophy originating from lichen planus. *Skinmed.* 2005;4(1):58–59.
33. Khandpur S, Reddy BS. An association of twenty-nail dystrophy with vitiligo. *J Dermatol.* 2001;28(1):38–42.

24

Transverse Overcurvature

Tracey C. Vlahovic

24.1 Introduction

Transverse overcurvature of the nail describes a deformity where the nail bed progressively pinches distally. Described by Cornelius and Shelley, a pincer nail (also known as a trumpet nail) is a result of transverse distal overcurvature.[1] This may occur in both toenails and fingernails; however, the great toenails are more commonly affected.[2] The pathophysiology of the pincer nail has not been established. Pincer nails may cause pain during ambulation, wearing shoes, application of light touch, and be cosmetically displeasing to the patient. It is important to distinguish that pincer nails and ingrown nails are not derived from the same pathology, as ingrown nails describe the symptoms of pain and discomfort produced at the nail distally, whereas pincer nails are a distinct morphological entity. Like pincer nails, ingrown nails contain a distal incurvated nail edge, but this symptomatic state is often attributed to improper nail trimming, heredity/the overall shape of the digit, biomechanical deformities such as bunion and hammertoe deformities, and physical forces from ill-fitting shoes.

Although toenails protect the distal phalanx and contribute to pedal biomechanics during ambulation, they are constantly subject to physical forces from the shoe and the gait cycle itself. The biomechanical forces on the toenail are unique and can be pathologic if the forces become excessive or misaligned. Mechanobiology is described as the way "physical forces and changes in cell or tissue mechanics contribute to development, physiology, and disease."[3,4] Toenails are consistently subject to physical forces from shoes and ground reaction forces from gait. The combination of these forces is a little described, often missed area of research that could explain the development of various nail deformities on the lower extremity. Sano and Ogawa hypothesized that toenails have an automatic curvature function that allows them to adapt to the ground reaction forces pushing them upward with each step.[4] For most people, the daily upward force exerted from the ground (ground reaction force) and the automatic curvature force are in balance; thus, giving the toenail its characteristic curve. They hypothesize that nail pathologies like pincer nails and koilonychia occur when those forces are not in balance.

24.2 How to Confirm the Diagnosis

Pincer nails may be hereditary or acquired. Acquired conditions that may create transverse overcurvature are onychomycosis, psoriasis, and biomechanical forces such as ill-fitting shoes or osteoarthritis at the first metatarsal phalangeal joint (Figures 24.1 and 24.2).[2] Acquired pincer nails are often asymmetrical, whereas hereditary cases are symmetrical. Shionaya reported that clinicians see a higher rate of pincer nails in the bedridden and nonambulatory community, which opposes the theory that the greatest cause of acquired pincer nails is ambulation in an ill-fitting shoe.[4,5] It is hypothesized that pincer nails may either be caused by the lack of ground reaction force on the digit during stance and ambulation or by an increase in the automatic curvature force.[4,5] If there is a lack of ground reaction force on the digit, as in a patient who is nonambulatory, it is plausible that the ventral and dorsal nail matrix grow in a mismatched state resulting in an inward curvature of the distal nail.[4] In the nail bed, Meissner's corpuscles and Merkel endings function as mechanoreceptors. Even though their roles are not completely elucidated, it

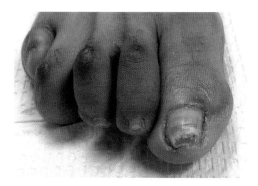

FIGURE 24.1   Painful great toe acquired-type pincer nail.

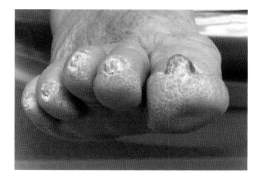

FIGURE 24.2   Significant pincer nail deformity in all toes in a patient with concomitant psoriasis.

is suggested that the way these mechanoreceptors respond to mechanical forces may help to shape nail configuration and stimulate nail cell growth and proliferation. This logic flows with the observation that some bedridden and nonambulatory patients still develop pincer nails. To show this relationship, Sano and Ichioka studied three groups of patients: (1) ambulatory volunteers, (2) those who were bedridden for 3 months or less, and (3) those who were bedridden for 3 months or more.[3] After measuring the curve index (a calculation of the nail height, width, and central thickness) of the volunteers, they concluded that the curve index increased significantly as the length of time bedridden progressed.

Even though fingernails are not subject to the same biomechanical loading forces as toenails, greater transverse nail plate overcurvature presented in fingernails of patients with hemiplegia on the palsy side compared to the nonpalsy side.[3,6] This suggests that mechanics (or lack thereof) and mechanoreceptors play a role in nail configuration and may lead to the development of nail pathologies.

Beyond mechanobiology, the shape of the underlying distal phalanx has been theorized to contribute to the overcurvature of the nail unit.[7] The distal tip of the phalanx is often described to have an osteophyte or upward protrusion of the boney tip when viewed on a lateral radiograph. Also, it has been thought that a widening of the base of the distal phalanx contributes to the pincer nail deformity.[8] Kosaka et al.'s study to determine the distal phalanx's influence on nail shape assessed 60 great toes from patients with "normal" nails, ingrown nails, and pincer nails.[7] Osteophytes of the distal phalanx were confirmed in 50%, 80%, and 100% of cases in the normal, ingrown and pincer nail groups, respectively.[7] The width and the height of pincer nails that were avulsed surgically were also measured. A statistically significant level between width and height of the nail plate was found compared to the same measurements in normal and ingrown nails. The distal narrowing of the pincer nail bed described in the literature is consistent with the width/height (or curvature) index in this study, but the investigators sought to explain the "shrinkage" of the nail bed. Ultimately, they theorized that an unknown cause creates nail bed shrinkage, which causes the ventral nail plate to shrink, but the dorsal nail plate continues to progress normally. This variation causes an inward twisting distally, and the lateral nail margins to roll inwardly. This "continuous traction" on the distal phalanx exerts force on the apex of the distal phalangeal tuft creating a secondary deformity to the primary nail deformity.[7] Ultimately, the distal phalanx does not seem to cause the pincer nail; rather the pincer nail causes the bone deformity, or osteophyte, to develop.

24.3 Evidence-Based Treatment

Conservative options seek to alleviate the symptoms of the distal lateral nail corners that are imbedded in the lateral nail folds. The distal tip of the pincer nail is often hypertrophic and grossly incurvated, which makes nail trimming difficult for the layperson. Using nail nippers, a practitioner can perform nail debridement starting at the center of the nail progressing laterally or medially along the nail plate, making sure the nail plate is in between the jaws of the nipper to ensure a pain-free patient experience. Attempting to debride the nail straight across without honoring the shape of the nail plate will often result in pain for the patient and may cause bleeding due to the proximity of the nail bed and nail plate. Softening agents such as urea 40% may assist in nail debridement as well before nail debridement or in lieu of it. For a mild overcurvature case, a thinning of the central nail plate may create relief.[8] This may be achieved with a burr. According to that same principle, flattening of the central portion of the nail plate while lifting the distal lateral nail edges may provide comfort.[8] Exerting tension on the transverse overcurvature may result in a flattened nail plate. This has been achieved with a metal brace that can be adjusted tension-wise over 6 months or more.[8] The chapter author has used plastic spring braces applied horizontally across the surface of the nail plate, which created temporary relief of corner pain, but the device must be readjusted consistently and has no guarantee of resolving the nail deformity. As seen with the plastic spring brace, Baran et al. also reported immediate relapse after removal of the metal brace.[8]

Arai et al. described using sterilized plastic IV tubing that is split on one side for the conservative treatment of an ingrown toenail; however, this technique can be applied to pincer nails.[9] One would apply the tubing to the entire length of the affected lateral nail margin in order to separate the skin from the nail plate. The tube would be affixed to the nail plate by application of an acrylic resin. Arai and colleagues related that patients experienced pain relief in 24 hours.[9] If the patient's main concern is distal lateral nail pain, the application of the gutter splint for weeks to months allows the skin and nail not to grow into each other and may provide relief from repeated surgical procedures or chronic slantback nail trimming (a noninvasive technique of trimming the nail plate on an angle toward the proximal nail fold to alleviate corner pressure).

Utilizing medical tape, Tsunoda et al. reported a conservative taping technique for patients to apply at home (Figure 24.3).[10] For 14 years, this study evaluated 541 patients who utilized this conservative

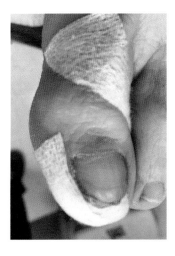

FIGURE 24.3 Conservative taping method to ease the discomfort of the lateral nail border in a nail with transverse overcurvature.

technique. Medical tape that has stretch was applied from one lateral nail corner, elongated, and pulled plantarly down and around the pulp of the digit to the other lateral nail corner. This was repeated once daily for 2 months or more. Some 44.5% of the patients involved had resolution of pain and deformity with consistent taping for 2 months. The remaining patients went on to have their nails surgerized or had a nail brace applied. Patients were given the following instructions: "Cut a 3–4-cm length of 2.5-cm wide mesh elastic adhesive tape. Place one end of the tape along the top of the lateral nail fold on the affected side and tuck it slightly inside the nail fold toward the nail. Carefully and gradually attach the tape along the upper nail fold. Then, pull the nail fold gently outward to make an insulated space between the side of the nail and nail fold and attach the tape to the side of the big toe. Finally, fix the other end of the tape (without pulling) to the toe pad without stretching the tape."[10] A drawback with this technique is the lack of patient adherence, as it can be difficult and time consuming to apply tape daily to the toes. Also, as it takes time to see any nail changes, many patients stop applying the tape after a short period of time instead of using the technique daily for 2 months or more.

As conservative treatments should be discussed and tried first, most physicians and patients agree the relief these procedures provide is temporary. Patients who have severely symptomatic nails or who have failed conservative therapy should be considered candidates for surgery. If onychomycosis is present, it should be treated prior to surgical intervention. When considering surgical management of a pincer nail, the physician should first rule out other pathologies such as nail tumors, bone tumors, onychomycosis, and psoriasis. Weight-bearing pedal radiographs should be ordered in order to assess the morphology of the foot in a more realistic manner. If the great toe is affected, a lateral radiographic view with the digit collimated, or isolated/hyperextended from the other digits, will provide a clearer view if an osteophyte is present on the distal phalanx (Figure 24.4).

Various surgical procedures that aim to flatten the distal nail have been described in the literature. The success of these procedures seems to involve not only flattening the distal nail tissue but also targeting the distal tuft of the phalanx. That said, chronic avulsion of the entire nail plate alone does not alleviate the deformity and may even contribute to its worsening of the curvature over time.[8] However, the procedures showing the most success do involve avulsion of the nail plate in order to expand the distal nail bed and give exposure to the distal phalanx (Figure 24.5). Plusjé described a technique where the nail plate is avulsed with a freer elevator, then phenol is applied to the lateral matrix horns, followed by an incision of the nail bed parallel the hyponychium extending all the way to the proximal nail fold.[11] The point of this is to expose the distal phalanx and any traction osteophytes, which can be removed with a bone rongeur or curette. The distal two-thirds of the lateral nail wall are excised; keeping in mind the width of tissue needed to stretch the nail unit flat in the horizontal plane.[11] The remaining tissue is coapted with nonabsorbable, simple, interrupted sutures; again, ensuring the distal nail unit is stretched distal and laterally/medially to create a flattened nail unit. Of the six patients treated with this technique, three had no recurrence, two had recurrence of the overcurvature but to a lesser extent and no pain, and one had total recurrence necessitating further procedures.

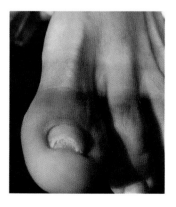

FIGURE 24.4   Preoperative pincer nail.

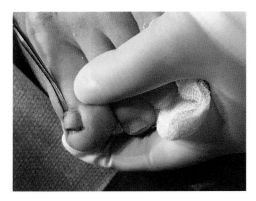

FIGURE 24.5 Nail avulsion prior to the soft tissue and bone work in pincer nail surgery.

Mutaf et al. proposed a new surgical technique that also required nail plate avulsion but did not involve phenolization of the matrix horns as many other authors have relayed.[12] This more complex approach involves two modified Z-plasties on each side of the nail tip. The central limb of the Z-plasty is lengthened transversely laterally and medially in order to widen the nail bed. This incision also allowed for exposure of the distal phalanx to be rongeured. The Z-plasties are then transposed in their typical manner and sutured. Eight patients exposed to this procedure had a mixture of hereditary and acquired pincer nail deformity. A 2-year follow-up revealed no recurrences of pain or deformity.[12]

Another nail matrix–sparing procedure is the zigzag method.[13] The process involves total nail avulsion, a modified fish-mouth incision distally that extended around the lateral nail folds with the apex of the incision pointing dorsally at the center of the pincer nail deformity. This produces a "W"-looking design. The nail bed flap is then dissected in order to expose the distal phalanx. Any osteophyte is removed with a bone rasp. Finally, the constricted hyponychium at the apex of the nail flap is excised into three portions by removal of a small portion medial and lateral to the apical aspect. This flap, when widened transversely, creates a zigzag pattern. The tissue can then be transposed into the zigzag flap and sutured (Figures 24.6 and 24.7). Follow-up of 90 nails ranged from 10 months to 4 years.[13] No major adverse events occurred. The authors also hypothesized the vicious cycle of the nail plate–nail bed–phalanx relationship in nails with transverse overcurvature and which techniques are imperative in having a successful surgical result. First, the nail plate must be removed since it is not pliable and for appropriate distal phalanx exposure. Second, the osteophyte must be flattened in order for the incoming nail to reach normal height. This cannot be achieved conservatively. Also, the shrunken distal nail bed must be cut and restored to its anatomical width for the nail to follow that pattern. The hardened hyponychium is severely compromised in pincer nails and needs to be incised in order to create a flat surface for new nail growth. The release of the hyponychium cannot be achieved with conservative methods.

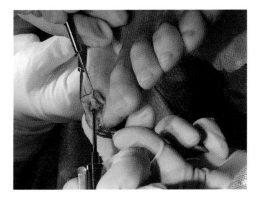

FIGURE 24.6 After the W incision has been made, the nail plate is totally avulsed, and the incision carried down to the bone, the exposed distal phalanx is reduced with a surgical burr.

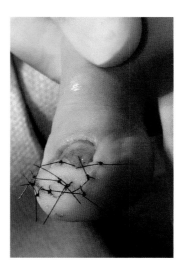

FIGURE 24.7   Immediately postoperative, following the zigzag procedure with 4-0 nylon sutures in place.

Jung et al. compared 20 cases of transverse overcurvature nail correction utilizing either the zigzag nail bed flap method or the inverted-T method.[14] They measured curvature index (width and height of the nail) and interphalangeal angle and base width of the distal phalanx on the anteroposterior radiographs to determine if there is a lateral deviation of the bone contributing to the deformity. They executed their zigzag method similarly to previously described, except they utilized a diamond burr to flatten the osteophyte. And, instead of transecting the nail bed flap apex into three sections, they deepithelialized the lateral nail borders in order to widen and flatten the flap transversely and distally. They also modified Haneke's median longitudinal incision into an inverted-T incision. The transverse bar of the T was made at the hyponychium and retained the median longitudinal incision in order to expose the osteophyte. The nail bed was simply repaired. Outcomes from both procedures were satisfactory from both a patient satisfaction score and visual improvement of the deformity. The interphalangeal angle was increased in the pincer nail group compared to a control group, and postoperative curvature index measurements were like the control group; thus, showing the success of the procedures. The base width of the distal phalanx was no different between the pincer nail group and control group.

Ultimately, the most successful surgical techniques for pincer nails consist of total nail avulsion to expose and modify the distal tip of the phalanx as well as widening and flattening of the distal nail bed. These elements allow for new nail growth to slide over the modified nail bed in a more anatomical shape and thickness. There is no standard surgical technique for this nail deformity, but adhering to the aforementioned steps seems to create a more normal curvature index and fortify a successful outcome. See further Table 24.1.

TABLE 24.1

Treatments and Levels of Evidence

Treatment for Pincer Nails	Level of Evidence
Conservative taping technique	B[10]
Avulsion of the nail with phenol of lateral matrix horns	C[11]
Nail avulsion with Z-plasties	C[12]
Zigzag method	B[13]
Zigzag method versus inverted-T method	B[14]

REFERENCES

1. Cornelius CE III, Shelley WB. Pincer nail syndrome. *Arch Surg.* 1968;96:321–322.
2. Jung DJ, Kim JH, Lee HY et al. Anatomical characteristics and surgical treatments of pincer nail deformity. *Arch Plast Surg.* 2015;42(2):207–213.
3. Sano H, Ichioka S. Influence of mechanical forces as a part of nail configuration. *Dermatology.* 2012;225:210–214.
4. Sano H, Ogawa R. Clinical evidence for the relationship between nail configuration and mechanical forces. *Plast Reconstr Surg Glob Open.* 2014;2(3):e115.
5. Shionaya K. Pincer nail and ingrown nail. *J Joint Surg.* 2009;28:91–97.
6. Kobayashi K, Kuroshima N. *Asymmetry of finger nails in hemiplegia.* Paper presented at 46th Annual Meeting of the Japanese Society for Surgery of the Hand, Nagoya, April 2003.
7. Kosaka M, Kusuhara H, Mochizuki Y, Mori H, Isogai N. Morphologic study of normal, ingrown, and pincer nails. *Dermatol Surg.* 2010;36(1):31–38.
8. Baran R, Haneke E, Richert B. Pincer nails: Definition and surgical treatment. *Dermatol Surg.* 2001;27(3):261–266.
9. Arai H, Arai T, Nakajima H, Haneke E. Formable acrylic treatment for in-growing nail with gutter splint and sculptured nail. *Int J Derm.* 2004;43(10):759–765.
10. Tsunoda M, Tsunoda K. Patient-controlled taping for the treatment of ingrown toenails. *Ann Fam Med.* 2014;12(6):553–555.
11. Plusjé LG. Pincer nails: A new surgical treatment. *Dermatol Surg.* 2001;27(1):41–43.
12. Mutaf M, Sunay M, Işk D. A new surgical technique for the correction of pincer nail deformity. *Ann Plast Surg.* 2007;58(5):496–500.
13. Kosaka M, Asamura S, Wada Y, Kusada A, Nakagawa Y, Isogai N. Pincer nails treated using zigzag nail bed flap method: Results of 71 toenails. *Dermatol Surg.* 2010;36(4):506–511.
14. Jung DJ, Kim JH, Lee HY, Kim DC, Lee SI, Kim TY. Anatomical characteristics and surgical treatments of pincer nail deformity. *Arch Plast Surg.* 2015;42:207–213.

25

Warts

Sonali Nanda, Rachel Fayne, and Martin N. Zaiac

25.1 Introduction

Verrucae vulgaris, or warts, are common cutaneous lesions caused by the human papilloma virus (HPV). The specific HPV subtypes of the warts dictate their varying morphologies, anatomic locations, and histopathology. Warts can occur on any part on the body. However, since they are transmitted via person-to-person contact, they have a predilection for exposed areas such as the hands and fingers.

Ungual warts, or warts affecting the nails, are typically caused by HPV subtypes 1, 2, 4, 27, and 57.[1] They are the most common tumor of the nail unit and are described as either periungual, referring to around the nail unit, or subungual, which refers to underneath the nail plate.[2] Rarely, premalignant subtypes 16 and 18 can cause ungual warts and, if these lesions are not treated, they may undergo malignant transformation to Bowen disease or squamous cell carcinoma (SCC).

Cutaneous viral warts typically affect children and young adults with prevalence ranging from 2% to 20%.[3] They develop through direct or indirect transmission of fomites. Close skin-to-skin contact and self-inoculation have been established to transmit warts.[4] There are also genetic conditions and immunodeficiency syndromes that can predispose patients to developing these viral lesions.[5]

Precise epidemiologic data on the occurrence and resolution of warts is not readily available. Ungual warts, in particular, are common in nail biters and meat workers.[6] Trauma associated with the nail or surrounding skin, such as in chronic nail biters, allows HPV entry into areas of the broken skin.

The pathogenesis of warts in meat workers, however, is not as clear.[7] It has been reported that about 23% of meat handlers present with warts compared to about 10% of non-meat handlers.[8] Butcher's warts typically present in a younger population, about 17–23 years of age, who have recently started handling meat.[9] The increased prevalence of warts in this group is largely due to HPV 7, a rare cause of warts in the general population. The source of HPV 7 is unknown and has not been found to be associated with trauma, damp environments, smoking, or handling any kind of meat in particular. However, Keefe and colleagues suggested that contact with an unidentified substance in meat might induce replication of HPV on the skin surface.[7]

Periungual and subungual warts typically present at nail folds such as the proximal nail fold, lateral nail fold, or hyponychium. They first appear as small, 1 mm hyperkeratotic, skin-colored papules that can grow into larger papules about 1 cm in diameter and eventually coalesce into plaques.[2] Warts of the nail folds may be painful unlike warts in other areas of the body.[10] Nail biters typically have warts involving multiple fingers. As a result, many patients experience pain due to tumor growth in the confined area of the nail unit.

Dermoscopy can help identify ungual warts, which usually present as scaly verrucous papules with rough surfaces and dilated capillaries in the papillary dermis.[11] Blood vessels may be seen as black dots on clinical exam or dermoscopy, which can help distinguish periungual warts from other tumors. A wart of the hyponychium or lateral nail folds can cause a hyperkeratotic nail bed if extension occurs to these areas. If the lesion is in the proximal nail fold, the cuticle may become hyperkeratotic as well.[1] Subungual warts can uproot the nail plate causing diffuse or linear onycholysis with splinter hemorrhages.[2] In the toenails, warts can cause distal nail thickening.[2] Warts can also cause compression of the underlying nail plate resulting in grooves and ridges.[1]

Histopathology reveals epithelial hyperplasia with acanthosis, papillomatosis, and hyperkeratosis with parakeratosis of the stratum corneum.[2] Prominent or thrombosed capillary vessels as well as mononuclear cells may be present in the dermis.[12]

The differential diagnosis for periungual and subungual warts includes squamous cell carcinoma or squamous cell carcinoma in situ (Bowen disease) of the nail, fibrokeratoma, glomus tumor, subungual exostoses, epithelial sarcomas, mucoid pseudocysts, foreign-body granulomas, periungual fibromas, mucous cysts, cutaneous horns, lichen planus, lichen nitidus, onychomatrichomas, and tuberculous verrucosa.[13,14]

Usually, clinical diagnosis of warts is straightforward and can be done without need for biopsy. However, if there is a long-standing history of recalcitrant warts despite repeated therapy, especially in an immunocompromised host, biopsy must be done to rule out Bowen disease or SCC.

There are many cases of Bowen disease or SCC mimicking periungual or subungual warts.[9,15] These tumors can present as periungual verrucous masses and can be ulcerated. If subungual, one can appreciate longitudinal melanonychia, subungual nodules, onycholysis, or paronychia similar to verrucae. The majority of these cases are associated with high-risk HPV subtypes, especially HPV 16, which can cause rare malignant transformation of viral warts.

Riddel and colleagues reported that out of 79 cases of HPV-associated digital SCC, 72% were located periungually or subungually. The third finger was most commonly involved, followed by the second finger at 26% and 25% prevalence, respectively.[16] Many of these patients were originally treated for viral warts for about 5 years in duration without improvement. In such cases, biopsy would help distinguish between SCC and warts.

Epithelioid sarcomas can present as erythematous, firm nodules of the lateral proximal fold. Histopathology reveals epithelioid tumor cells that stain strongly positive for vimentin. Subungual exostoses are firm, bony tumors of the distal phalanx that can present with hyperkeratosis and lifting of the nail plate with growth.[17] Although these lesions are not difficult to diagnose clinically, radiography can help confirm diagnosis of exostoses if necessary. Glomus tumors are usually solitary and cause severe, localized pain.[18] Lichen planus and lichen nitidis of the nail is uncommon and can imitate warts if located in the proximal nail fold or hyponychium.[2] Swelling and discoloration may be seen. Onychomatricomas are typically indolent and painless, usually occurring in Caucasian women in their 40s.[19]

25.2 How to Confirm the Diagnosis

The diagnosis of periungual or subungual warts is usually clinical. The most classic clinical sign of verrucae includes pinpoint bleeding after paring the surface as a result of trauma to the capillaries.[2] However, the clinical appearance may vary from site to site, so dermoscopy and biopsy are helpful in establishing the correct diagnosis (Figure 25.2a). One can also subtype the HPV virus on Papanicolaou smears, but this is not commonly done as it does not change treatment decisions.

25.3 Evidence-Based Treatment

When compared to cutaneous warts, periungual and subungual warts are challenging to treat due to their recalcitrance and high recurrence rate as well as the discomfort associated with treatment. There are a whole host of treatment options ranging from topical immunotherapy to laser therapy to surgery. There is not one specific treatment that is significantly better than other options and the lack of double-blinded clinical trials makes treatment decisions difficult. Combination therapy, such as cryotherapy in addition to topical salicylic acid, is generally more successful in achieving clearance than monotherapy.[20] Each therapy involves unique mechanisms to target these viral lesions and will be discussed in the following order: topical, systemic, and surgical.

25.3.1 Topical Treatments

Although recent epidemiologic data is lacking, in 1985, it was reported that up to 65% of warts spontaneously resolve in 2 years.[21] Spontaneous resolution is more common in young children, and thus, conservative treatment is recommended initially for this age group. Lesions in older children and adults typically do not clear without treatment. In addition, warts in the nail unit are particularly hard to treat and ignoring these lesions can lead to a more extensive lesion and greater morbidity.

Topical agents include keratolytic drugs; destructive or caustic agents such as cantharidin, monochloroacetic (MCA), trichloroacetic (TCA), and pyruvic acid; virucidal agents; and immunomodulators (Table 25.1).

25.3.1.1 Keratolytic Agents

Keratolytics are the most popular first-line agents used to treat warts. They act by causing local destruction and irritation of the virally infected keratinocytes in the epidermis.[22] Salicylic acid is the most commonly used agent, and products ranging in concentration from 16%–50% can be found over the counter at local drugstores and used to treat warts at home. Topical keratolytics are especially good options for young children as they are safe, painless, and applied topically. These medications are inexpensive and can be applied as creams, ointments, or lacquers.[2]

Currently, there are no double-blind randomized controlled trials involving keratolytic agents. Most of the clinical studies are prospective trials with greater than 20 subjects and have shown that treatment of common warts with salicylic acid is less efficacious than cryotherapy (15% versus 49%), but better than placebo (8% cure rate).[23] Another study reported salicylic acid to be just as effective as gentle cryotherapy, with both resulting in clearance rates of only 14%.[24] The studies typically soaked the wart in warm water or pared it down before application. However, these agents need to be applied consistently for days to weeks in order to effectively treat the lesion, as studies have shown that application for 5–7 days per week for 12 weeks incurs a higher clearance rate than treating with placebo.[22]

25.3.1.2 Cantharidin

Cantharidin is a terpenoid isolated from the blister beetle, *Cantharis vesicatoria*. Its application leads to activation of proteases, triggering acantholysis and eventually, apoptosis of treated cells.[25] Cantharidin

TABLE 25.1

Topical Wart Treatments and Evidence Levels

Topical Treatments	Evidence Level
Keratolytic Agents	B
Cantharidin	B
Monochloroacetic acid (MCA)	B
Trichloroacetic acid (TCA)	B
Formic acid	B
Pyruvic acid	B
Zinc oxide	A
5-Fluorouracil	B
Retinoids	B
Podophyllin and podophyllotoxin	B
Virucidal Agents	
Glutaraldehyde	B
Formaldehyde	B
Cidofovir	C
Topical Immunotherapy	
Imiquimod	B
Diphenylcyclopropene	B
Squaric acid dibutyl ester	B
Measles, mumps, rubella (MMR) vaccine	C

0.7% is typically applied directly to the lesion, taking care to avoid unaffected skin, as it leads to blistering. Patients should keep the area covered for 4–8 hours, and then thoroughly clean it with soap and water. They should be instructed that a blister will form in the area and resolve in 1–2 weeks. Side effects include pain and tenderness at the treated site.

The efficacy of cantharidin has been reported as 80%.[26] In 1960, 40 patients affected with digital and periungual warts were treated with cantharidin. Only 1 of 29 digital warts recurred and none of the periungual warts recurred after treatment.[27] A more recent trial by Kacar and colleagues determined that cantharidin was particularly useful in treating long-standing warts and required less treatments than cryotherapy in order to achieve clearance.[28] The painless application and minimal side effects of cantharidin make it one of the best options of treatment for children.

25.3.1.3 Trichloroacetic Acid (TCA)

High concentrations (80%–90%) of trichloroacetic acid have been used to treat warts. In a recent study, treatment with TCA was compared to cryotherapy. The cure rate was higher in the cryotherapy group as only 20% of TCA-treated patients achieved cure.[29] The only side effect noted with this treatment was hyperpigmentation.

25.3.1.4 Formic Acid

Formic acid is an irritant first isolated from red ants.[12] The mechanism of action is unknown but thought to be similar to the virucidal agent, formalin, by drying out and destroying the affected tissue. Topical puncture with 85% formic acid in water led to a 91% cure rate in a double-blind, randomized controlled trial with 34 participants by Faghihi and colleagues.[30] Side effects included mild burning. However, one case of burning requiring extensive debridement and reconstruction was reported after inappropriate application.[31]

25.3.1.5 Pyruvic Acid

Pyruvic acid is a chemical peeling agent used for its keratolytic properties. It has been used in chemical peels for cosmetic purposes, but also recently studied in a clinical trial comparing its effectiveness with salicylic acid for plantar wart treatment. Based on this study, 70% pyruvic acid and salicylic acid were similar in efficacy and recurrence and also shared a similar side effect profile.[32]

25.3.1.6 Zinc Oxide

Zinc is well-known for its immune-mediating properties. Oral zinc sulfate was used in one study to treat recalcitrant warts and achieved a clearance of 86.9%.[33] A double-blind, randomized, controlled trial compared the efficacy of zinc oxide 20% ointment with salicylic acid 15% + lactic acid 15%, and reported a 50% cure rate with zinc oxide compared with 42% in the salicylic acid group.[34] Side effects reported included swelling (85.7%), erythema (71.6%), and scaling (50%).

Less commonly used topical medications that have been studied include monochloroacetic acid (MCA), retinoids, 5-fluorouracil, and podophyllin or podophyllotoxin.

Virucidal agents such as glutaraldehyde, formaldehyde, and cidofovir have also been reported to treat warts. Glutaraldehyde and formaldehyde (formalin) are two topical treatments that lead to viral destruction. Typically used are 10%–25% glutaraldehyde and 0.7% gel or 3% solution of formaldehyde.[12] Their efficacies have been shown to be comparable to salicylic acid with around a 67%–70% cure rate. Cidofovir is an acyclic nucleoside phosphonate that inhibits DNA replication through competitive inhibition of DNA polymerase. The 3% cream has shown to be effective for the treatment of periungual warts in a retrospective study with a 56.1% cure rate.[35] However, cidofovir is very expensive and treatment with low-cost methods should be employed first. However, clinicians typically do not reach for these medications when searching for second- or third-line treatment options.

25.3.1.7 Topical Immunotherapy

25.3.1.7.1 Imiquimod

Imiquimod acts as an immunomodulator that stimulates the production of cytokines and mediators to trigger a robust immune response. Originally approved by the U.S. Food and Drug Administration (FDA) to treat anogenital warts, the efficacy of imiquimod 5% cream for cutaneous warts was assessed in 2000. After 9 weeks of treatment, 56% of patients achieved wart clearance.[36] In a small study focusing on imiquimod for subungual and periungual warts, 80% of patients showed complete resolution.[37] Side effects include a local erythema, itching, and pain.

Other immunotherapeutic agents such as diphenylcyclopropene (DPCP or DCP), squaric acid dibutyl ester (SADBE), and intralesional vaccinations of the MMR vaccine, *Candida albicans* antigen, tuberculin, and *Mycobacterium welchii* have been reported.[38] DPCP 1% in acetone and SADBE 2% cause a local sensitization reaction that stimulates a local immune response in the target region.[39] A recently conducted study comparing a subset of patients with *C. albicans* antigen with a subset of patients who received cryotherapy reported a 77% cure rate with immunotherapy compared to 57% with cryotherapy.[40] In addition, *C. albicans* antigen administration has been shown to induce resolution of distant warts, suggesting that immunotherapeutic agents may create a systemic response and induce HPV-directed immunity.[41]

25.3.2 Systemic or Intralesional Treatments

25.3.2.1 Bleomycin

Bleomycin is an antimitotic agent that has been reported to be safe and effective in treating periungual warts with a success rate as high as 92%–96%.[14,42,43] The study reporting a 94% cure rate for periungual warts used up to two intralesional injections to achieve cure.[44] Application includes placing 1 mg/mL bleomycin onto the target lesion and then pricking the wart with a needle to allow penetration of the treatment. Superficial intralesional bleomycin at 0.5–1 mg/cc is also used successfully.[45] In this case, bleomycin is injected into the epidermal–dermal junction to create a blanching (Figures 25.1 and 25.3). The technique of bleomycin delivery is important and bifurcated needles may provide better results.[46]

After treatment, an eschar forms in the treated area and is scraped off to reveal healthy tissue. Side effects include pain with infection, burning, erythema, and swelling. Raynaud phenomenon has also been reported as a late side effect of intralesional bleomycin injection and can lead to nail dystrophy or loss.[47] This method of treatment should be avoided in patients with collagen and vascular diseases.

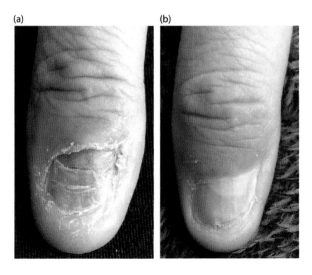

(a)   (b)

FIGURE 25.1   (a) Periungual wart on the thumbnail. (b) Periungual wart on thumbnail 5 months after treatment with intralesional bleomycin 0.5 mg/cc.

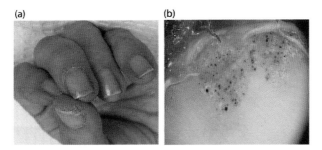

FIGURE 25.2 (a) Clinical image of periungual verruca on the thumbnail. (b) Thumbnail periungual verruca under videoscopy showing pinpoint vessels.

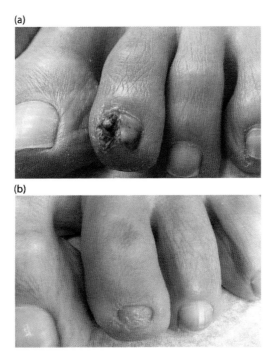

FIGURE 25.3 (a) Verruca on the second toenail. (b) Second toenail after three treatments with intralesional bleomycin 0.5 mg/cc.

25.3.2.2 Oral Cimetidine

Oral cimetidine is an H_2 antagonist with a variable efficacy in treating warts. It has been reported to increase T-cell activity and cause a cell-mediated response.[14] One double-blind, randomized, controlled trial in 1996 reported a 32% clearance rate with 25–40 mg/kg/day cimetidine compared to 31% with placebo.[48] However, in 1999, another well-designed trial showed a 25% clearance rate with 2400 mg/day cimetidine compared with 5% clearance with placebo.[49]

Intravenous administration of interferon-beta and oral acyclovir have also been reported to cure subungual and periungal warts.[50] Due to the necessary mode of treatment of IFN-beta as well as the high cost, it is not recommended for regular use. In 2016, a 49-year-old women with persistent plantar warts who had undergone wart therapy without improvement was prescribed a 10-day course of oral acyclovir treatment for herpes zoster and complete resolution of her warts were noted.[51] Currently, there are no clinical trials to support these treatments. See further Table 25.2.

TABLE 25.2

Systemic Wart Treatments and Evidence Levels

Systemic/Intralesional Treatments	Evidence Level
Bleomycin	A
Cimetidine	A
Interferons	E
Acyclovir	E

TABLE 25.3

Surgical Wart Treatments and Evidence Levels

Surgical Treatments	Evidence Level
Cryotherapy	A
Surgical excision	N/A
Electrosurgery/infrared coagulation	N/A
Localized heating	B
CO_2 laser	C
Pulsed dye laser	B
Er:YAG laser	B

25.3.3 Surgical Treatments

Surgical treatments should be performed cautiously as to prevent permanent iatrogenic nail dystrophy (Table 25.3).

25.3.3.1 Cryotherapy

Cryotherapy, commonly used in dermatologic practice for the treatment of precancerous actinic keratoses and other cutaneous lesions, is a fast, noninvasive technique that may also be used in the treatment of warts, including ungual warts. It involves freezing the lesion with liquid nitrogen for approximately 10–15 seconds. For thick, hyperkeratotic periungual warts, superficial layers of the lesion should be removed with a blade prior to freezing to allow for penetration of the liquid nitrogen to more active regions of the wart.[2] Cryotherapy may induce edema of the nail bed, resulting in blister formation and localized pain for up to 72 hours.[14] As such, it is contraindicated in children.[2] Topical EMLA, a local anesthetic, can be used to reduce pain of many cutaneous procedures but is not useful in reducing pain from cryotherapy in the treatment of warts and should not be used.[52]

Cryotherapy has been shown to have a cure rate as high as 70.7% and is generally well-tolerated.[53] Compared to topical salicylic acid, cryotherapy demonstrates a superior cure rate (39% vs. 24%) in the treatment of cutaneous warts, but also results in more side effects, including pain, blistering, scarring, skin irritation, pigmentation and crust formation.[23] For warts close to the proximal nail fold, cryotherapy should be used with caution, as damage to the nail matrix may result in leukonychia, Beau's lines, and onychomadesis. Severe damage to the matrix can result in irreversible nail atrophy.[54]

25.3.3.2 Surgical Excision

Excision of warts of the nail unit is generally not recommended, as in almost all cases it would require partial or even total removal of the nail matrix.[14] Surgical excision may also result in damage to other structures within the nail unit and the distal phalanx, and exposes patients to the potential risks associated with surgical intervention, including infection and scarring. These patients may be left with complete nail loss and digital disfigurement, in addition to significant scarring.[2,14] Excision may also create an environment in which lesions recur, as viral particles may spread to the scar or residual tissue during excision.

25.3.3.3 Electrosurgery and Infrared Coagulation

Electrosurgery, in which an electrical charge is sent through the tip of a needle, and infrared coagulation, in which a small probe delivers infrared light to induce coagulation, are two additional surgical techniques that are not recommended in the treatment of ungual warts. These techniques are destructive and may cause scarring in the area of treatment or even permanent damage to the structures of the nail unit. Use of electrosurgery and infrared coagulation in the treatment of ungual warts should be avoided.[2]

25.3.3.4 Localized Heating

While electrosurgery and infrared coagulation induce thermal damage sufficient to cause scarring and permanent changes to the nail unit, controlled localized heating has shown promising results with a minimal side effect profile. In the treatment of common hand warts, one to four treatment sessions at 50°C for 30–60 seconds yielded an 86% clearance rate, compared to 41% in controls, with no regression observed in 3-month follow-up.[55] While this has not yet been studied in warts of the nail unit, its low potential for adverse effects make localized heating an attractive potential alternative for these difficult-to-treat lesions.

25.3.3.5 CO$_2$ Laser

The mechanism of action of the 10,600 nm laser is to target water as the chromophore and induce localized thermal tissue damage, thus vaporizing layers of HPV-infected epidermis. For warts with extension into the nail fold or nail bed, the nail should be avulsed prior to laser treatment to improve penetration.[2] When studied at 3–15 W with spot size 2 mm, the CO$_2$ laser yielded an overall cure rate of 57.4% over 10 months.[56] In another study with similar energy settings, 71% of patients demonstrated clearance at 12-month follow-up. Common side effects are pain associated with treatment and, more rarely, nail changes like distal onycholysis, nail thickening, and temporary sensory changes.[57] A significant number of patients who were successfully treated with CO$_2$ laser therapy for ungual warts had previously failed treatment with cryotherapy or other topical therapies; as such, CO$_2$ laser is typically reserved as a secondary treatment option for recalcitrant warts.[2,56,57]

Additional safety precautions should be taken when using the CO$_2$ laser, as studies have shown intact HPV DNA to be present in the plume present after CO$_2$ laser use for cutaneous warts, placing patients and providers at risk for respiratory papillomatosis.[58,59] Smoke evacuation with suction as well as gloves and face masks should always be used.[60]

25.3.3.6 Pulsed Dye Laser

Pulsed dye laser (PDL) acts by causing thermal damage to the vasculature supplying the wart as well as direct damage causing cell death and possibly stimulating cell immunity.[61]

The typical pulsed dye laser session consists of treatment with PDL 585–595 nm with a 5–7 mm spot diameter at energy fluencies between 8–10 J/cm^2 and delivers two pulses with 1 to 2 mm overlap.[61]

PDL is a well-studied treatment for common and plantar warts with efficacy similar to cryotherapy or cantharidin.[60] However, PDL is most successful in warts such as verruca plana compared to thick and hyperkeratotic warts, which may be difficult for PDL to penetrate. A recent review regarding the use of pulsed dye laser in the treatment of warts found that PDL resulted in variable efficacy for peripheral warts on the hands or feet. In addition, periungual warts were less responsive to this treatment than palmar or plantar warts.[2] The response rates ranged from 48% to 95% throughout four studies specifically testing it on hands and feet, and complications included discomfort and erythema of the treated area. Usually, postoperative pain is minimal and patients can return to work directly after the procedure.[2] Compared to the CO$_2$ laser, PDL has been shown to be safer and have a much lower risk of scarring.[61]

25.3.3.7 Er:YAG Laser

At a wavelength of 2940 nm, the Er:YAG laser is 10 times more selective in its induction of thermal damage than the previously described CO$_2$ laser, particularly when used with a short pulse duration

TABLE 25.4

Alternative Wart Treatments and Evidence Levels

Alternative Treatments	Evidence Level
Tea tree oil	E
Sandalwood oil	C
Duct tape	B
Hot water treatment/exothermic patches	E

(approximately 250 μs).[62] Further, it has been shown that plumes after Er:YAG laser therapy for warts do not contain viable HPV DNA, as seen with the CO_2 laser.[63] As such, its safety profile makes this laser an attractive option for precise ablation and to avoid damage to the nail unit.

In a study of difficult-to-treat warts, including periungual and plantar warts, 72.5% of patients demonstrated complete response after a single treatment with the Er:YAG laser. Only 5.9% of the patients with periungual warts were nonresponders. However, by 3-month follow-up, 24% of patients who showed a complete response demonstrated relapse.[64] In general, Er:YAG treatment is very well-tolerated. Laser-induced wounds healed within approximately 7–10 days and common adverse effects like infection, pigment changes, or scarring are almost never reported.[64] This laser may be used safely in patients with periungual warts, but patients should be followed-up long term to observe for potential recurrence.

25.3.4 Alternative Therapies

25.3.4.1 Essential Oils

Tea tree oil and sandalwood oil are two alternative essential oil treatments used to treat warts. Tea tree oil (TTO) is a known antimicrobial agent and has been reported to clear warts after topical application.[65] Sandalwood oil is thought to decrease incorporation of thymidine in epidermal DNA. In a recent study with 10 participants, 80% of lesions resolved after twice daily application for 12 weeks with no side effects.[66] The authors did not specify whether any of these warts involved the nails.

25.3.4.2 Duct Tape

Duct tape has also been shown to be efficacious in the treatment of warts.[67] In the trial, tape, approximately the size of the target lesion, was applied and removed 6 days later. The lesion was then soaked in water, filed down, and duct tape was applied again. After 2 months, duct tape not only demonstrated a higher clearance rate than six treatments of 10 s cryotherapy, but also induced clearance of cutaneous warts at distant sites with no reported side effects.[67]

25.3.4.3 Hot Water Treatment and Exothermic Patches

Hot water treatment (45–48°C) as well as exothermic patches that release thermal energy have also been employed to treat warts at an anecdotal level.[68,69]

Although the efficacy of alternative therapies is not well-established, they are generally safe and well-tolerated and therefore may be good alternative options for children who do not respond to standard treatment. See previous Table 25.4.

REFERENCES

1. Herschthal J, McLeod MP, Zaiac M. Management of ungual warts. *Dermatol Ther.* 2012;25(6):545–550.
2. Tosti A, Piraccini BM. Warts of the nail unit: Surgical and nonsurgical approaches. *Dermatol Surg.* 2001;27(3):235–239.
3. Kilkenny M, Marks R. The descriptive epidemiology of warts in the community. *Australas J Dermatol.* 1996;37(2):80–86.

4. Stock I. [Molluscum contagiosum—A common but poorly understood "childhood disease" and sexually transmitted illness]. *Med Monatsschr Pharm.* 2013;36(8):282–290.
5. Leiding JW, Holland SM. Warts and all: Human papillomavirus in primary immunodeficiencies. *J Allergy Clin Immunol.* 2012;130(5):1030–1048.
6. Tosti A, Piraccini BM. Nail Disorders. In: Bolognia JL, Jorizzo JJ, Schaffer JV (eds), *Dermatology,* vol. 1, 3rd ed: Elsevier; 2012, pp. 1141–1142.
7. Keefe M, al-Ghamdi A, Coggon D et al. Cutaneous warts in butchers. *Br J Dermatol.* 1994;130(1):9–14.
8. Finkel ML, Finkel DJ. Warts among meat handlers. *Arch Dermatol.* 1984;120(10):1314–1317.
9. Melchers W, de Mare S, Kuitert E, Galama J, Walboomers J, van den Brule AJ. Human papillomavirus and cutaneous warts in meat handlers. *J Clin Microbiol.* 1993;31(9):2547–2549.
10. Huilgol SC, Barlow RJ, Markey AC. Failure of pulsed dye laser therapy for resistant verrucae. *Clin Exp Dermatol.* 1996;21(2):93–95.
11. Piraccini BM, Bruni F, Starace M. Dermoscopy of non-skin cancer nail disorders. *Dermatol Ther.* 2012;25(6):594–602.
12. Lipke MM. An armamentarium of wart treatments. *Clin Med Res.* 2006;4(4):273–293.
13. Rastrelli M, Mosconi M, Tosti G. Epithelioid sarcoma of the thumb presenting as a periungual warty lesion: Case report and revision of the literature. *J Plast Reconstr Aesthet Surg.* 2011;64(8):e221–e222.
14. Moghaddas N. Periungual verrucae diagnosis and treatment. *Clin Podiatr Med Surg.* 2004;21(4):651–661, viii.
15. Kaiser JF, Proctor-Shipman L. Squamous cell carcinoma in situ (Bowen's disease) mimicking subungual verruca vulgaris. *J Fam Pract.* 1994;39(4):384–387.
16. Riddel C, Rashid R, Thomas V. Ungual and periungual human papillomavirus-associated squamous cell carcinoma: A review. *J Am Acad Dermatol.* 2011;64(6):1147–1153.
17. Russell JD, Nance K, Nunley JR, Maher IA. Subungual exostosis. *Cutis.* 2016;98(2):128–129.
18. Lee JK, Kim TS, Kim DW, Han SH. Multiple glomus tumours in multidigit nail bed. *Handchir Mikrochir Plast Chir.* 2017;49(5):321–325.
19. Kamath P, Wu T, Villada G, Zaiac M, Elgart G, Tosti A. Onychomatricoma: A rare nail tumor with an unusual clinical presentation. *Skin Appendage Disord.* 2018;4(3):171–173.
20. Kwok CS, Gibbs S, Bennett C, Holland R, Abbott R. Topical treatments for cutaneous warts. *Cochrane Database Syst Rev.* 2012;(9):CD001781.
21. Laurent R, Kienzler JL. Epidemiology of HPV infections. *Clin Dermatol.* 1985;3(4):64–70.
22. Sterling J. Treatment of warts and molluscum: What does the evidence show? *Curr Opin Pediatr.* 2016;28(4):490–499.
23. Bruggink SC, Gussekloo J, Berger MY et al. Cryotherapy with liquid nitrogen versus topical salicylic acid application for cutaneous warts in primary care: Randomized controlled trial. *CMAJ.* 2010;182(15):1624–1630.
24. Cockayne S, Hewitt C, Hicks K et al. Cryotherapy versus salicylic acid for the treatment of plantar warts (verrucae): A randomised controlled trial. *BMJ.* 2011;342:d3271.
25. Prasad SB, Verma AK. Cantharidin-mediated ultrastructural and biochemical changes in mitochondria lead to apoptosis and necrosis in murine Dalton's lymphoma. *Microsc Microanal.* 2013;19(6):1377–1394.
26. Baumbach JL, Sheth PB. Topical and intralesional antiviral agents. In: Wolverton SE, *Comprehensive Dermatologic Drug Therapy.* Philadelphia, PA: W. B. Saunders Company; 2001, pp. 524–536.
27. Epstein JH, Epstein WL. Cantharidin treatment of digital and periungual warts. *Calif Med.* 1960;93:11–12.
28. Kacar N, Tasli L, Korkmaz S, Ergin S, Erdogan BS. Cantharidin-podophylotoxin-salicylic acid versus cryotherapy in the treatment of plantar warts: A randomized prospective study. *J Eur Acad Dermatol Venereol.* 2012;26(7):889–893.
29. Abdel Meguid AM, Abdel Motaleb AA, Abdel Sadek AMI. Cryotherapy vs trichloroacetic acid 90% in treatment of common warts. *J Cosmet Dermatol.* 2018 October 24 [Epub].
30. Faghihi G, Vali A, Radan M, Eslamieh G, Tajammoli S. A double-blind, randomized trial of local formic acid puncture technique in the treatment of common warts. *Skinmed.* 2010;8(2):70–71.
31. Tong E, Dorairaj J, O'Sullivan JB, Kneafsey B. Deep full thickness burn to a finger from a topical wart treatment. *Ir Med J.* 2015;108(9):283–284.
32. Shahmoradi Z, Assaf F, Al Said H, Khosravani P, Hosseini SM. Topical pyruvic acid (70%) versus topical salicylic acid (16.7%) compound in treatment of plantar warts: A randomized controlled trial. *Adv Biomed Res.* 2015;4:113.

33. Al-Gurairi FT, Al-Waiz M, Sharquie KE. Oral zinc sulphate in the treatment of recalcitrant viral warts: Randomized placebo-controlled clinical trial. *Br J Dermatol.* 2002;146(3):423–431.

34. Khattar JA, Musharrafieh UM, Tamim H, Hamadeh GN. Topical zinc oxide vs. salicylic acid-lactic acid combination in the treatment of warts. *Int J Dermatol.* 2007;46(4):427–430.

35. Padilla Espana L, Del Boz J, Fernandez Morano T, Arenas-Villafranca J, de Troya M. Successful treatment of periungual warts with topical cidofovir. *Dermatol Ther.* 2014;27(6):337–342.

36. Hengge UR, Esser S, Schultewolter T et al. Self-administered topical 5% imiquimod for the treatment of common warts and molluscum contagiosum. *Br J Dermatol.* 2000;143(5):1026–1031.

37. Micali G, Dall'Oglio F, Nasca MR. An open label evaluation of the efficacy of imiquimod 5% cream in the treatment of recalcitrant subungual and periungual cutaneous warts. *J Dermatolog Treat.* 2003;14(4):233–236.

38. Na CH, Choi H, Song SH, Kim MS, Shin BS. Two-year experience of using the measles, mumps and rubella vaccine as intralesional immunotherapy for warts. *Clin Exp Dermatol.* 2014;39(5):583–589.

39. Silverberg NB, Lim JK, Paller AS, Mancini AJ. Squaric acid immunotherapy for warts in children. *J Am Acad Dermatol.* 2000;42(5 Pt 1):803–808.

40. Khozeimeh F, Jabbari Azad F, Mahboubi Oskouei Y et al. Intralesional immunotherapy compared to cryotherapy in the treatment of warts. *Int J Dermatol.* 2017;56(4):474–478.

41. Horn TD, Johnson SM, Helm RM, Roberson PK. Intralesional immunotherapy of warts with mumps, Candida, and Trichophyton skin test antigens: A single-blinded, randomized, and controlled trial. *Arch Dermatol.* 2005;141(5):589–594.

42. Munn SE, Higgins E, Marshall M, Clement M. A new method of intralesional bleomycin therapy in the treatment of recalcitrant warts. *Br J Dermatol.* 1996;135(6):969–971.

43. Soni P, Khandelwal K, Aara N, Ghiya BC, Mehta RD, Bumb RA. Efficacy of intralesional bleomycin in palmo-plantar and periungual warts. *J Cutan Aesthet Surg.* 2011;4(3):188–191.

44. Shumer SM, O'Keefe EJ. Bleomycin in the treatment of recalcitrant warts. *J Am Acad Dermatol.* 1983;9(1):91–96.

45. Singh Mehta KI, Mahajan VK, Chauhan PS, Chauhan S, Sharma V, Rawat R. Evaluation of efficacy and safety of intralesional bleomycin in the treatment of common warts: Results of a pilot study. *Indian J Dermatol Venereol Leprol.* 2019;85(4):397–404.

46. Shelley WB, Shelley ED. Intralesional bleomycin sulfate therapy for warts. A novel bifurcated needle puncture technique. *Arch Dermatol.* 1991;127(2):234–236.

47. Vanhooteghem O, Richert B, de la Brassinne M. Raynaud phenomenon after treatment of verruca vulgaris of the sole with intralesional injection of bleomycin. *Pediatr Dermatol.* 2001;18(3):249–251.

48. Yilmaz E, Alpsoy E, Basaran E. Cimetidine therapy for warts: A placebo-controlled, double-blind study. *J Am Acad Dermatol.* 1996;34(6):1005–1007.

49. Rogers CJ, Gibney MD, Siegfried EC, Harrison BR, Glaser DA. Cimetidine therapy for recalcitrant warts in adults: Is it any better than placebo? *J Am Acad Dermatol.* 1999;41(1):123–127.

50. Schofer H, Sollberg S. [Systemic treatment of common warts with beta-interferon]. *Hautarzt.* 1991;42(6):396–398.

51. Bagwell A, Loy A, McFarland MS, Tessmer-Neubauer A. Oral acyclovir in the treatment of verruca. *J Drugs Dermatol.* 2016;15(2):237–238.

52. Lee SH, Pakdeethai J, Toh MP, Aw DC. A double-blind, randomised, placebo-controlled trial of EMLA® cream (Eutectic Lidocaine/Prilocaine Cream) for analgesia prior to cryotherapy of plantar warts in adults. *Ann Acad Med Singapore.* 2014;43(10):511–514.

53. Walczuk I, Eertmans F, Rossel B et al. Efficacy and safety of three cryotherapy devices for wart treatment: A randomized, controlled, investigator-blinded, comparative study. *Dermatol Ther (Heidelb).* 2018;8(2):203–216.

54. Dawber R, Colver G, Jackson A. Viral warts, cryosurgical technique. In: Dawber R, Colver G, Jackson A (eds), *Cutaneous Cryosurgery Principles and Clinical Practice,* 2nd ed. London: Martin-Dunitz; 1997, p. 43.

55. Stern P, Levine N. Controlled localized heat therapy in cutaneous warts. *Arch Dermatol.* 1992;128(7):945–948.

56. Lim JT, Goh CL. Carbon dioxide laser treatment of periungual and subungual viral warts. *Australas J Dermatol.* 1992;33(2):87–91.

57. Street ML, Roenigk RK. Recalcitrant periungual verrucae: The role of carbon dioxide laser vaporization. *J Am Acad Dermatol.* 1990;23(1):115–120.

58. Garden JM, O'Banion MK, Shelnitz LS et al. Papillomavirus in the vapor of carbon dioxide laser-treated verrucae. *JAMA*. 1988;259(8):1199–1202.

59. Gloster HM, Jr., Roenigk RK. Risk of acquiring human papillomavirus from the plume produced by the carbon dioxide laser in the treatment of warts. *J Am Acad Dermatol*. 1995;32(3):436–441.

60. Nguyen J, Korta DZ, Chapman LW, Kelly KM. Laser treatment of nongenital verrucae: A systematic review. *JAMA Dermatol*. 2016;152(9):1025–1034.

61. Veitch D, Kravvas G, Al-Niaimi F. Pulsed dye laser therapy in the treatment of warts: A review of the literature. *Dermatol Surg*. 2017;43(4):485–493.

62. Langdon RC. Erbium:YAG laser enables complete ablation of periungual verrucae without the need for injected anesthetics. *Dermatol Surg*. 1998;24(1):157–158.

63. Hughes PS, Hughes AP. Absence of human papillomavirus DNA in the plume of erbium:YAG laser-treated warts. *J Am Acad Dermatol*. 1998;38(3):426–428.

64. Wollina U, Konrad H, Karamfilov T. Treatment of common warts and actinic keratoses by Er:YAG laser. *J Cutan Laser Ther*. 2001;3(2):63–66.

65. Millar BC, Moore JE. Successful topical treatment of hand warts in a paediatric patient with tea tree oil (*Melaleuca alternifolia*). *Complement Ther Clin Pract*. 2008;14(4):225–227.

66. Haque M, Coury DL. Topical sandalwood oil for common warts. *Clin Pediatr (Phila)*. 2018;57(1):93–95.

67. Focht DR, 3rd, Spicer C, Fairchok MP. The efficacy of duct tape vs cryotherapy in the treatment of verruca vulgaris (the common wart). *Arch Pediatr Adolesc Med*. 2002;156(10):971–974.

68. Dvoretzky I. Hyperthermia therapy for warts utilizing a self-administered exothermic patch. Review of two cases. *Dermatol Surg*. 1996;22(12):1035–1038; discussion 8–9.

69. Kang S, Fitzpatrick TB. Debilitating verruca vulgaris in a patient infected with the human immunodeficiency virus. Dramatic improvement with hyperthermia therapy. *Arch Dermatol*. 1994;130(3):294–296.

26

Yellow Nail Syndrome

Michela Starace, Aurora Alessandrini, and Bianca Maria Piraccini

26.1 Introduction

Yellow nail syndrome (YNS) is an uncommon disorder of unknown etiology characterized by the triad of yellow nails, lymphedema, and pleural effusion. The complete triad is seen in 25% of patients, lymphedema in 40%, and pleural effusions in only 2% of patients with yellow nails. The presence of typical nail alterations is an absolute requirement of the diagnosis.

YNS is a rare disorder in which the nail alterations are often the symptom that leads to medical consultation. Due to its association with potential serious comorbidity, physicians should be able to diagnose and order further investigations to assess the presence of lymphedema or lung disease. The etiology is unknown.[1,2]

The pathogenesis of the nail and systemic changes of yellow nail syndrome remains obscure. Anatomic and functional lymphatic abnormalities have been proposed as the underlying cause. Impaired lymphatic drainage appears to play a central role in the various clinical findings seen, with the presence of abnormal findings such as atresia, hypoplasia, and varicose abnormalities of peripheral lymphatics at lymphangiograms. In a study of quantitative lymphoscintigraphy in subjects with yellow nail syndrome, the authors underlined that the lymphatic impairment is not due to anatomical abnormalities, but rather to a functional disorder due to the reversibility of lymphedema in this condition.[3] While this hypothesis might explain lymphedema and pleural effusions, yellow nails and other respiratory manifestations are more difficult to understand. Capillaroscopic observation of dilated and tortuous nail fold capillary loops suggests microangiopathy as the cause for the nail changes.[1] Another possible explanation recently described is titanium exposure, but this hypothesis is not confirmed.[4,5,6]

Yellow nail syndrome is a rare disorder and epidemiologically it involves 0.13% of middle-aged adults, both female and males equally affected,[7] it can rarely occur in pediatric patients,[8–14] and congenital cases are rarely reported.[15,16]

While the syndrome was initially classified as hereditary with familial cases reported,[16–18] contemporary literature recognizes a predominance of acquired cases.[2]

Dermatologic signs diagnostic for YNS are arrested or slowed nail growth rate, nail plate thickening, lack of cuticles, yellow-green discoloration, and increased transverse curvature of the nail plate. Paronychia and onycholysis can be observed[7] (Figure 26.1).

The diagnosis of YNS is usually made clinically by dermatologists. Early diagnosis is very important to detect as well as monitor respiratory problems and other associated disorders.

The differential diagnosis of nail alterations includes nail diseases associated with an increase in thickness of the nail plate, which is frequent at the level of the feet: onychogryphosis, acquired pachyonychia, and onychomycosis. On the hands, the absence of the cuticle poses the differential diagnosis with chronic paronychia.

According to the literature, pleuropulmonary symptoms and lymphedema are found in 63% and 80%, respectively, of patients with yellow nail syndrome.[19,20]

Nail changes may precede the development of lymphedema or respiratory manifestations by years. When it occurs, lymphedema usually begins on the ankles and legs but the hands or even the face can be affected. It can rarely be generalized.[3,20,21,23] Congenital lymphedema has also been reported in

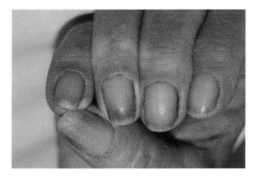

FIGURE 26.1 Clinical picture of YNS fingernails: Nail plate thickening, lack of cuticles, yellow-green discoloration and increased transverse curvature of the nail plate are typical nail signs of the disease.

association with yellow nail syndrome. A possible association of YNS with intestinal lymphangiectasis has rarely been reported.[24,25]

Pleuropulmonary symptoms are present in 63% of cases.[19] Respiratory manifestations are variable and include rhinosinusitis, chronic cough, chronic inflammatory/infective disorders such as asthma, chronic sinusitis,[26,27] bronchiectasis,[28] chronic bronchitis, pulmonary fibrosis, giant cell interstitial pneumonitis, pneumonia, tuberculosis, chronic obstructive pulmonary disease, chylothorax and thoracic tumors including thoracic nonmalignant lymphatic disorders,[29] and lung cancer.[30,31]

Pleural effusion is reported in 36% of YNS cases,[32] usually it is the last manifestation of YNS to appear; in 50% of cases it is bilateral. Yellow nail syndrome may involve not only the pleura, but also other serous membranes: pericardial effusions[33] and chylous ascites with intestinal lymphangiectasia have been described.[34] Together with fingernails and respiratory problems, lymphedema is the third major component of the syndrome. It is present in 80% of the cases in the literature,[19] but it is only reported in one-third of the cases as a symptom of onset. The pathophysiology of YNS remains indefinite. Among the various pathogen hypotheses, the most followed is an abnormality of lymphatic drainage, anatomical and functional, as an underlying cause. In fact, patients with YNS have a shorter lifespan than the general population.

YNS is linked to a variety of underlying diseases.[19,20,35,36] Eighteen of our patients (85.1%) had concomitant diseases. Malignant tumors were present in two (9.2%). In one case the neoplasia developed at same time of nail alterations; in the other case, several years before. Considering the age of the population affected by YNS and the frequency of malignant tumors, it is difficult to claim increased tumor susceptibility in the patients affected by YNS. Patients with carcinomas of the respiratory system can develop paraneoplastic yellow nail syndrome. This occurrence has been described in lung carcinoma[30,31] and in carcinoma of the larynx.[37] YNS has been associated with various types of diseases. However, these associations are often reported in clinical cases, and it is therefore difficult to establish their significance. Patients with yellow nail syndrome have several comorbidities other than the respiratory ones, possibly due to their old age, and they generally have a lower life expectancy when compared to the average population.[1]

Removal of the tumor may or may not be associated with improvement of the nail signs.

Improvement or spontaneous resolution of nail changes associated with improvement of the systemic manifestations of YNS has been reported in up to 30% of the cases.[7] Nail abnormalities have also been reported to improve or regress when the associated respiratory disease is successfully treated.

26.2 How to Confirm the Diagnosis

Diagnosis of YNS is clinical. Coexistence of all three symptoms is not always present. According to Hiller's definition,[38] the presence of two of the three symptoms (nail involvement, lymphedema, and pleural effusion) is enough to establish the diagnosis, but it is now accepted that the typical nail alterations are a sufficient requirement.[39] Individual manifestations of the syndrome can appear at different times, even with intervals of several years, but nail changes usually follow pulmonary abnormalities. Nail changes in yellow nail syndrome are pathognomonic. All nails are usually affected, both fingernails and toenails, with different degrees of severity (Figures 26.2 through 26.4). Nail signs diagnostic for YNS included yellow-green to brown discoloration, arrested or slowed nail growth rate, increased transverse curvature of the nail plate, nail plate thickening, hardness and opaqueness, onycholysis with possible shedding of the nail due to excessive transverse curvature may be very severe and cause a total nail loss, lack of cuticles, and nail fold swelling. Despite the adjective "yellow" that can indicate the typical color of the nail plate, the most characteristic nail symptom is a considerably slowed or arrested growth rate (<0.25 mm/week) that can explain the clinical appearance of the nail. Patients report not cutting them off for months.[21,40] Nail signs and symptoms were quite severe, with color changes and onycholysis that caused considerable cosmetic and functional impairment and frequently the patients remarked that their nails stopped growing. Comparing the normal nail growth (0.46 mm/week) with the nail growth of YNS, the difference was approximately 50% and the nail plate was twice as thick. With the resolution of the nail changes, there is usually a resumption of normal nail growth. The fingernails have a growth rate twice that of the toenails. In most cases of YNS, all 20 nails are affected. The typical symptoms of YNS are more easily identified in the fingernails, in how many nails, and in the elderly it is frequent to observe thickened nails and yellowishness in toenails as a result of repeated trauma and peripheric circulatory deficit.

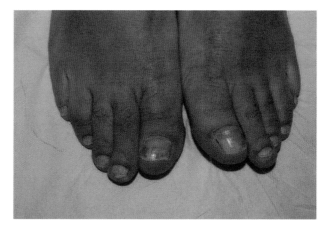

FIGURE 26.2   Clinical picture of mild YNS.

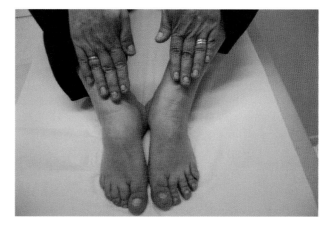

FIGURE 26.3   Clinical picture of moderate YNS.

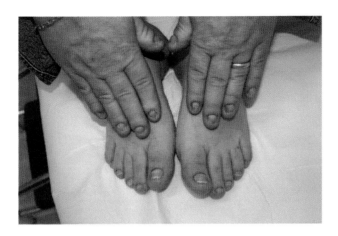

FIGURE 26.4   Clinical picture of severe YNS.

Most of the patients that do not show diagnostic signs of YNS on histological examination or nail histology is normal with no demonstrable changes in small vessels and dermal lymphatic function.[41] Since the diagnosis is clinical, histology is very rarely performed, but in past literature, histopathology of the nail matrix and bed demonstrated dense, fibrous tissue replacing subungual stroma with numerous ectasic, endothelium-lined vessels that are similar to the histology in the pleura in yellow nail syndrome.[35] Sclerosis of the subungual tissue is postulated as leading to lymphatic obstruction. On electron microscopy, keratohyalin granules are seen in the nail matrix and have been postulated to be associated with slow nail growth.[42]

In front of a patient with YNS nail marks, a laboratory and instrumental control is recommended in order to exclude associated diseases, especially respiratory diseases, to eliminate the strong suspicion of neoplasms. The exams include glucose, liver enzymes, creatinine, urea, complete cell count, hematocrit, hormones, immunoglobulins, and urine test, and must also require instrumental examinations (e.g., chest radiography, ultrasound of the abdomen). To exclude the lymphedema, the volume of the lower limbs and upper limbs is determined, measuring the circumference at intervals of 4 cm to compare them with one another. Lymphoscintigraphy may show slowed lymphatic drainage in the upper and lower limbs. Capillaroscopy of the proximal nail fold is a nonessential examination, but shows dilated and tortuous capillary loops.

26.3 Evidence-Based Treatment

Although YNS may resolve spontaneously, treatment is often sought by sufferers. There are no large series or randomized trials in the treatment of yellow nail syndrome. Therapy of YNS is reviewed in Table 26.1 with the different level of evidence.

Often there is a spontaneous improvement of nail changes: more than 30% of patients according to Samman et al.,[21] but only in 10% of cases according to a review of 70 patients in a publication by Norton.[43] Nail abnormalities improve or regress when the respiratory diseases are successfully treated. YNS therapy includes treatments for associated diseases: bronchopulmonary hygiene (e.g., postural drainage, thoracic physiotherapy), inhaled steroids and antibiotics to control symptom exacerbations, and serial thoracentesis or pleurodesis for the control of pleural effluxion. Lymphedema can be managed in the majority of patients with a regimen consisting of the use of gradual pressure devices, exercises, bandages, manual lymphatic drainage, and possibly diuretics. In patients with paraneoplastic YNS, the nails often return to normal with tumor eradication. Three cases of YNS remission after tumor treatment have been described in the literature. In one case it is a breast cancer,[44] another case of remission after the treatment of cholangiocarcinoma,[45] and a case of healing after the resection of the larynx carcinoma.[37] These cases indicate that the nail changes are reversible. A possible explanation of this tumor-healing regression phenomenon of YNS could be a direct involvement of the tumor of the lymphatic vessels, already deficient.[44]

TABLE 26.1

Treatments and Levels of Evidence

Treatment	Level of Evidence
α-Tocopherol + fluconazole	B[2,7,43,46–51]
Treatment of the concomitant disorder	E[37,44,45]
Intradermal triamcinolone injections in the proximal nail matrix (PNM)	B[54]
Clarithromycin	E[55–57]
Physiotherapy	E[22,58]
Oral zinc supplementation	E[55,56,57]
Dietary treatment	E[55,56,57]
Octreotide treatment	E[55,56,57]

Patients with yellow nail syndrome require treatment because the nail changes cause pain, the fingers lose part of their functionality, and there is psychological discomfort related to the aesthetic appearance of the nail. Various therapeutic regimens are cited in the literature, but without consistent results.

26.3.1 Systemic Treatment

26.3.1.1 α-Tocopherol

Oral α-tocopherol (vitamin E) at high doses, 600–1200 international units (IU) daily, is the only treatment that has been utilized in a large number of patients despite mixed results.[2,7,43,46,47] Even though it has been reported to clear the respiratory manifestations of the syndrome, vitamin E: high-dose vitamin E, 1200 mg/day, was the only treatment to be used in a large number of patients, even though it did not have good results in all cases. The treatment has a duration of 6–18 months and has been used as monotherapy (Figure 26.5). The mechanism of action of vitamin E in YNS is still unknown, its effectiveness could be linked to antioxidant properties from α-tocopherol.

Although the mechanism of action of vitamin E in yellow nail syndrome is not known, the antioxidant properties of α-tocopherol may account for its efficacy. Vitamin E has been postulated to restore lymphatics to normal function.

26.3.1.2 Antifungals

The use of systemic antifungals is described by Luyten and colleagues in a patient suffering from YNS and onychomycosis, in which the YNS nail changes recovered after systemic itraconazole therapy.[48] The efficacy of itraconazole may be due to its ability to increase the speed of nail growth; the same capacity has also been reported for fluconazole. The oral azole antifungals itraconazole and fluconazole have also been reported to be effective alone or in combination with vitamin E. The combination of fluconazole and vitamin E is certainly the best treatment for curing the nail unit. This was confirmed by some anecdotal reports that supplement our own statistics.[49] Pulse therapy with itraconazole 400 mg per day for 1 week a month for 6 months, reported with or without vitamin E, is effective, although the real benefit of this azole, whose mechanism of action in the YNS is thought to be stimulation of nail growth, is yet to be proven.[7,50] Combination treatment of oral fluconazole pulse therapy and oral vitamin E is another possible option often cited as the best option in the treatment of YNS.[51]

The arrested nail growth and the local immunodepression due to the lymphatic deficit may explain a predisposition to fungal infection in YNS.

26.3.2 Topical Treatment

Topical vitamin E solution in dimethyl sulfoxide (DMSO) has been successful in the treatment of nail changes in yellow nail syndrome in one study[52] and unsuccessful in another study.[53]

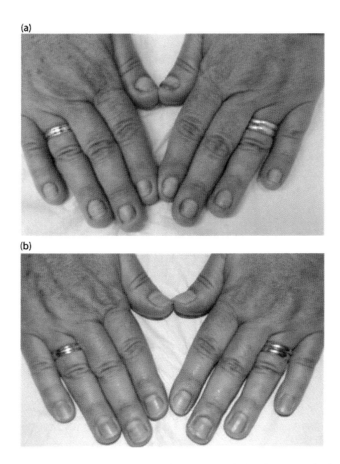

FIGURE 26.5 Clinical picture of YNS (a) before and (b) after 6 months of high-dose systemic vitamin E.

26.3.2.1 Intralesional Steroid Injections

Repeated nail matrix steroid injections have been successfully employed.[54]

26.3.2.2 Others

Octreotide, zinc, and medium-chain fatty acid triglyceride supplements as well as clarithromycin have been used in anecdotal reports.[55–57]

26.3.3 Physiotherapy

A manual lymphatic drainage or physiotherapy with bronchial drainage are described in patients with respiratory alterations where these methods induced disappearance of nail abnormalities.[58,22] In summary, treatment of underlying disease (or concomitant disorder) is mandatory but does not always bring resolution of YNS, and cure of the nail is not always accompanied by disappearance of the other signs.

26.4 Prognosis

The long-term evolution of YNS is variable and correlates with the type and severity of the associated conditions. There may be healing and relapses of the syndrome. The progression of respiratory manifestations up to respiratory failure is rare.[1] The largest YNS series published in the literature concerns

41 patients in a study done by a group of U.S. pulmonologists. In this study the associated diseases of 41 patients with YNS were highlighted and their overall survival was estimated, compared to the general population, using Kaplan-Maier methods. It was found that the syndrome of yellow nails is associated with a slight reduction in the duration of life.[1]

26.5 Conclusion

Although rare, YNS is a multidisciplinary pathology, where nail alterations are often the symptom that leads the patient to go to the doctor, even if it is not the most serious. The diagnosis of the nail marks of YNS should be within the reach of general practitioners and dermatologists. Only in this way can the patient be subjected to laboratory and instrumental examinations to evaluate any associated diseases affecting the respiratory system and other organs/systems. In fact, YNS is associated with an increased prevalence of serious systemic diseases compared to the general population. In the face of these patients, it is a good idea not to neglect a complete examination of the nails, because YNS is associated with an increased incidence of onychomycosis. About 50% of patients with YNS benefit from systemic treatment with high-dose vitamin E.

REFERENCES

1. Maldonado F, Tazelaar HD, Wang CW, Ryu JH. Yellow nail syndrome. *Chest.* 2008;134:375–378.
2. Hoque SR, Mansour S, Mortimer PS. Yellow nail syndrome: Not a genetic disorder? Eleven new cases and a review of the literature. *Br J Dermatol.* 2007;156:1230–1234.
3. Bull RH, Fenton DA, Mortimer PS. Lymphatic function in the yellow nail syndrome. *Br J Dermatol.* 1996;134:307–312.
4. Baran LR. Yellow nail syndrome and nail lichen planus may be induced by a common culprit. Focus on dental restorative substances. *Front Med (Lausanne).* 2014;1:46.
5. Ataya A, Kline KP, Cope J, Alnuaimat H. Titanium exposure and yellow nail syndrome. *Respir Med Case Rep.* 2015;16:146–147.
6. Dos Santos VM. Titanium pigment and yellow nail syndrome. *Skin Appendage Disord.* 2016;1:197.
7. Piraccini BM, Urciuoli B, Starace M, Tosti A, Balestri R. Yellow nail syndrome: Clinical experience in a series of 21 patients. *J Dtsch Dermatol Ges.* 2014;12:131–137.
8. Cecchini M, Doumit J, Kanigsberg N. Atypical presentation of congenital yellow nail syndrome in a 2-year-old female. *J Cutan Med Surg.* 2013;17:66–68.
9. Cebeci F, Celebi M, Onsun N. Nonclassical yellow nail syndrome in six-year-old girl: A case report. *Cases J.* 2009;2:165.
10. Göçmen A, Küçükosmanoğlu O, Kiper N et al. Yellow nail syndrome in a 10-year-old girl. *Turk J Pediatr.* 1997;39:105–109.
11. Yalçin E, Doğru D, Gönç EN et al. Yellow nail syndrome in an infant presenting with lymphedema of the eyelids and pleural effusions. *Clin Pediatrics.* 2004;43:569–572.
12. Al Hawsawi K, Pope E. Yellow nail syndrome. *Pediatr Dermatol.* 2010;27:675–676.
13. Dessart P, Deries X, Guérin-Moreau M, Troussier F, Martin L. Yellow nail syndrome: Two pediatric case reports. *Ann Dermatol Venereol.* 2014;141:611–619.
14. Kamatani M, Rai A, Hen H, Hayashi K, Aoki T, Umeyama K, Takebayashi J. Yellow nail syndrome associated with mental retardation in two siblings. *Br J Dermatol.* 1978;99:329–333.
15. Nanda A, Al-Essa FH, El-Shafei WM, Alsaleh QA. Congenital yellow nail syndrome: A case report and its relationship to nonimmune fetal hydrops. *Pediatr Dermatol.* 2010;27:533–534.
16. Semiz S, Dagdeviren E, Ergin H, Kilic I, Kirac S, Cimbis M, Semiz E. Congenital lymphoedema, bronchiectasis and seizure: Case report. *East Afr Med J.* 2008;85:145–149.
17. Kuloğlu Z, Üstündağ G, Kirsaçlioğlu CT et al. Successful living-related liver transplantation in a child with familial yellow nail syndrome and fulminant hepatic failure: Report of a case. *Pediatr Transplant.* 2008;12:906–909.
18. Razi E. Familial yellow nail syndrome. *Dermatol Online J.* 2006;12:15.
19. Norklid P, Kroman-Andersen H, Struve-Christensen E. Yellow nail syndrome—The triad of yellow nails, lymphedema and pleural effusions. *Acta Med Scand.* 1986;219:221–227.

20. Beer DJ, Pereira W Jr, Snider GL. Pleural effusion associated with primary lymphedema: A perspective on the yellow nail syndrome. *Am Rev Respir Dis.* 1978;117:595–599.
21. Samman PD, White WF. The yellow nail syndrome. *Br J Dermatol.* 1964;76:153–157.
22. Szolnoky G, Lakatos B, Husz S, Dobozy A. Improvement in lymphatic function and partial resolution of nails, after complete decongestive physiotherapy in yellow nail syndrome. *Int J Dermatol.* 2005;44:501–503.
23. Solal-Celigny P, Cormier Y, Fourmier M. The yellow nail syndrome: Light and electron microscopic aspect of the pleura. *Arch Pathol Lab Med.* 1983;107:183–185.
24. Malek NP, Ocran K, Tietge UJ et al. A case of the yellow nail syndrome associated with massive chylous ascites, pleural and pericardial effusions. *Zeitschrift für Gastroenterologie.* 1996;34:763–766.
25. Ocana I, Bejarno E, Ruiz I et al. Intestinal lymphangiectasia and the yellow nail syndrome (letter). *Gastroenterology.* 1988;94:858.
26. Imadojemu S, Rubin A. Dramatic improvement of yellow nail syndrome with a combination of intralesional triamcinolone, fluconazole, and sinusitis management. *Int J Dermatol.* 2015;54:e497–e499.
27. Letheulle J, Deslée G, Guy T et al. The yellow nail syndrome: A series of five cases. *Rev Mal Respir.* 2012;29:419–425.
28. Woodfield G, Nisbet M, Jacob J et al. Bronchiectasis in yellow nail syndrome. *Respirology.* 2016 August 23 [Epub].
29. Itkin M, McCormack FX. Nonmalignant adult thoracic lymphatic disorders. *Clin Chest Med.* 2016;37:409–420.
30. Thomas PS, Sidhu B. Yellow nail syndrome and bronchial carcinoma. *Chest.* 1987;92:191.
31. Carnassale G, Margaritora S, Vita ML et al. Lung cancer in association with yellow nail syndrome. *J Clin Oncol.* 2011;29:e156–e158.
32. Hersko A, Hirshberg B, Nahir M, Friedman G. Yellow nail syndrome. *Postgrad Med J.* 1997;73:466–468.
33. Wasaka M, Imaizumi T, Suyama A et al. Yellow nail syndrome associated with chronic pericardial effusion. *Chest.* 1987;97:366–367.
34. Duhra PM, Quigley EM, Marsh MN. Chylous ascites, lymphangiectasia and yellow nail syndrome. *Gut.* 1985;26:1266–1269.
35. Marks R, Ellis JP. Yellow nails: A report of six cases. *Arch Dermatol.* 1970;102:619–623.
36. David-Vaudey E, Jamard B, Hermant C, Cantagrel A. Yellow nail syndrome in rheumatoid arthritis: A drug-induced disease? *Clin Rheumatol.* 2004;23:376–378.
37. Guin JD, Elleman JH. Yellow nail syndrome possible association with malignancy. *Arch Dermatol.* 1979;115:734–735.
38. Hiller E, Rosenow EC, Olsen AM. Pulmonary manifestations of the yellow nail syndrome. *Chest.* 1972;61:452–458.
39. Bourcier T, Baudrimont M, Borderie V et al. Conjunctival changes associated with yellow nail syndrome. *Br J Ophtalmol.* 2002;86:930.
40. Moffitt DL, de Berker DA. Yellow nail syndrome: The nail that grows half as fast grows twice as thick. *Clin Exp Dermatol.* 2000;25:21–23.
41. DeCoste SD, Imber MJ, Baden HP. Yellow nail syndrome. *J Am Acad Dermatol.* 1990;22:608–611.
42. Pavlidakey GP, Hashimoto K, Blum D. Yellow nail syndrome. *J Am Acad Dermatol.* 1984;11:509–512.
43. Norton L. Further observations on the yellow nail syndrome with therapeutic effects of oral alpha-tocopherol. *Cutis.* 1985;36:457–462.
44. Iqbal M, Rossoff LJ, Marzouk KA et al. Yellow nail syndrome: Resolution of yellow nails after successful treatment of breast cancer. *Chest.* 2000;117:1516–1518.
45. Di Stefano F, Verna N, Balatsinou L et al. Genetic hemochromatosis with normal transferrin saturation in a man with cholangiocarcinoma and yellow nail syndrome. *J Gastroentereol Hepatol.* 2003;18:1221–1222.
46. Tosti A, Guidetti MS, Lorenzi S et al. La sindrome delle unghie gialle. Esperienza di nove casi. *Giornale Italiano di Dermatologia e Venereologia.* 1997;132:255–258.
47. Banta DP, Dandamudi N, Parekh HJ et al. Yellow nail syndrome following thoracic surgery: A new association? *J Postgrad Med.* 2009;55:270–271.
48. Luyten C, André J, Walraevens C, De Doncker P. Yellow nail syndrome and onychomycosis. Experience with itraconazole pulse therapy combined with vitamin E. *Dermatol.* 1996;192:406–408.
49. Hawasie K, Pope E. Yellow nail syndrome. *Pediatr Dermatol.* 2010 Nov-Dec;27(6):675–676.

50. Tosti A, Piraccini BM, Iorizzo M. Systemic itraconazole in the yellow nail syndrome. *Br J Dermatol.* 2002;146:1064–1067.
51. Held JL, Chew S, Grossman ME et al. Transverse striate leukonychia associated with acute rejection of renal allograft. *J Am Acad Dermatol.* 1989;20:513–515.
52. Williams BC, Buffham R, du Vivier A. Successful use of topical vitamin E solution in the treatment of nail changes in yellow nail syndrome. *Arch Dermatol.* 1991;127:1023–1028.
53. Lambert EM, Dziura J, Kauls L et al. Yellow nail syndrome in three siblings: A randomized double-blind trial of topical vitamin E. *Pediatric Dermatol.* 2006;23:390–395.
54. Samman PD. The yellow nail syndrome (report on 55 cases). *Trans St John's Hosp Dermatol Soc.* 1973;59:37–38.
55. Arroyo JF, Cohen ML. Yellow nail syndrome cured by zinc supplementation. *Clin Exp Dermatol.* 1992;18:62–64.
56. Makrilakis K, Pavlatos S, Giannikopoulos G et al. Successful octreotide treatment of chylous pleural effusion and lymphedema in the yellow nail syndrome. *Ann Intern Med.* 2004;141:246–247.
57. Lotfollahi L, Abenini A, Darazam I et al. Yellow nail syndrome: Report of a case successfully treated with octreotide. *Tanaffos.* 2015;14:67–71.
58. Fournier C, Just N, Leroy S, Wallaert B. Syndrome des ongles jaunes d'évolution favorable: Role de la kinésithérapie respiratoire?. *Rev Mal Resp.* 2003;20:969–972.

Appendix A: Practical Procedures

Nilton Gioia Di Chiacchio, Cristina Diniz Borges Figueira de Mello, and Nilton Di Chiacchio

A.1 Anesthesia of the Nail Apparatus

A.1.1 Introduction

The needle stick is the most apprehensive moment for the patient in any procedure. Anesthesia of the nail apparatus is a painful procedure, and we should consider the emotional experience of the patient. Premedication may be useful in some situation, such as for very anxious patients.[1] Knowledge of the techniques and anatomy of the nail apparatus is mandatory, and makes the procedure more comfortable, both for the patient and surgeon. History of allergy to lidocaine or bupivacaine or parabens must be checked before the procedure, and local anesthetics may be contraindicated in patients with cardiac disease such as heart block.[2]

A.1.2 Anesthetic Products

Lidocaine 1%–2% is considered the reference of local anesthetic. Plain 2% should be preferred as it seems slightly more efficient.[3]

Lidocaine with epinephrine is considered safe for nail surgery.[4–9] Be careful in cases of vascular disease, smoking patients, and fingers. Take into account that its benefits do not overmatch the risks, since most surgical nail procedures require a completely bloodless field that is only achieved when a tourniquet is used.

Bupivacaine 0.5% has a duration of action of 8 hours.[10] Injecting 0.5–1 mL of bupivacaine immediately postoperatively will ensure very comfortable postoperative pain relief for the patient.[1]

Ropivacaine has the same quick onset as lidocaine, provides better postoperative pain relief (up to 9–20 hours),[11–13] and is less cardiotoxic than bupivacaine.[14] Concentrations over 5 mg/mL may increase the pain during infiltration.[1] A recent study injected 1 mL of an "antipain solution" (0.5 mL of ropivacaine and 0.5 mL of triamcinolone) into the surgical wound just after the nail surgical procedure and achieved better analgesia during the postoperative period when compared with lidocaine alone. This is explained by the association of the extended analgesia of ropivacaine to the anti-inflammatory power of triamcinolone.[15]

A.1.3 Materials

Luer lock syringes: Avoid the detachment of the needle from the syringe. This is very important for nail surgery, since the nail apparatus has high resistance to injections (Figure A.1).

Thin needles: 30G needles are preferred, especially for fingers and children. 27G needles may be used for toes. A thin needle decreases pain from puncture and limits the anesthetic flow, thus performing a very slowly progressive swelling of the soft tissues.[1]

A.1.4 Procedures

Remember to inform the patient about the needle stick to avoid a reflex jerk.

A reclining position should be preferred during the hole procedure to prevent a vasovagal event.

Thin needles, ice, anesthetic creams, massage, vibration, or pressure are useful tools to minimize the pain from the needle stick.[1]

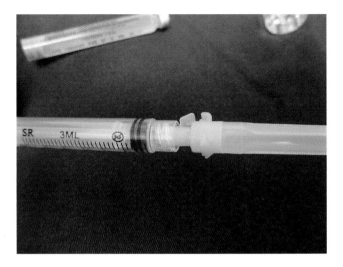

FIGURE A.1   Luer lock syringe: Useful in nail surgery to avoid the detachment of the needle from the syringe.

Pain during the injection of the anesthetic product can be minimized using thin needles, keeping the product temperature close to the body temperature, and adding bicarbonate to the anesthetic solution (alkalinization 1:9).[1]

A.1.4.1 Proximal Digital Block

See Figure A.2.

Less pain during infiltration.

Takes 10–15 minutes to start the procedure. Sometimes a distal digital block should the performed to complement the block.

Since the nerve branches are thicker in the proximal phalanx when compared to distal, nervous trauma are more common.

Punctures reach the skin in the midline of the lateral aspect of the proximal phalanx, with an angle of 45°, 1 cm distal to the interdigital web. The needle touches bone, where 1.5–2 mL of anesthetic is deposited.[1]

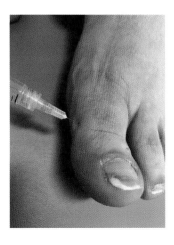

FIGURE A.2   Proximal digital block.

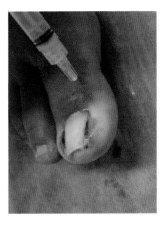

FIGURE A.3   Distal digital block.

A.1.4.2 Distal Digital Block (Wing Block)

See Figure A.3.

The most useful since it acts immediately.

More pain during infiltration.

Acts as a volumetric tourniquet.

Injection site is at a point about 5–10 mm proximal and lateral to the junction of the proximal nail fold and the lateral nail fold, directing the needle at a 45° angle directed distal down to the bone, slow injection of about 0.5 mL, and it will distend and blanch the nail folds, and sometimes the lunula. An injection into the lateral nail fold up to the hyponychium will ensure a complete anesthesia of the tip of the digit (0.5 mL of anesthetic can be deposited into the lateral nail fold). This will provide anesthesia to half of the nail apparatus. For a complete anesthesia, the procedure should be repeated on the opposite side.[1]

The procedure requires about 1.0–1.5 mL/side.

A.1.4.3 Matricial Block

See Figure A.4.

Moderate pain during infiltration.

Allows an immediate anesthesia of the proximal nail fold, the matricial area, and the proximal half of the nail bed (the same as performed for intramatricial injection of steroids).

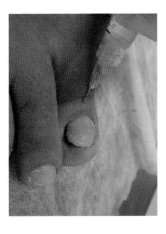

FIGURE A.4   Matricial block.

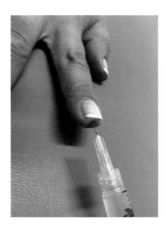

FIGURE A.5   Hyponychial block.

The needle touches the skin in the midline of the proximal nail fold (5 mm proximal to the cuticle, at 60° angle).

Since the needle touches the bone, pull approximately 1 mm backward, then inject very slowly, and observe a progressive blanching of the lunula and the proximal nail bed.[1]

A.1.4.4 Hyponychial Block

See Figure A.5.

Very painful procedure. Not recommended.

Can be used to inject steroids into the nail bed, but after a transthecal block.

The needle touches the hyponychium about 1–2 mm under the nail plate (midline), and then placed laterally to avoid hitting the distal phalangeal ungual process.[1]

A.1.4.5 Transthecal Digital Block

See Figure A.6.

It is a single palmar percutaneous injection of the anesthetic (3 mL of 2% plain lidocaine) into the space of the flexor tendon sheath. A centrifugal anesthetic diffusion and complete anesthesia of the digital nerves of the finger is achieved in about 3–5 minutes.[16]

Useful block especially for intralesional injection of steroids at the nail complex.

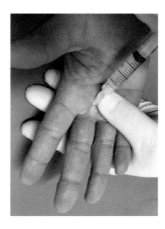

FIGURE A.6   Transthecal digital block.

Works for the index, middle, and ring fingers.

There is the risk of trauma of the neurovascular bundles.

The hand is placed supinated, and the needle is inserted at the palmar digital crease, straight to the bone, perpendicular to the volar skin. The needle is then slowly withdrawn from the bone while gentle pressure is applied on the plunger of the syringe. While the needle tip lumen is against the bone or within the substance of the tendon, there is almost complete resistance to anesthetic flow. Immediately as the needle tip lumen clears the tendon on slow pullback of the needle, the anesthetic solution flows easily at low pressure into the tendon sheath. The patient should keep his limb hanging downward to help diffusion of the anesthetic distally.[1,17]

A.2 Biopsy of the Nail Apparatus

Biopsy of the nail apparatus is mostly a simple procedure and is considered a useful tool for the diagnosis of inflammatory, tumoral, and infectious diseases. Knowledge of nail anatomy and biology is a prerequisite for a successful nail biopsy. It can confirm clinical diagnosis before prescribing systemic treatments, facilitate the diagnosis of some unusual benign tumors, establish early diagnosis of malignant lesions, and sometimes can result in the treatment of the disease.[18]

A nail biopsy is not always performed by dermatologists due to the unfamiliarity of the techniques and the correct location of the biopsy, and fear of nail dystrophy.

The surgeon must have a clear and direct communication with the pathologist to ensure correct handling of the specimen and provide as much information as possible as to what part of the nail unit has been sampled, orientation, type of biopsy, and information about the patient and the disease.[18]

Although it is a simple procedure, patients should always be prepared, and some considerations are relevant, such as local anesthesia, hemostasis, and possibility of surgical complications. Preserving the proximal area of the nail matrix decreases the risk of nail dystrophy.

The type of nail biopsy depends largely on the location of the pathology in the nail unit, in addition to the necessity of nail avulsion, tissue to be studied, and potential risk of nail dystrophy.

Partial or total nail avulsion should be considered for tumors of the nail bed or matrix. On the other hand, for inflammatory diseases (psoriasis, lichen planus, and others) the retention of the nail plate must be considered, since the detachment of the nail plate from the nail bed could compromise the histology analysis due to the firm attachment of the nail plate to the nail bed.[19,20]

For example, pitting is a nail matrix lesion of nail psoriasis, so a nail biopsy should be performed on the matrix (proximal), and "oil drop spots" are a nail bed lesion, so a biopsy should be performed in the nail bed within the nail plate.

A.2.1 Nail Plate Biopsy

Also known as nail clipping, it is the simplest diagnostic technique performed and consists of the histopathological exam of the nail plate. Benefits of nail clipping for diagnostic purposes: minimal risk to the patient, increased diagnostic information about a nail disorder, and rapid completion in the office.[21]

It is indicated for the diagnosis of onychomycosis, onychomatricoma, psoriasis, and subungual hematoma. The technique is able to confirm and localize melanocytic pigmentation in the nail plate, and it is also used for forensics, as well as in distinguishing nail cosmetics from other dermatoses.[21,22]

A nail clipper is required for this technique (Figure A.7), and it is important to obtain a sample that is at least 3–4 mm in length. The nail should be clipped as far back as possible without causing pain or bleeding. If onycholysis is present, the nail should be clipped back to the most proximal attachment of the nail plate to the nail bed. The clipped nail plate can be put into a formalin-filled bottle and sent to the pathology laboratory.[21]

Although we have many indications for this modality, onychomycosis is the most useful one. It is a very frequent condition that all dermatologists encounter every day, and nail clipping can give us the diagnosis

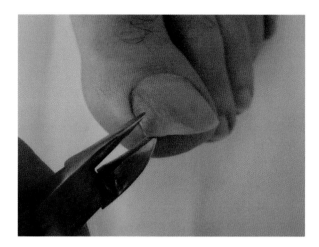

FIGURE A.7   Nail clipping.

in a faster way (2–7 days), with higher sensibility and specificity rates when compared to culture or direct microscopy.[23] Although it is possible to examine the morphology of pathogens, histologic evaluation of nail clippings cannot precisely identify pathogens and their susceptibilities, or whether the organisms were viable at the time of sampling.[21]

A.2.2 Nail Bed Biopsy

Simple and safe techniques indicated for diseases of the nail bed presented as onycholysis, subungual hyperkeratosis, and tumors.[18]

For inflammatory lesions, do not detach the nail plate from the nail bed. A punch with a lateral hole is preferred in order to facilitate the removal of the specimen. The punch should not exceed 4 mm for second intention healing, and it must be pushed perpendicular to the nail bed, through the nail plate in a rotation motion to the bone (Figures A.8 and A.9). Hemostasis could be performed with cotton or hemostatic foam, and a compressive dressing is applied for 24 h.

Tumors can be removed with an elliptical excision after the detachment of the nail plate (total or partial). Longitudinal orientation is preferred for nail bed tumors, and the specimen must be detached from the bone. The defect is reapproximated (primary closure) with 5-0 absorbable sutures (Figures A.10 and A.11). The nail plate should the placed back as a biological dressing (Figure A.12). A double-set

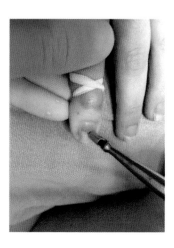

FIGURE A.8   Nail bed punch biopsy.

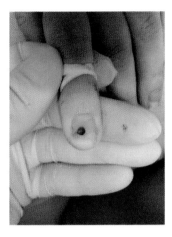

FIGURE A.9   Nail bed punch biopsy defect.

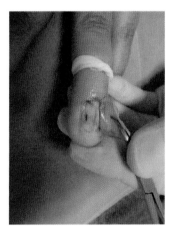

FIGURE A.10   Longitudinal incisional for the removal of a tumor from the nail bed.

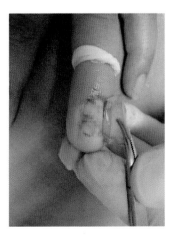

FIGURE A.11   Primary closure with 5-0 absorbable suture.

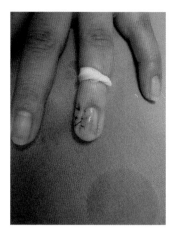

FIGURE A.12   The nail plate is placed back as a biological dressing.

punch technique is another way to remove smaller tumoral lesions from the nail bed.[24] A 6 mm diameter incisional is performed only into the nail plate with a sharp punch. The detached 6 mm nail plate is removed, and a smaller punch of 3 mm is performed on the nail bed to the bone. The keratin disk may be replaced and secured with adhesive strips and will act as a dressing.[25]

A.2.3 Nail Matrix Biopsy

Nail matrix biopsies can be used in many situations, but are more useful for longitudinal melanonychias.

Nail psoriasis clinically presented by pittings can be confirmed by histologically biopsying the proximal nail matrix with a 2–3 mm punch. It is important to know that any trauma in the proximal nail matrix area is more frequently related with nail dystrophy (Figure A.13). Tumors located underneath the matrix, such as a glomus tumor, can be removed using a transverse elliptical excision (Figure A.14). In both situations it is recommended to recline the proximal nail fold and detach the nail plate for better visualization of the lesion to be biopsied. In cases where the defect is around 2 mm, a second intention can be considered; on the other hand, in cases that are more than 3–4 mm wide, stitches with 6-0 absorbable sutures are recommended.

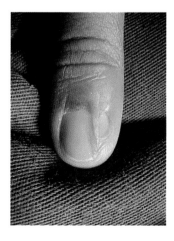

FIGURE A.13   Nail dystrophy after a punch biopsy of the proximal nail matrix.

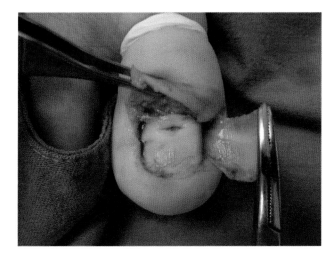

FIGURE A.14   Removal of a glomus tumor from the nail matrix using a transverse elliptical incisional.

Many techniques are described for a good biopsy of the nail matrix in cases of longitudinal melanonychias, especially for a lesion that is less than 3 mm.[26,27]

Tangential excisions are very well-indicated for pigmented lesions of the nail matrix.[28] It allows the total removal of the lesion with a low risk of nail dystrophy, treats benign lesions, and enables the diagnosis of malignance pigmented lesions (Figure A.15).[29] After the nail matrix is exposed, intraoperative dermoscopy should be performed, helping in the delimitation of the pigmented lesion and improving the diagnostic accuracy of in situ melanoma.[30] The wound can be reanalyzed with dermoscopy to make sure that the entire lesion has been removed, and the nail proximal nail fold and the nail plate are placed back with 4-5/0 nylon suture (Figure A.16). Variations of the technique have been described, such as the use of local anesthetic (lidocaine or ropivacaine) in order to elevate the pigmented lesion of the matrix, making the excision easier and with less chance of dystrophy.[31,32]

Incisional biopsy using a 2–3 punch for wider and worrisome pigmented lesions can be considered in some situations.[26,27]

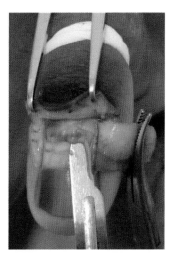

FIGURE A.15   Tangential excision of a pigmented lesion of the nail matrix.

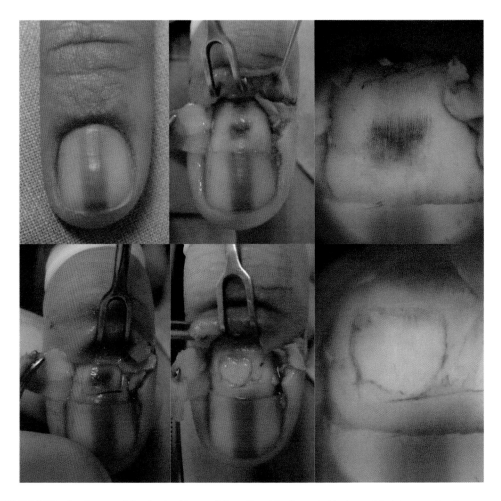

FIGURE A.16   Step by step of the shaving biopsy of the nail matrix pigmented lesion and its intraoperative dermoscopy.

A.2.4 Lateral Longitudinal Nail Biopsy

Lateral longitudinal nail biopsy of the whole nail unit includes tissue from the lateral and proximal nail folds, the nail bed, nail matrix, and nail plate. It is well-indicated in inflammatory diseases, melanonychias, and tumors that affect the lateral part of the nail apparatus.[18] It is the most useful biopsy technique for the pathologist, since it gives information over the entire period of the growth of the biopsied nail.[33]

The incision must reach the bone and special attention must be taken to cut the nail plate, in repeated oblique up-and-down movements with distal progression to avoid accidents. The specimen should have an "S" shape, so the lateral horn of the matrix can be reached, avoiding the remaining nail plate spiculae (Figure A.17). A 4-0 nylon is used for direct closure of the defect.

A.3 Injecting Medication

Treatment of nail disorders is challenging due to the anatomical properties of the nail unit that acts as a barrier to drug penetration and the naturally slow rate of nail growth that slows the therapeutic response for months.[34] Intralesional therapy is the injection of drugs directly into or near the specific structure of the nail unit: the nail bed or nail matrix.[35] Intralesional administration of drugs offers some advantages: it

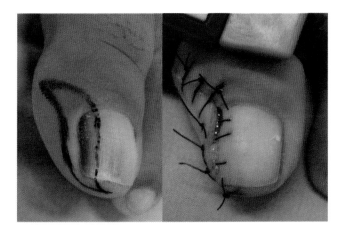

FIGURE A.17 Lateral longitudinal biopsy of the nail unit in an "S" shape.

minimizes the potential side effects of systemic administration and topical therapies, which have limited effectiveness.[3]

A.3.1 Drugs

One of the most commonly used drugs for intralesional infiltration is triamcinolone acetonide suspension. Studies utilize different doses and outcome assessments, with varying results depending on onychopathy and some possible side effects (Table A.1).[35–40] Recent studies show that intralesional methotrexate appears to be a promising medication for the treatment of nail psoriasis, with no significant side effects (Table A.1).[41–44] Bleomycin is an off-label option in treating resistant periungual warts. Studies revealed a high cure rate even in cases refractory to other therapies, in lesions on difficult-to-handle sites, and in immunosuppressed patients, with some considerable adverse effects (Table A.1).[44–47]

A.3.2 Techniques for Intralesional Therapy

There are many methods that can be used to inject drugs. Doses, concentrations, and frequency of injections have not yet been standardized. Periodic photography is used to monitor the progress. The site of injection depends on the targeted area of drug administration, for example, pitting or onychorrhexis are a result of inflammation affecting the nail matrix, thus intralesional injection into the area of the nail

TABLE A.1 Drugs Used in Nail Disease Therapy

Drug	Indication	Side Effects	Dosage
Triamcinolone[35–40]	Nail psoriasis, nail lichen planus, trachyonychia, nail lichen striatus, ingrown nails	Pain, atrophy, hypopigmentation, transient postinjection numbness, subungual hematoma, acute paronychia	• Concentration: 2.5–10 mg/mL • 0.1 mL per digit
Methotrexate[39–43]	Nail psoriasis	Pain, hyperpigmentation, pinpoint nail bed hemorrhage, transient postinjection numbness	• Concentration: 25 mg/mL • 0.1–0.2 mL per digit
Bleomycin[44–47]	Subungual warts	Extravasation into normal skin, extensive necrosis, scarring, pigmentary changes, nail damage, and Raynaud phenomenon	• Concentration: 1.0–5 U/mL • Average 0.1 mL/ periungual wart

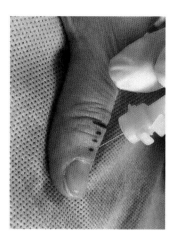

FIGURE A.18   The site of injection is approximately 2 to 3 mm proximal to the cuticle.

matrix is indicated in these cases.[3] For other nail changes like oil drop of psoriasis, distal onycholysis, and subungual hyperkeratosis, the ideal location for intralesional injection is the nail bed.

Local anesthesia may be given in the form of a local or digital block. The need for local anesthetic will depend on the patient, the site of injection, the technique, and the patient's pain tolerance.[48] Topical anesthetics, vibration devices, precooling the digit with an ice pack, liquid nitrogen, or a refrigerant spray may help with the discomfort of injection.

The injections are preferably given with the patient in a lying down position, preferentially with 28G–30G needle, and a 1 mL Luer lock syringe to enable injection under pressure, preventing any needle dislodgement or backsplash.[3] For nail matrix and proximal nail bed injections, the site is approximately 2 to 3 mm proximal to the cuticle (Figure A.18) into the proximal nail fold. The needle is inserted superficially, bevel up, and generally perpendicular or slightly angled, directly into the proximal nail fold dermis, creating a blanched wheal during injection.[36] No more than 0.1–0.2 mL of the drug can usually be administered in an average-sized nail.[3] The doses depend on the drug of choice. The injections are generally repeated at 4 weekly intervals, until a desired improvement is seen.

Nail bed injections are expectedly more painful than nail matrix injections, and may be used under digital anesthesia. The injection sites are the lateral nail folds and directing the needle medially toward the nail bed, bilaterally (Figure A.19).

Hyponychial injections are even more painful and are not routinely recommended.[3]

Translesional injection is indicated for periungual or subungual warts. The needle is injected strictly intralesionally until blanching of the lesion.[45] The amount of drug to be infiltrated is dependent on the size of the lesion being injected (Table A.1). For larger warts, multiple injections may be needed.[3]

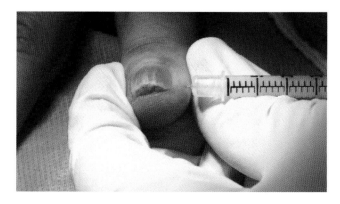

FIGURE A.19   Lateral approach for nail bed infiltration.

REFERENCES

1. Richert B. Anesthesia of the nail apparatus. In: Richert B, Di Chiacchio N, Haneke E (eds), *Nail Surgery*, 1st ed. London: Healthcare; 2010, pp. 24–30.
2. Zook EG, Baran R, Haneke E et al. Nail surgery and traumatic abnormalities. In: Baran R, Dawber RPR, de Berker DAR et al. (eds), *Nail Diseases and Their Management*. Oxford: Blackwell Scientific Publications; 2001, pp. 425–514.
3. Abimelec P. Tips and tricks in nail surgery. *Semin Cutan Med Surg.* 2009;28:55–60.
4. Sylaidis P, Logan A. Digital blocks with adrenaline. An old dogma refuted. *J Hand Surg Br.* 1998;23:17–19.
5. Thomson CJ, Lalonde DH, Denkler KA et al. A critical look at the evidence for and against epinephrine use in the finger. *Plast Reconstr Surg.* 2007;119:260–266.
6. Sylaidis P, Logan A. Epinephrine in digital blocks: Revisited. *Ann Plast Surg.* 1999;43:572.
7. Whilelmi BJ, Blackwell SJ, Miller JH et al. Do not use epinephrine in digital blocks: Myth or thuth? *Plast Reconstr Surg.* 2001;107:393–397.
8. Andrades PR, Olguin FA, Calderon W. Digital blocks with or without epinephrine. *Plast Reconstr Surg.* 2003;111:1769–1770.
9. Richert B. Anesthesia of the nail apparatus: Techniques and tips. *Dermatol Online.* 2005;11(1).
10. Reichl M, Quinton D. Comparison of 1% lignocaine with 0.5% bupivacaine in digital ring blocks. *J Hand Surg Br.* 1987;12:375–376.
11. Peng PW, Coleman MM, McCartney CJ et al. Comparison of anesthetic effect between 0.375% ropivacaine versus 0.5% lidocaine in forearm intravenous regional anaesthesia. *Reg Anesth Pain Med.* 2002;27:595–599.
12. Moffit DL, de Berker DAR, Kennedy CTK et al. Assessment of ropivacaine as a local anaesthetic for skin infiltration in skin surgery. *Dermatol Surg.* 2001;27:437–440.
13. Keramidas EG, Rodopoulou SG. Ropivacaine versus lidocaine in digital nerve blocks: A prospective study. *Plast Reconstr Surg.* 2007;119:2148–2152.
14. Fayman M, Beeton A, Potgieter E et al. Comparative analysis of bupivacaine and ropivacaine for infiltration analgesia for bilateral breast surgery. *Aesthetic Plast Surg.* 2003;27:100–103.
15. Di Chiacchio N, Ocampo-Garza J, Villarreal-Villarreal CD, Ancer-Arellano J, Noriega LF, Di Chiacchio NG. Post-nail procedure analgesia: A randomized control pilot study. *J Am Acad Dermatol.* 2019 September;81(3):860–862.
16. Chiu DT. Transthecal digital block: Flexor tendon sheath used for anesthetic infusion. *J Hand Surg Am.* 1990;15A:471–473.
17. Whetzel TP, Mabourakh S, Barkhordar R. Modified transthecal digital block. *J Hand Surg Am.* 1997;22A:361–363.
18. Richert B, Haneke E, Zook EG, Baran R. Nail surgery. In: Baran R, de Berker R, Haneke E, Holzberg M, Piraccini BM, Richert B, Thomas L (eds), *Baran & Dawber's Diseases of the Nails and their Management*, 5th ed. Hoboken, NJ: Wiley-Blackwell Science; 2019, pp. 825–895.
19. Krull EA. Biopsy techniques. In: Krull ED, Zook EG, Baran R, Haneke E (eds), *Nail Surgery – a Text and Atlas*, 1st ed. Philadelphia: Lippincott Williams & Wilkins; 2001, pp. 55–81.
20. Haneke E. Surgical anatomy of the nail apparatus. In: Richert B, Di Chiacchio N, Haneke E (eds), *Nail Surgery*, 1st ed. London: Informa Healthcare; 2010, pp. 1–10.
21. Stephen S, Tosti A, Rubin AI. Diagnostic applications of nail clippings. *Dermatol Clin.* 2015 April;33(2):289–301.
22. Grover C, Bansal S. The nail as an investigative tool in medicine: What a dermatologist ought to know. *Indian J Dermatol Venereol Leprol.* 2017 November-December;83(6):635–643.
23. Wilsmann-Theis D, Sareika F, Bieber T et al. New reasons for histopathological nail-clipping examination in the diagnosis of onychomycosis. *J Eur Acad Dermatol Venereol.* 2011;25(2):235–237.
24. Siegle RJ, Swanson NA. Nail surgery: A review. *J Dermatol Surg Oncol.* 1982;8:659–666.
25. Bertrand R, Haneke E, Di Chiacchio N. Surgery of the nail bed. In: Richert B, Di Chiacchio N, Haneke E (eds), *Nail Surgery*, 1st ed. London: Informa Healthcare; 2010, pp. 55–84.
26. Jellinek N. Nail matrix biopsy of longitudinal melanonychia: Diagnostic algorithm including the matrix shave biopsy. *J Am Acad Dermatol.* 2007 May;56(5):803–810.
27. Richert B, Theunis A, Norrenberg S, André J. Tangential excision of pigmented nail matrix lesions responsible for longitudinal melanonychia: Evaluation of the technique on a series of 30 patients. *J Am Acad Dermatol.* 2013 Jul;69(1):96–104.

28. Haneke E, Baran R. Longitudinal melanonychia. *Dermatol Surg.* 2001;27:580–584.
29. Di Chiacchio N, Loureiro WR, Michalany NS, Kezam Gabriel FV. Tangential biopsy thickness versus lesion depth in longitudinal melanonychia: A pilot study. *Dermatol Res Pract.* 2012;2012:353864.
30. Hirata SH, Yamada S, Enokihara MY, Di Chiacchio N, de Almeida FA, Enokihara MMSS, Michalany NS, Zaiac M, Tosti A. Patterns of nail matrix and bed of longitudinal melanonychia by intraoperative dermatoscopy. *J Am Acad Dermatol.* 2011 August;65(2):297–303.
31. Zaiac MN, Ocampo-Garza J. Modified tangential excision of the nail matrix. *J Am Acad Dermatol.* 2018 August 3. pii: S0190–9622(18)32338–7.
32. Xue S, Pradhan S. Ropivacaine for modified tangential excision of nail matrix. *Dermatol Ther.* 2019 May;32(3):e12889.
33. Haneke E, Bertrand R, Di Chiacchio N. Surgery of the whole nail unit. In: Richert B, Di Chiacchio N, Haneke E (eds), *Nail Surgery*, 1st ed. London: Informa Healthcare; 2010, pp. 133–148.
34. Kivelevitch D, Frieder J, Watson I, Paek SY, Menter MA. Pharmacotherapeutic approaches for treating psoriasis in difficult-to-treat areas. *Expert Opin Pharmacother.* 2018;19(6):561–575.
35. Piraccini BM, Starace M. Optimal management of nail disease in patients with psoriasis. *Psoriasis (Auckl).* 2015 January 9;5:25–33.
36. Clark A, Jellinek NJ. Intralesional injection for inflammatory nail diseases. *Dermatol Surg.* 2016 February;42(2):257–260.
37. Boontaveeyuwat E, Silpa-Archa N, Danchaivijitr N, Wongpraparut C. A randomized comparison of efficacy and safety of intralesional triamcinolone injection and clobetasol propionate ointment for psoriatic nails. *J Dermatolog Treat.* 2019 March;30(2):117–122.
38. Vílchez-Márquez F, Morales-Larios E, Del Río de la Torre E. Nonsurgical treatment of ingrown nails with local triamcinolone injections. *Actas Dermosifiliogr.* 2019 March 13. pii: S0001–7310(19)30068–7.
39. Mittal J, Mahajan BB. Intramatricial injections for nail psoriasis: An open-label comparative study of triamcinolone, methotrexate, and cyclosporine. *Indian J Dermatol Venereol Leprol.* 2018 July–August;84(4):419–423.
40. Piraccini BM, Saccani E, Starace M, Balestri R, Tosti A. Nail lichen planus: Response to treatment and long term follow-up. *Eur J Dermatol.* 2010;20:489–496.
41. Grover C, Daulatabad D, Singal A. Role of nail bed methotrexate injections in isolated nail psoriasis: Conventional drug via an unconventional route. *Clin Exp Dermatol.* 2017 June;42(4):420–423.
42. Mokni S, Ameur K, Ghariani N, Sriha B, Belajouza C, Denguezli M, Nouira R. A case of nail psoriasis successfully treated with intralesional methotrexate. *Dermatol Ther (Heidelb).* 2018 December;8(4):647–651.
43. Sarıcaoglu H, Oz A, Turan H. Nail psoriasis successfully treated with intralesional methotrexate: Case report. *Dermatology.* 2011 February;222(1):5–7.
44. Di Chiacchio NG, Di Chiacchio N, Criado PR, Brunner CHM, Suaréz MVR, Belda Junior W. Ungual warts: Comparison of treatment with intralesional bleomycin and electroporation in terms of efficacy and safety. *J Eur Acad Dermatol Venereol.* 2019 July 17 [Epub].
45. Soni P, Khandelwal K, Aara N, Ghiya BC, Mehta RD, Bumb RA. Efficacy of intralesional bleomycin in palmo-plantar and periungual warts. *J Cutan Aesthet Surg.* 2011;4:188–191.
46. Singh Mehta KI, Mahajan VK, Chauhan PS, Chauhan S, Sharma V, Rawat R. Evaluation of efficacy and safety of intralesional bleomycin in the treatment of common warts: Results of a pilot study. *Indian J Dermatol Venereol Leprol.* 2019;85(4):397–404.
47. Noriega L, Valandro LS, Di Chiacchio NG, Vieira ML, Di Chiacchio N. Treatment of viral warts with intralesional bleomycin. *Surg Cosmet Dermatol.* 2018 January;10(1):16–20.
48. Piraccini BM, Holzberg M, Pasch M, Rigopoulos D. Dermatological Disorders. In: Baran R, de Berker DAR, Holzberg MJ, Piraccini BM, Richert B, Thomas L (eds), *Diseases of the Nails and Their Managements*, 5th ed. Hoboken, NJ: Wiley-Blackwell; 2019, p. 457.

Appendix B: Preparing a Biopsy Specimen

Curtis T. Thompson

B.1 Introduction

Since there are only a few esoteric neoplasms particular to the nail unit (Figure B.1),[1] the primary challenge in nail pathology is in securing and processing an adequate specimen for analysis. Much of the trepidation that pathologists have about nail pathology is centered on this challenge, particularly when a pigmented lesion is being sampled. One major challenge of processing is centered on the fact that the nail plate is hard and difficult to section and adhere to a glass slide. In contrast, the nail matrix/bed specimens are usually small and delicate. In addition, orientation is challenging, particularly when the biopsy is from an abnormal or diseased nail unit. A few simple techniques employed by the nail surgeon and by the pathology laboratory can greatly simplify the process and produce high-quality histologic sections.

This appendix aims to present simple protocols for submission and processing of nail unit specimens. For submission of a nail matrix/bed biopsy, the technique described incorporates concepts from previous protocols, particularly those associated with ophthalmologic pathology, wherein small, delicate specimens are submitted to pathology on a paper cartoon, in a manner that preserves anatomic orientation (Figure B.2).[2] Margin assessment is easier with this technique. By submitting the specimen on a paper cartoon drawing of a nail, the delicate matrix/bed tissue becomes fixed flat, while maintaining orientation for proximal/distal and medial/lateral anatomy.

The following concepts are important in submitting nail specimens to pathology:

- Submitting an oriented, intact specimen to the laboratory for precise grossing, sectioning, and embedding.
- Providing a clinical history with a differential, which guides the pathologist and the laboratory in the preparation and analysis of each specimen.
- Deciding whether to submit the nail plate and submitting it separately from the delicate matrix/bed specimen.
- Using a protocol for nail plate processing for better adherence of the plate to the glass slide.

B.2 Nail Plate Processing

One of the greatest challenges in nail specimen analysis is processing the nail plate so that it remains adhered to the glass slide. A wide variety of techniques exist, though most of these techniques are developed in individual histologic laboratories, and the protocols are rarely assessed in a controlled manner. As such, a plethora of these homebrew techniques exist. Some techniques use either a strong acid or base to pretreat the tissue.[3] Laboratories also precoat the glass slides with a variety of products, such as gelatin. In my experience, gelatin coating significantly improves nail plate adherence (Figure B.3).

When nail plate alone is submitted, usually for fungal or blood identification, the following items should be considered:

- Submit the nail plate dry and include subungual debris.
- Process larger nail plate fragments for H&E (hematoxylin and eosin stain) and PAS (periodic acid-Schiff) sections using a special protocol.

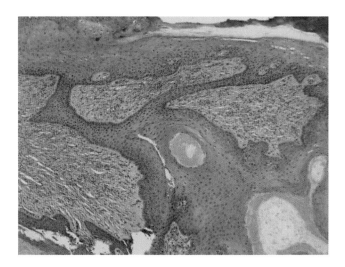

FIGURE B.1   An H&E section of an uncommon nail tumor, onychomatricoma, showing the epithelial and the dermal component.

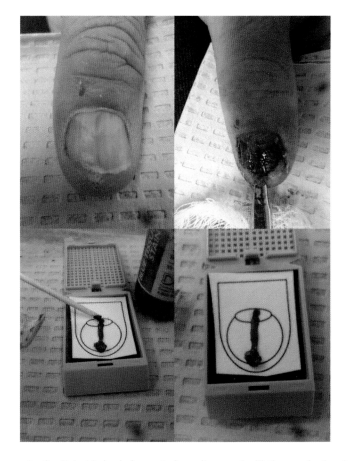

FIGURE B.2   An example of a clinical lesion before and after nail removal with the sample placed on a paper cartoon, inked for orientation and set in a cassette. (Photo courtesy of Phoebe Rich, MD.)

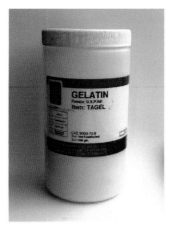

FIGURE B.3   A bottle of gelatin used in the water bath to assist in adherence of the nail plate to charged glass slides.

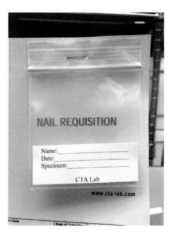

FIGURE B.4   A ziplock bag attached to a requisition for deposition of nail plate fragments, which should especially include subungual debris.

- Use a cytospin PAS-staining technique for analysis of subungual debris.
- Reserve nail culture or PCR (polymerase chain reaction) identification for dermatophyte speciation or mold identification.

When submitting a dry nail plate sample, it is important to include subungual debris for fungal identification.[4] A small ziplock bag is particularly useful, because subungual debris is less likely to be lost as can happen when an empty specimen bottle is used (Figure B.4). The larger nail fragments should undergo usual overnight or rapid histologic processing, and the subungual debris is reserved for a possible cytospin or fungal identification with culture of PCR.[5]

B.3 Protocol for Nail Plate Fragments Histologic Processing and PAS Staining

1. Place a small amount (pinch) of gelatin in the water bath so that it spreads across the surface of the water.
2. Using positively charged slide, pick up desired sections.

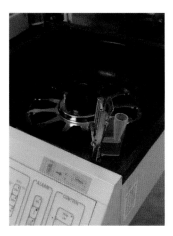

FIGURE B.5   A cytospin centrifuge that is used for isolating subungual debris and adhering it to a charged glass slide.

3. Place in 60°C oven for 30–60 minutes. Larger specimens should be heated longer. If the nail falls off the slide during staining, subsequent repeat sections should also be heated longer.

4. Deparaffinize the slides using xylene or a xylene substitute and then hydrate through an alcohol series.

5. Gently rinse the slide in running tap water.

6. Gently rinse the slide in distilled water.

7. Do not use digestion (i.e., diastase).

8. Place the slide in 1% periodic acid for 12 minutes.

9. Gently and quickly rinse the slide in distilled water.

10. Place the slide in Schiff's reagent for 15 minutes.

11. Rinse the slide in warm tap water for 5 minutes.

12. Place the slide in light green stain as needed to reach desired background intensity. This is usually 30 seconds.

13. Dehydrate the slide through 3 changes of absolute alcohol.

14. Clear the slide through three changes of xylene or xylene substitute.

15. Coverslip using permanent mounting media.

If the PAS stain is negative on the larger nail fragments, it is necessary to analyze the subungual debris. It is possible to isolate subungual debris from a sample in 10% formalin, however, this requires centrifugation of all of the formalin, a process that is burdensome and not necessary if the specimen is submitted dry (Figure B.4). A cytospin protocol for detecting subungual debris is quite easy in the laboratory as long as the proper centrifuge system is used (Figure B.5). It is important to note that the cytospin places all of the subungual debris from the sample onto the glass slide, so only a PAS stain can be performed. An easy protocol for the cytospin is presented next.

B.4 Cytospin Protocol for PAS Staining of Subungual Debris

B.4.1 Materials Needed (Other Than Usual Histology Supplies)

Calibrated pipette (1–5 ml)
Disposable pipette
Cytospin centrifuge

Cytospin funnel/holder

Culture test tube

Charged plus slide

1. Using the calibrated pipette, dispense 1 mL of 10% neutral buffered formalin into the debris container and agitate to suspend the nail debris.
2. Using the disposable pipette, dispense the debris/formalin solution into a labeled culture test tube.
3. Place capped culture test tube into the centrifuge and spin for 5 minutes.
4. Using the disposable pipette, draw off some of the supernatant (about half of it), taking care not to disturb the debris pellet at the bottom of the test tube.
5. Replace the cap and centrifuge for another 5 minutes.
6. Assemble the cytospin funnel with the labeled slide and holder.
7. Using a disposable pipette, dispense the remaining supernatant and the nail debris pellet from the test tube into the cytospin funnel.
8. Centrifuge 11 minutes to completion.
9. Remove the funnel/holder with the slide and air-dry the slide 5 minutes.
10. Place in 95% alcohol for 1 minute in a Coplin jar.
11. Air-dry the slide for 10 minutes.
12. Stain with PAS using the nail PAS protocol (see earlier).

Microscopic analysis of the cytospin PAS slide can be burdensome, especially for a dermatopathologist who is not routinely performing analysis of cytologic preparations. If possible, a cytotechnologist may be engaged to screen the cytospin PAS slide to ensure a thorough analysis for fungal forms. It is not uncommon to identify a single focus of hyphal forms with this method (Figure B.6).

B.4.2 Fungal/Yeast Speciation and Assessment for a Mold Using Culture or PCR

Tissue culture should not be used as a primary screen for a fungal infection, since it is much less sensitive than a PAS stain.[6] PCR detection, while highly specific and much more sensitive than culture, is still not as sensitive as a PAS stain. PCR detection does allow for highly specific identification of the fungus, including mold and yeast species, but this is generally not needed for initial treatment and adds

FIGURE B.6 Hyphal forms identified in a cytospin preparation of subungual debris (PAS stain).

significantly to the cost of treatment.[7] Thus, culture and PCR identification are best reserved for cases in which there has been positive identification of fungus using a PAS stain and in which the following information is needed for patient treatment as follows:

- If speciation of the dermatophyte if needed; or
- If a mold infection is suspected.

For culture it is important to notify the microbiology laboratory that a mold is a consideration, so that the culture may be performed using a cycloheximide-free medium. Unfortunately, there is high variability among microbiology laboratories in their ability to culture fungus. Laboratories performing PCR for fungus are not yet common, though PCR, while not quite as sensitive as a PAS stain, appears to be much more sensitive than traditional culture techniques.[8] At the time of this writing, the only laboratory known to perform PCR for identification and speciation of dermatophytes, mold, and yeast is Bako Diagnostics (Alpharetta, Georgia).

B.4.3 Identification of Blood in the Nail Plate

One of the most common reasons that the nail plate is sampled is when the patient presents with a black lesion, and the clinician wants to identify the source of the black color, particularly to rule out melanoma. Trauma is the cause of nail plate hemorrhage, but the patient often does not report a history of overt trauma. Often, the trauma results from poor-fitting shoes. Of particular note is that the blood in the nail plate does not degrade easily, and the iron remains a part of the heme group. Thus, iron stains, such as the Perl's iron stain, do not work on nail plate.[9] A benzidine stain may be used, but this is not necessary, since the blood is identifiable on H&E sections as blood (Figure B.7).

B.4.4 Nail Matrix/Bed Biopsy Submission

After a biopsy or excision, skin specimens are routinely placed free floating in a container of 10% formalin. If orientation is needed, a suture may be placed on the tissue, or the tissue may be marked with a cut or ink. With nail unit specimens, however, especially shave specimens of the delicate nail matrix/ bed, simply placing the specimen free floating in formalin leads to the specimen becoming fixed in an awkward shape with loss of orientation. One particular challenge in nail matrix/bed sampling arises when the clinician observes various, irregular areas of pigmentation upon reflecting the nail plate (Figure B.8).

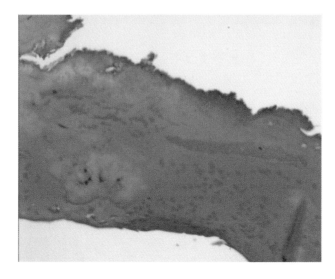

FIGURE B.7   Blood within a nail plate, identifiable on H&E sections. A special stain is unnecessary.

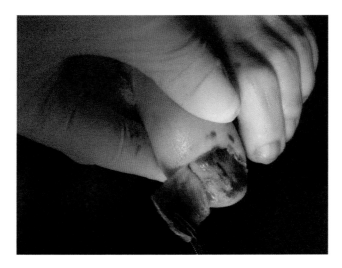

FIGURE B.8   A pigmented lesion in vivo before a biopsy. (Photo courtesy of Phoebe Rich, MD.)

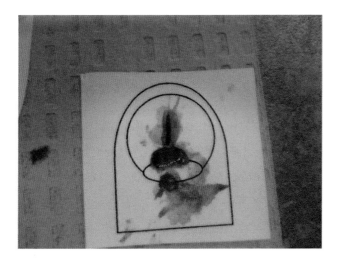

FIGURE B.9   A pigmented lesion of the matrix/bed, sampled in multiple pieces and placed in an oriented manner on the paper cartoon. (Photo courtesy of Phoebe Rich, MD.)

In cases like this, the shave specimen of the matrix/bed is often removed in multiple pieces (Figure B.9). The techniques and protocols described later help overcome these limitations. By maintaining the integrity of the nail unit specimen, the process of grossing and sectioning is greatly streamlined, and the pathologist has a much better chance at arriving at a precise diagnosis.

A laboratory that regularly processes nail specimens is ideal, but medical systems are now quite large and varied, so submission of the specimen in a way that allows for precise processing in different laboratories is ideal. Communication between the clinician and the laboratory is important as both need to pay close attention to all of the fragments of tissue removed. This is particularly important when sampling a pigmented lesion, since histologic identification of the pigmentation may be focal and subtle.

Because small nail matrix/bed specimens are often depleted with initial sectioning, it is important for the laboratory to perform initial H&E level sections with intervening unstained sections. Refacing of the tissue block for later sections is not ideal. Also, ensuring that the clinician has provided a clear clinical history with a differential is important, so that grossing and initial sections can attempt to show specific features of the different nail lesions. Without a differential, such as "rule-out onychopapilloma," a pathologist may end up incorrectly rendering a diagnosis of "verruca/wart," since benign epithelial neoplasm of the nail unit often have hyperkeratosis and hypergranulosis features of a verruca.

For preservation of specimen orientation, a couple of methods have previously been proposed. The epithelial surface may be inked and then dipped in glacial acetic acid to fix the ink before being placed in formalin for transport.[10] This technique alone, however, still promotes placing the specimen free-floating in formalin. The specimen can also be placed on cardboard with a nail diagram and covered with a sheet of filter paper, before being stapled together and placed in formalin.[11]

B.4.5 A Simple Technique for Submission of Nail Matrix/Bed Samples

Using a nail cartoon and simple equipment from the histopathology laboratory (Figure B.10), a clinician can submit a specimen in a protected and oriented manner. Borrowing from ophthalmologic specimen processing,[12] the specimen is oriented by placing it on a paper cartoon printout of a nail, with the specimen in the same location as its in vivo location (Figure B.2). Any type of paper may be utilized for the cartoon, and the cartoon may even be drawn by hand with a pencil. A cartoon printout may be found at www.cta-lab.com/nail_resources.html. The cartoon paper should be wetted before the specimen is placed on it to prevent histologic artifact drying. The cartoon with the specimen should fit easily within the tissue cassette, so the cassette does not pop open.

Orientation may be maintained by inking one or more edges of the specimen and the corresponding cartoon paper. Precise inking is best achieved using the wooden end of a cotton swab rather than the cotton end. Because many lesions are pigmented, avoiding black ink is important to prevent confusion of ink with melanin. Thus, green or blue ink are best.

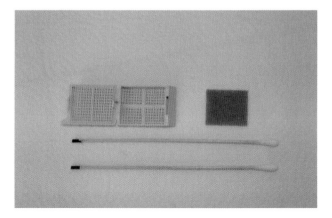

FIGURE B.10   Tools from the histopathology laboratory that are necessary for submitting an oriented matrix/bed biopsy.

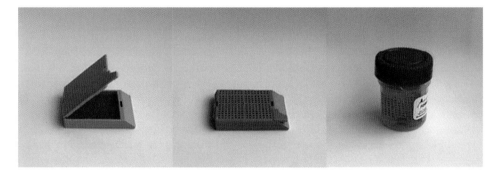

FIGURE B.11   A cassette with the cartoon, specimen, and sponge closed and placed in a larger specimen bottle.

The specimen on the cartoon printout is then placed in a tissue cassette (Figure B.11). Request a supply of tissue cassettes and sponges from a local histopathology laboratory since these can only be purchased in bulk. Place a tissue sponge over the cartoon with the specimen in the cassette, because the tissue will float off the cartoon if the sponge is not used. The cassette can then be placed in an appropriately sized container with formalin for fixation and transportation to the laboratory. Nail fragments may be placed in the same container outside of the tissue cassette so that only one specimen is submitted, thereby lowering the number of specimens submitted and, thus, the overall charge for the case.

B.4.6 Tips for Laboratory Processing of Nail Specimens

- Prior to sectioning, an initial assessment of the specimen by the pathologist is ideal. The clinical differential should guide grossing and sectioning.
- Consider sending the entire cassette with the specimen on the cartoon and the sponge through overnight processing prior to sectioning, so the specimen becomes firmer and can be more precisely sectioned.
- Submit matrix/bed pieces in separate blocks if the specimen is fragmented.
- Cut initial H&E level sections with intervening unstained charged slides.

B.4.7 Submission of a Specimen of a Pigmented Band

The most common diagnosis for a pigmented band in the nail unit is "benign activation of junctional melanocytes," also known as "melanotic macule" or "benign lentigo" of the nail unit.[13,14] The findings in this specific benign lesion are often focal and subtle. If the tissue is not processed carefully, the source of the clinical pigmentation may not be found. The laboratory should perform the following initial H&E and special stains when a pigmented band has been sampled.

B.4.8 Protocol for Initial Laboratory Workup of a Pigmented Band

- Level H&E sections (3 slides)
- MelanA (Mart-1) or SOX-10 immunohistochemical stains to characterize melanocyte density
- Fontana-Masson stain to identify melanin
- PAS stain to identify pigmented fungus
- A few unstained sections on charged slides, taken between each H&E slide for possible additional H&E and special stains

Immunohistochemical staining is quite helpful in assessing the melanocyte density in the epithelium, a feature that may not be evident on H&E sections. MelanA/Mart-1 or SOX-10 may both be used, since one of these may work better than the other one in different laboratories (Figure B.12). It is optimal to have the nail plate for analysis since nail unit epithelium may remain adhered to the plate.[15] However, if the clinician is adept at reflecting the nail plate, this is generally not the case.[16] In addition, even though the plate will not readhere to the nail matrix/bed, clinicians often prefer to use the nail plate as a postsurgical protective barrier. If the epithelium remains attached to the nail plate and the plate is not submitted, there may be an inadequate sample. As mentioned earlier, trauma-associated blood in the nail plate may also produce pigmentation.

B.5 Conclusion

By submitting and processing nail unit specimens using the specific protocols described herein, significantly better H&E and special stain sections of both the nail plate and matrix/bed are produced.

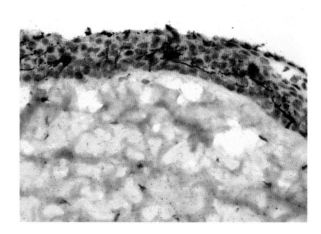

FIGURE B.12   MelanA/Mart-1 immunohistochemical stain of a pigmented band matrix/bed specimen.

With better processing, the pathologist can more accurately diagnose the variety of tumors, dermatitides, and infections of the nail unit.

REFERENCES

1. Baran R, Kint A. Onychomatricoma. Filamentous tufted tumour in the matrix of a funnel-shaped nail: A new entity (report of three cases). *Br J Dermatol.* 1992;126:510–515.
2. Reinig E, Rich P, Thompson CT. How to submit a nail specimen. *Dermatol Clin.* 2015;33:303–307.
3. Lewin K, DeWit SA, Lawson R. Softening techniques for nail biopsies. *Arch Dermatol.* 1973;107(2):223–224.
4. Jordan CS, Stokes B, Thompson CT. Subungual debris cytopathology increases sensitivity of fungus detection in onychomycosis. *J Am Acad Dermatol.* 2016; 75:222–224.
5. Bock M, Maiwald M, Kappe R, Nickel P, Näher H. Polymerase chain reaction-based detection of dermatophyte DNA with a fungus-specific primer system. *Mycoses.* 1994;37(3–4):79–84.
6. Weinberg JM, Koestenblatt EK, Tutrone WD, Tishler HR, Najarian L. Comparison of diagnostic methods in the evaluation of onychomycosis. *J Am Acad Dermatol.* 2003;49(2):193–197.
7. Verrier J, Monod M. Diagnosis of dermatophytosis using molecular biology. *Mycopathologia.* 2017;182(1–2):193–202.
8. Spiliopoulou A, Bartzavali C, Jelastopulu E, Anastassiou ED, Christofidou M. Evaluation of a commercial PCR test for the diagnosis of dermatophyte nail infections. *J Med Microbiol.* 2015;64(Pt 1):25–31.
9. Hafner J, Haenseler E, Ossent P, Burg G, Panizzon RG. Benzidine stain for the histochemical detection of hemoglobin in splinter hemorrhage (subungual hematoma) and black heel. *Am J Dermatopathol.* 1995;17(4):362–367.
10. George R, Clarke S, Ioffreda M, Billingsley E. Marking of nail matrix biopsies with ink aids in proper specimen orientation for more accurate histologic evaluation. *Dermatol Surg.* 2008;34(12):1705–1706.
11. Richert B, Theunis A, Norrenberg S, André J. Tangential excision of pigmented nail matrix lesions responsible for longitudinal melanonychia: Evaluation of the technique on a series of 30 patients. *J Am Acad Dermatol.* 2013;69(1):96–104.
12. Torczynski E. Preparation of ocular specimens for histopathologic examination. *Ophthalmology.* 1981;88(12):1367–1371.
13. Theunis A, Richert B, Sass U, Lateur N, Sales F, André J. Immunohistochemical study of 40 cases of longitudinal melanonychia. *Am J Dermatopathol.* 2011;33(1):27–34.
14. Ruben BS. Pigmented lesions of the nail unit: Clinical and histologic features. *Semin Cutan Med Surg.* 2010;29:148–158.
15. Ruben BS, McCalmont TH. The importance of attached nail plate epithelium in the diagnosis of nail apparatus melanoma. *J Cutan Pathol.* 2010;37(10):1027–1029.
16. Daniel CR III. Basic nail plate avulsion. *J Dermatol Surg Oncol.* 1992;18:685–688.

Index